Islet Transplants: Hope for T1D Cure

Furguson

Table of contents

1 Motivation

Diabetes mellitus type 1 is an autoimmune disease during which the insulin-producing β-cells of the pancreas are irreversibly destroyed. The exact causes of the immune-mediated destruction of the β-cells are as of yet not sufficiently identified. The disease usually develops in childhood or adolescence, affects about one out of 700 children of up to 14 years of age in Germany, and has shown a continuously increasing incidence (+3.4 % between 1999 and 2008) (Bendas et al., 2015). The consequence of β-cell loss is a lack of insulin and thereby a deficient blood-glucose regulation with potentially dramatic acute and long-term complications. Patients depend on life-long substitution of insulin and despite major improvement in diabetes therapy over the last decade, exogenous insulin therapy remains a huge challenge and burden. Short term, a lack of glucose in the blood (hypoglycaemia) can be acutely life-threatening due to an insufficient supply of body- and especially brain cells. Long-term, recurring episodes of high blood-glucose levels (hyperglycaemia) lead to multiple organ and tissue injuries such as cardiovascular diseases, retinopathy, neuropathy, kidney failure, and cognitive impairments through microvascular complications (Opara & Kendall, 2002; DiMeglio et al., 2018; Riddl et al., 2018; Harding et al., 2019).

The conventional therapy consists of a life-long regime of multiple daily injections of insulin and a thorough continuous monitoring of blood-glucose levels by the patient, which is associated with a lower quality of life and a shortened life-expectancy. Furthermore, especially in patients with labile metabolic control, dangerous hypo- and hyperglycaemic episodes cannot be completely prevented despite a strict and intensive treatment regimen.

A promising approach to avoid these uncontrollable situations as well as lasting systemic injuries is the (allogenic) transplantation of islets of Langerhans, the pancreatic cell clusters which contain β-cells, from a donor organ. Thereby, pancreatic islets are isolated from donor pancreata and infused into the liver of diabetic patients via the portal vein. These cell clusters contain up to 60 % β-cells and may functionally replace the destroyed endogenous ß-cells at least in part, and help to stabilize glycaemic control.

Crucial limitations of this procedure are the critical shortage of donor organs, the necessity of a life-long immune suppression to prevent transplant rejection and an insufficient survival of the transplanted islets. The direct, non-physiological contact of islets with blood in the portal vein evokes an inflammatory reaction which results in a dramatic loss of islet mass directly after transplantation. Additionally, in the liver the islets are exposed to a high dose of the mandatory immunosuppressants and toxins which also contributes to a progressive loss of viability and function. Only 20 % of the recipients remain independent of exogenous insulin five years after transplantation (Welsch et al., 2019). Allogenic islet transplantation is thus far restricted to patients with recurring dangerous hypoglycaemic episodes and labile glucose-control as well as patients who received a kidney transplant due to diabetes-associated kidney failure (DiMeglio et al., 2018; Pepper et al., 2018).

In recent years, multiple research activities have focused on means to address those limitations by the development of micro- and macroencapsulation systems in order to protect the transplanted islets from the immune system and therefore allow for transplantation without immunosuppression and potentially enable safe utilization of alternative cell sources (De Vos & Marchetti, 2002; Calafiore et al., 2006; Farney et al., 2016). Of those two main strategies, microbeads have the considerable advantage of minimal diffusion distances through a favourable surface-to-volume ratio which supports viability and functionality of encapsulated islets, but are almost impossible to retrieve in case of graft failure and tend to clump when transplanted in close vicinity. Macroencapsulation devices on the other hand, contain a large number of islets within one single device, which can easily be transplanted to extra-hepatic sites or removed in case of graft failure. They have the intrinsic disadvantage of increased diffusion distances though, which limits broader clinical use (Korsgren, 2017; Ryan et al., 2017; Hwa & Weir, 2018; Dimitrioglou et al., 2019).

Aim of this book

Against the background of a conventional clinical islet transplantation program at the University Hospital Carl Gustav Carus in Dresden and long-standing experience in experimental work with cell encapsulation approaches, the present book aimed at developing a strategy to com-bine the advantages of microencapsulation, specifically short diffusion distances, with those of macroencapsulation, i.e. the enclosure of a high number of islets within a single construct. 3D bioprinting (bioplotting) is an extrusion-based additive manufacturing technique whereby a highly viscous material is deposited strand by strand and layer by layer to create scaffolds with a defined geometry. With this technique scaffolds in clinically relevant dimensions with defined macropores can be fabricated, which increases the surface-to-volume ratio. Extrusion-based bioprinting also allows for the incorporation of cells into the material prior to scaffold fabrication. In the present book the specific aim was to employ the technique of 3D bioprinting to encap-sulate pancreatic islets in semi-permeable macroporous structures with the potential for up-scaling to clinically relevant sizes. Within this framework the different objectives were to modify a cell-compatible alginate/ methylcellulose hydrogel blend with an alginate of clinical-grade purity and to characterise said blend concerning its crosslinking density as an indicator for stability, and its composition over time. Further aims were to analyse compatibility with an endocrine cell line and to demonstrate the survival and function of primary adult murine islets (from rat) as proof-of-concept for the feasibility of the 3D bioprinting of pancreatic islets. In a further step towards clinical relevance these results were to be validated in a preliminary study with potentially clinically translatable but more sensitive neonatal porcine islet-like clusters.

2 Introduction and state of the art

2.1 Pancreatic islets and diabetes mellitus type 1

2.1.1 Anatomy and function of the pancreas and pancreatic islets

The pancreas (Figure 1 A), a digestive organ interspersed with blood vessels located in the back of the abdomen behind the stomach and connected to the duodenum, is an exocrine as well as an endocrine gland. The main bulk of the organ is comprised of clustered exocrine acinar cells which secrete digestive enzymes such as proteases and lipases. Scattered among the exocrine tissue, at about 1-2 % of the total tissue mass, are the endocrine islets of Langerhans, also called pancreatic islets, closely associated with the vasculature. Within pancreatic islets, the majority of cells are the insulin-producing β-cells followed by the glucagon-producing α-cells. Further cell types that can be found in human pancreatic islets are δ-, PP-, and ε-cells which produce somatostatin, pancreatic polypeptide (PP), and ghrelin, respectively. (Da Silva Xavier, 2018; Pape et al., 2018)

Gross anatomy and function of the pancreas are conserved across species to a large part, and independent of species and size of pancreas, islet size can range from 50-400 µm but typically lies between 100-200 µm in diameter (Jo et al., 2007). In islet microarchitecture on the other hand, inter- but also intra-species differences, such as during pregnancy or obesity, become readily apparent. In terms of cell distribution, β-cells constitute 50-70 % of human islets, α-cells and δ-cells approximately 30 % and 10 %, respectively (Rorsman & Braun, 2013; Da Silva Xavier, 2018), all of which are scattered randomly throughout the islets. Rodent islets have a core of β-cells surrounded by a discontinuous mantle of α-cells, which make up only 15-20 % of islet mass with up to 85 % β-cell mass (Cabrera et al., 2006; Kim et al., 2009). Porcine islets have been described as seemingly comprised of smaller subunits comparable to rodent islets but with a cell distribution closer to human islets (Cabrera et al., 2006; Kim et al., 2009). (Figure 1 B&C)

The function of the pancreatic hormones is to regulate blood glucose levels within a narrow range between 70-140 mg/dl (≙ 0.7-1.4 g/l or 4-8 mM) (Marshall et al., 2014). Amongst them, insulin lowers the blood glucose level and glucagon leads to an elevation, while somatostatin, PP and ghrelin regulate secretion of pancreatic hormones and appetite. Overall, blood glucose levels arise from the controlled addition and removal of glucose to the circulation. Briefly, an increase in blood-glucose levels leads to glucose uptake by skeletal muscle and liver cells as well as fat cells, which store glucose in form of glycogen and triglycerides, respectively. A decrease on the other hand, results in hepatic glucose output through the breakdown of glycogen or gluconeogenesis. Since glucose is the main energy source for neurons and a severe lack of it in the circulation therefore acutely life-threatening, the body has a number of mechanisms to increase blood-glucose-levels, among them for example the pancreatic hormone glucagon but also adrenalin, cortisol and somatotropin (growth hormone). On the contrary, a decrease in blood-glucose levels can almost exclusively be achieved via insulin. (Aronoff et al., 2004; Pape et al., 2018; Petersen & Shulman, 2018)

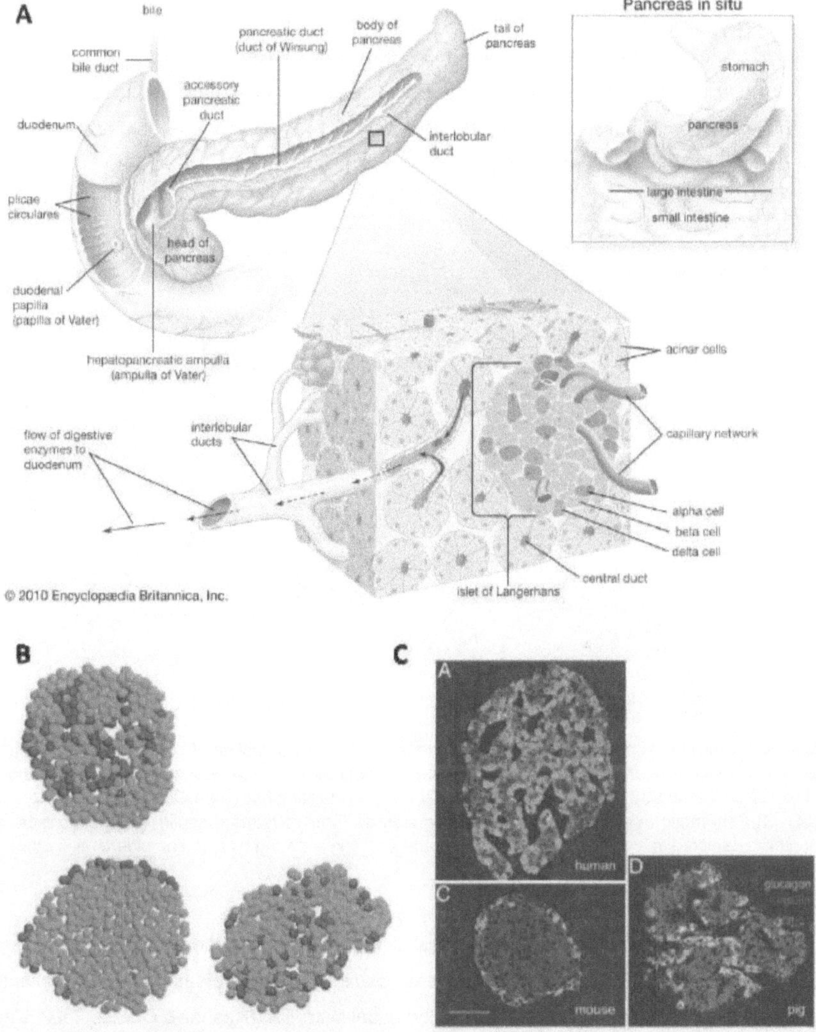

Figure 1: Anatomy of the pancreas. A) Schematic depiction of the location and anatomy of the human pancreas (top) and a magnified view of the pancreatic tissue (bottom) with a pancreatic islet of Langerhans interspersed with blood vessels and surrounded by exocrine tissue (Encyclopædia Britannica, 2010). B) Schematic depiction of species differences of pancreatic islets with β-cells shown in green and α-cells shown in red. Represented are human (top), murine (lower left), and porcine (lower right) islets (adapted from Hoang *et al.* (Hoang et al., 2014)). C) Immunofluorescently stained sections of human (top), murine (lower left), and porcine (lower right) islets (adapted from Cabrera *et al.* (Cabrera et al., 2006)).

2.1.2 Insulin biosynthesis, release and function

Insulin is a peptide hormone of 5.8 kDa, which consists of an A- and a B-chain connected by disulphide bonds. The hormone is synthesised as preproinsulin, cleaved and folded into pro-insulin, and packed into secretory vesicles, where the C-peptide ("connecting" peptide) is cleaved from the chain and the insulin peptides are assembled into the hexameric storage form clustered around a central Zn^{2+} ion (Figure 2) (Weiss et al., 2014).

The amino acid sequence of insulin is conserved across most mammalian species and human insulin only differs from the two murine insulin subtypes in three and four, from porcine insulin in one single amino acid (Smith, 1966).

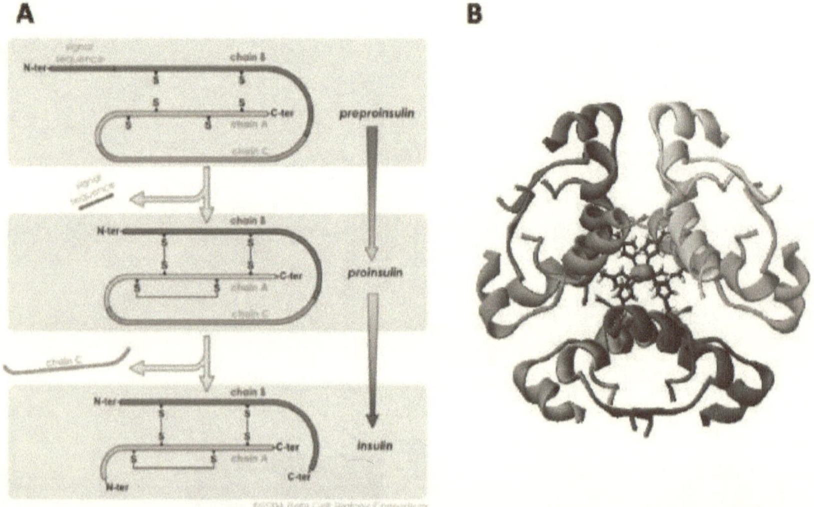

Figure 2: Insulin biosynthesis and 3D structure. A) Schematic depiction of insulin biosynthesis from preproinsulin with a hydrophobic signal sequence at the N-terminus, to proinsulin with the A- and B-chains still connected by the C-peptide and finally the insulin monomer (Beta Cell Biology Consortium, 2004). B) Schematic depiction of the hexameric storage form of human insulin with each of the six monomers depicted in a different colour. The central Zn^{2+}-ion is bound by histidine side chains depicted in detail (Wikipedia, 2007).

The main trigger for a strong increase in insulin levels in the blood is the rise of glucose through intestinal uptake, but from the healthy pancreas, insulin is not only released after a meal but in regular intervals of several minutes, also called basal secretion (Nesher & Cerasi, 2002; Pape et al., 2018). This pulsatile manner of release is thought to prevent desensitization of insulin receptors on somatic cells, as a pulsatile delivery of insulin to cells has been shown to lead to improved function compared to a constant exposure of equal amounts. The rate of basal secretion in humans is about 20-30 pM and increases up to 50-fold after glucose uptake, especially delivered in form of dietary carbohydrates. The nutrient dependent release of insulin ensues in two phases, an acute spike followed by a more muted but longer-lasting sustained phase (Figure 3 B). If glucose-dependent insulin secretion is evaluated by an intra-venous glucose tolerance test, the acute phase begins as little as 1 min after exposure and lasts approximately 10 min whereas the sustained phase follows after and persists for the entire duration of hyperglycaemia. (Scheen, 2004; Fu et al., 2012)

On the cellular level, release of insulin triggered by elevated levels of blood glucose is initiated by the facilitated transport of glucose into β-cells through insulin-independent glucose transporters where it is metabolized. In β-cells, the glycolytic breakdown is initiated by the enzyme glucokinase. Compared to hexokinase, which initiates glycolysis in most somatic cells, glucokinase has a lower affinity for glucose but an increased capacity and is not inhibited by glucose-6-phosphate, the first reaction product of the glycolysis which enables glucose concentration dependent regulation of glycolysis in β-cells and thereby concentration dependent release of insulin. The direct trigger for insulin release is the rise in the ATP/ADP (adenosine-triphosphate / adenosine-diphosphate) ratio which induces closure of membrane-bound ATP-sensitive K^+-channels. The following depolarization of the cell membrane leads to the opening of voltage-dependent Ca^{2+}-channels, and the influx of Ca^{2+} ions into the cytosol in turn triggers the fusion of insulin-containing vesicles with the cell membrane, leading to exocytosis of insulin and C-peptide in equimolar amounts (Figure 3 A) (Pape et al., 2018).

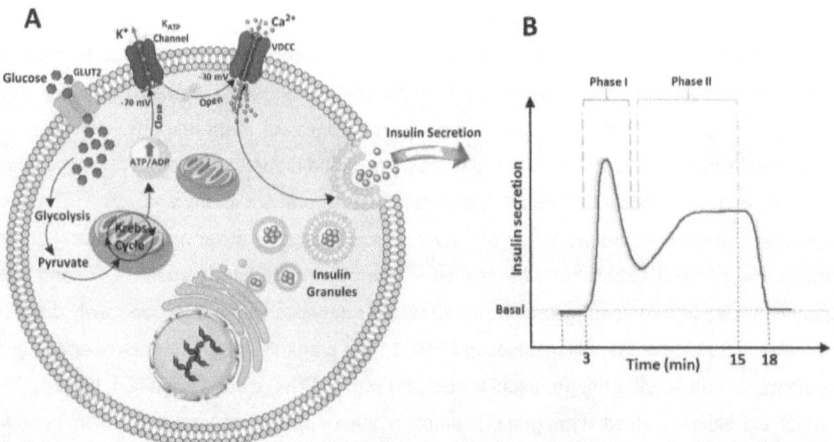

Figure 3: Glucose-dependent insulin release from β-cells. A) Schematic depiction of the mechanism. Glucose enters the β-cell through insulin-independent transport (GLUT2) and is metabolised. The resulting rise in ATP induces closure of ATP-sensitive K^+-channels and leads to membrane depolarization which in turn opens voltage-dependent Ca^{2+}-channels. The influx of Ca^{2+} into the β-cell triggers exocytosis of insulin-containing granules. B) Schematic depiction of the biphasic release pattern of insulin from β-cells in reaction to elevated blood-glucose levels. (Castiello et al., 2016)

During the acute phase, exocytosis occurs from primed vesicles forming approximately 1 % of all vesicles which are co-localised with Ca^{2+}-channels in the cell membrane, and can thereby sense a local elevation of Ca^{2+} ions (Soria et al., 2010; Rorsman & Braun, 2013). The remaining vesicles undergo modifications for release after the primed vesicles are depleted and are used during the sustained release and to replenish the pool of vesicles for immediate release. Even during maximum stimulation, release of insulin is therefore not limited by storage of insulin (Weiss et al., 2014) but by modification of vesicles. Further modulators of the strength of insulin release are nutrient signals whereby carbohydrates lead to a higher rate of release than proteins and fat, and oral ingestion additionally triggers the release of gastroenteral hormones. Such hormones, also called non-glucose secretagogues, like the Glucagon-like peptide 1 (GLP-1) from L-cells located in the lining of the stomach, are active at even picomolar concentrations and potentiate the insulin response from β-cells (Fu et al., 2012; Rorsman & Braun, 2013).

Insulin hexamers, which are separated into monomers (Weiss et al., 2014) with a half-life of 5 min after entering the bloodstream, are released into the portal vein. The acute phase is thought to mainly downregulate hepatic glucose output (Scheen, 2004) whereas during the sustained phase, insulin is distributed through the body and initiates removal of glucose from the blood.

2.1.3 Diabetes mellitus type 1 (T1D)

A lack of insulin in the body due to a reduced or absent production is called diabetes mellitus type 1. T1D is considered to be an immune-mediated disease which is characterised by the destruction of pancreatic β-cells until no endogenous basal or meal-responsive insulin secretion can be detected. Commonly thought of as "childhood diabetes" because of a large peak in incidence in early childhood and adolescence, T1D can present at any age.

In general, prevalence and incidence of T1D vary considerably between geographical areas such as Finland and China but also between neighbouring countries such as Finland and Estonia. Incidence has been increasing worldwide for decades with 4.4 million newly diagnosed cases in 2000 and 5.4 million cases in 2010. T1D is primarily an autoimmune disease and to date more than 40 different gene loci associated with T1D have been identified, the majority of which are either involved in antigen presentation or immune function and regulation. In addition to genetic risk factors, there is a high likelihood that environmental risk factors play a role as well since firstly T1D can also occur idiopathically, secondly there is a strong rise in incidence which cannot be explained genetically, and thirdly a seasonal synchronisation of both, the development (spring births are correlated with a higher likelihood for the development of T1D) and the symptomatic onset (diagnoses are more frequent in autumn and winter) can be observed. In contrast to genetics, environmental cues have proven to be more difficult to pin down. Presently, a large focus of research lies on factors such as early infant diet and hygiene standards as well as factors influencing the gut microbiome which has shown a reduced diversity in different human studies of young T1D patients. (Fu et al., 2012; Atkinson et al., 2014; Warshauer et al., 2020)

Although the symptomatic onset of T1D is generally abrupt, the disease itself begins months to years before with the development of autoimmune antibodies. At least one type of auto-immune antibody is present in 90 % of all T1D cases. The antibodies themselves are not directly pathogenic but their number is clearly correlated with the speed of disease progression. Further characteristics of disease progression are the inflammatory infiltration of pancreatic islets by immune cells (CD8⁺ T-cells, macrophages, CD4⁺ T cells, B cells, and plasma cells in declining order) and selective T-cell-mediated apoptosis of β-cells. In healthy adult mammals, the rate of β-cell-turnover is very low but evidence exists that during obesity, pregnancy and the early stages of T1D, the rate can be transiently increased by β-cell proliferation, differentiation from stem cells, and trans-differentiation from α-cells leading to a balance between loss and generation of functional β-cells and normal blood-glucose levels. With progressive loss of β-cells, islets first lose the ability to react to non-glucose secretagogues followed by an impaired first phase of insulin response to glucose stimulation. During this second stage, blood-glucose levels are already abnormal, and this chronic hyperglycaemia possibly promotes disease progression through further apoptosis of remaining β-cells. With clinical onset, approximately 80 % of β-cells have been destroyed or lost function and the sustained 2ⁿᵈ phase of insulin response is impaired as well but some reaction can still be detected, while in patients with long-standing T1D almost the entirety of pancreatic islets is insulin-deficient (Figure 4). (Atkinson & Eisenbarth, 2001; Scheen, 2004; Fu et al., 2012; Atkinson et al., 2014; DiMeglio et al., 2018; Pape et al., 2018; Warshauer et al., 2020)

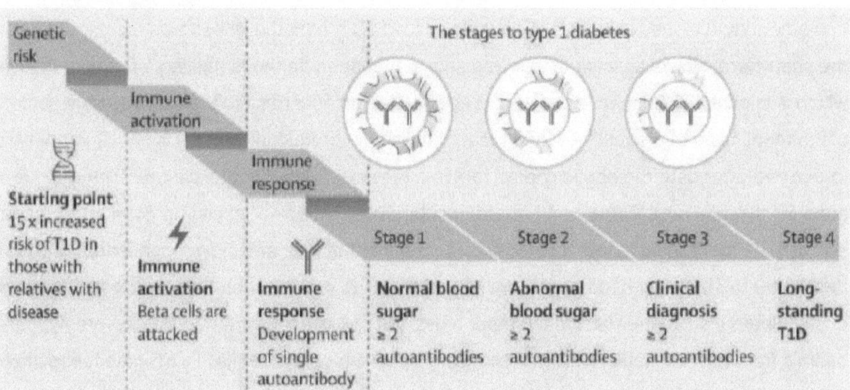

Figure 4: Schematic depiction of the progression of T1D. Disease progression from risk factors to the destruction of pancreatic β-cells along with complete lack of insulin (DiMeglio et al., 2018).

With clinical onset, symptoms of disease are polydipsia and polyuria due to an increased concentration of glucose in the blood and increased renal clearance; polyphagia due to a lack of glucose reaching the somatic cells; and strong hyperglycaemia. Main diagnostic criteria are a fasting blood glucose of > 7 mM, any blood glucose values > 11.1 mM, an impaired reaction to oral glucose tolerance testing, impaired secretion of C-peptide, and high values of glycosylated haemoglobin (HbA1c). As mentioned, C-peptide is released equimolar to insulin but its lesser hepatic extraction (Polonsky et al., 1986), greater biochemical stability, and longer half-life in the blood predispose it as diagnostic marker to test for remaining functionality of β-cells in diabetes patients. At clinical onset, the amount of secreted C-peptide is about 20 % of that found in healthy individuals, coinciding with the finding that approximately 80 % of β-cells are destroyed when T1D becomes symptomatic. The other prevalent metabolic marker, HbA1c, is an indicator for abnormally high blood-glucose levels in the preceding 3 months since the stable binding of glucose to the haemoglobin only occurs during strongly elevated blood-glucose levels and remains for the entire duration of erythrocyte survival. (Atkinson & Eisenbarth, 2001; Atkinson et al., 2014; Pape et al., 2018; Warshauer et al., 2020)

2.1.4 Current treatment options for T1D

The conventional therapy for T1D is a life-long treatment with multiple daily injections of exogenous insulin which was historically isolated from different mammalian species while today different human insulin analogues can be produced recombinantly. While there had been concerns in the past about a higher immunogenicity of bovine and porcine insulin than of the human variant, a meta-analysis of controlled trials disproved this with no detectable difference concerning metabolic control (determined by HbA1c values), fasting plasma glucose values, required insulin dose, and presence of antibodies. Instead of species of origin, immunogenicity of insulin was influenced mainly by the purity of the preparation. (Richter et al., 2002)

Implementation of insulin injections as therapy for T1D meant the illness was no longer fatal in the short-term. However, over time it was shown that subcutaneous delivery of regular insulin, which is injected 30-60 min before a meal and calculated according to the carbohydrate content of the meal, is no true substitute for endogenous insulin production since it is nearly impossible to achieve adequate metabolic control to avoid disease-related complications. The main reasons for this are on the one hand, that subcutaneously injected insulin, in contrast to insulin secreted by the pancreas into the portal vein, reaches the liver at far lower concentrations than necessary to suppress hepatic glucose output which is usually controlled by the acute phase of stimulated insulin release. On the other hand, the risk of acutely dangerous severe hypoglycaemia from excess insulin limits the chance of reaching euglycaemia. To mitigate these drawbacks, over time many different insulin analogues with adapted pharmacogenetics as well as supporting technologies were developed. Improvement of pharmacogenetics concentrated on time-controlled and less variable absorption for example with amino acid modifications interfering with multimer formation. To date, insulin analogues ranging from ultra-fast (effective within minutes) to ultra-long (effective for up to 42 h with minimal peaks) are available. With a combination of ultra-long insulin analogues to cover the basal requirements, ultra-fast acting analogues which are given shortly before a meal and continuous real-time glucose monitoring via subcutaneous sensors, in a rising number coupled to autonomous insulin pumps, metabolic control has improved by far with lower HbA1c values and less (nocturnal) hypoglycaemia. (Atkinson & Eisenbarth, 2001; Atkinson et al., 2014; Warshauer et al., 2020)

Nevertheless, even with these improvements only a minority of patients reach HbA1c levels comparable to healthy individuals (Foster et al., 2019), episodes of severe hypoglycaemia and diabetic coma cannot be ruled out completely (Miller et al., 2015), and overall life expectancy of individuals with long-standing T1D is reduced by 8-13 years (Livingstone et al., 2015; DiMeglio et al., 2018;).

In general terms, acute hypoglycaemia is immediately life-threatening, and recurrent hypoglycaemic episodes can lead to hypoglycaemic unawareness which increases the risk of further episodes. In addition, long-term hypoglycaemia is associated with reduced cognitive function. While acute hyperglycaemia can also result in a diabetic coma, hyperglycaemia-induced complications are more prevalent as long-term effects on the vasculature as a result of frequent episodes of increased blood-glucose levels. On a microvascular level, this can result in retinopathy, nephropathy, and neuropathy; on a macrovascular level, complications primarily manifest atherosclerosis and cardiovascular diseases. While the occurrence of these complications can be reduced with intensive insulin therapy, the disease remains a medical, but also psychological and financial burden. (Atkinson & Eisenbarth, 2001; Atkinson et al., 2014; Pape et al., 2018; Warshauer et al., 2020)

As the vast majority of T1D cases are immune-mediated and a later onset and extended presence of C-peptide are associated with fewer complications, many efforts have been undertaken to preserve the function of the remaining β-cells after symptomatic onset and possibly replenish β-cell-mass over time through immunosuppression or immunomodulatory measures. Research in this area has focused on engineered antibodies against activated islet-specific T- and B-cells, generation of immunomodulatory T regulatory cells to restore immune-tolerance, desensitisation with immunogenic peptides, and even bone-marrow transplants – all with varying amounts of success but no clear breakthrough yet. (Atkinson & Eisenbarth, 2001; Atkinson et al., 2014; Warshauer et al., 2020)

The only truly functionally curative treatment remains the replacement of functional β-cells which can be achieved only via organ or islet / tissue transplantation. In future, it could also be possible to restore glucose-dependent insulin response through the transplantation of *in vitro* differentiated insulin-producing cells from stem cells (Rezania et al., 2014).

2.2 <u>Surgical replacement of β-cells</u>

To date, restoration of β-cell mass is possible through either whole pancreas or isolated islet transplantation, whereby the surgical procedure for whole organ transplantation is riskier than the far less invasive islet transplantation. Both procedures increase the glycaemic control of patients by far, but for a long time whole pancreas transplantation has had a higher likelihood of resulting in insulin-independence while the vast majority of patients receiving islet transplantations remained dependent on external insulin. However, with growing experience and improved protocols in islet transplantation centres around the world, clinical outcomes between the procedures are levelling out. (Ludwig et al., 2010; Shapiro et al., 2017).

2.2.1 Islet transplantation

For islet transplantation, pancreatic islets from cadaveric donors are isolated with collagenase digestion, purified, kept in cell culture medium for at least 24 h for quality control and further purification, transferred to a sterile infusion bag with heparin to reduce the risk of coagulation and transplanted into the portal vein of the recipient by gravity infusion (Shapiro et al., 2017). With refined protocols for increased safety and efficacy, the procedure has been declared a standard therapy for selected patients in a number of North American and European countries since 2001 (Welsch et al., 2019). After infusion into the portal vein, ideally the islets settle into small capillaries and are revascularised over a time of 10-14 days. Infusion into the portal vein had shown early success and is now an established method so that today up to 70 % of the recipients achieve insulin-independence initially (Shapiro et al., 2017). It has been shown over the years however, that the liver is not an ideal transplantation site for islets anatomically, physiologically and immunologically. Mainly due to early hypoxia, coagulation, and an instant blood mediated inflammatory reaction (IBMIR), a considerable number of islets are lost shortly after transplantation (Van Der Windt et al., 2007; Pepper et al., 2018;), so in many cases islets from two donors are required to achieve euglycaemia in the recipient (Emamaullee et al., 2006). IBMIR is a result of the direct non-physiological contact of the islets with blood in the hepatic capillaries which initiates complement activation and clotting. This, in turn, can result in thrombosis and ischemia of hepatic tissue due to blocking of capillary ends. A high loss of transplanted β-cell-mass is critical, since the transplantation outcome mainly depends on the number of functional islets in the recipient (Shapiro et al., 2017), yet the number of transplanted islets cannot be increased without restriction to prevent an inner-hepatic rise of blood pressure and an increased clogging of capillaries (Cantarelli & Piemonti, 2011). Furthermore, the placement within the liver chronically exposes the transplanted islets to unphysiologically high levels of nutrients but also to many toxic substances and a high level of immunosuppressive drugs (Cantarelli & Piemonti, 2011).

Alternative transplantation sites such as the gastric submucosa, skeletal muscle, omentum or bone marrow have been tested in preclinical studies, some with promising results (Cantarelli & Piemonti, 2011). Despite this, the liver remains the sole transplantation site at which insulin-independence could be achieved clinically so far (Pepper et al., 2018), likely because of prolonged hypoxia at alternative sites (De Groot et al., 2004).

As with any transplantation, immunosuppression is mandatory in case of allogeneic islet transplantation to prevent allo-rejection even with a high level of Major Histocompatibility Complex / Human Leucocyte Antigen (MHC/HLA) compatibility. Immunosuppressive regimens for early islet transplantations in the 1990ies relied on the use of corticosteroids which are effective immunosuppressants but toxic to islets. Transplantations were only sporadically successful until the publication of the so-called Edmonton protocol which introduced a corticoid-free immunosuppressive regimen in 2000 (Shapiro et al., 2000; Bruni et al., 2017; Rickels & Robertson, 2019). Since then, protocols have been refined further so that success rates for islet transplantation are now comparable to those of whole pancreas transplantation, with 50-70 % of patients becoming insulin-independent initially (Shapiro et al., 2017). However, long-term immunosuppression remains challenging since many immunosuppressive agents, especially calcineurin inhibitors which block interleukin 2 (IL-2) mediated T-cell activation, lead to a reduction in insulin secretion, can interfere with angiogenesis and β-cell-proliferation, and are directly toxic to the kidneys which are already affected by continual hyperglycaemia in T1D (Cantarelli & Piemonti, 2011; Shapiro et al., 2017). In addition, long-term immunosuppression results in a strongly increased risk for infectious diseases and the development of tumours (Shapiro et al., 2017; Rickels & Robertson, 2019; Warshauer et al., 2020).

Even in case of successful engraftment and initial insulin-independence, in a not insignificant number of patients there is a progressive loss of function of transplanted islets resulting in recurring dependence on exogenous insulin (Welsch et al., 2019). In light of these disadvantages, transplantations for T1D patients are only performed in case of pancreas resection, concurrent or prior kidney transplantation due to diabetes-induced nephropathy which require immunosuppression in any case, or for patients with severely labile glucose control (Warshauer et al., 2020).

However, even with a return to insulin-dependence, the vast majority of recipients still retain endogenous secretion of C-peptide. As a direct result these patients still exhibit a far greater glycaemic control even 10 years after transplantation and fewer complications than patients treated with improved sensor / pump systems (Shapiro et al., 2017; Pepper et al., 2018). It would therefore be preferable to extend this therapeutic option to a far wider range of patients which necessitates an alleviation of the disadvantages and the procurement of alternative sources of insulin-producing cells as even with the present select group of recipients there is a severe shortage of donors. Potential unlimited sources of insulin-producing cells are embryonic stem cells that can be differentiated into β-cells, and xenogeneic pancreatic islets. However even in case of differentiated stem cells the fact remains, that T1D is an auto-immune disease selectively destroying β-cells. The use of xenogeneic islets on the other hand almost inevitably results in hyperacute rejection due to xeno-reactive components of the innate immune system, the intensity of which increases the less related the species are (Van Der Windt et al., 2012; Cooper et al., 2016).

2.2.2 Xenotransplantation

Xenogeneic transplantation provides a very attractive alternative due to the near limitless source of donor organs. So far, this approach has been hampered by immunological incompatibilities between species that surpass those present in allotransplantation.

In xenotransplantation with human recipients, the most closely related and most similar in terms of anatomy, physiology and immunology are of course different primate species. The use of such species as organ donors, apart from questions of ethics, has a number of disadvantages though, such as low availability due to slow growth and low number of offspring, high cost, oftentimes inadequate organ size, as well as lack of experience with genetic engineering (Cooper et al., 2015). Less similar, but adequate in terms of anatomy, physiology and immunological protection, in addition to quicker growth, a much higher number of offspring and a more adequate organ size, and therefore a more realistic donor species are domestic pigs (Korbutt et al., 1996; Cooper et al., 2015). Especially relevant for the transplantation of pancreatic islets are the similarities in blood glucose ranges and the insulin molecule. Porcine islets cover a comparable range of metabolic fluctuations to human islets (Pellegrini et al., 2016) with fasting blood glucose values of 4-5 mM in humans (Fu et al., 2012) and 5-6 mM in pigs (Manell et al., 2016). Additionally, as mentioned, porcine insulin differs from human insulin in only a single amino acid (Richter et al., 2002).

However, the immunological differences between donor and recipient are more severe in xeno- than in allotransplantation. In general, one major barrier to the use of xenogeneic organs are natural, or pre-formed, human antibodies against a number of antigenic surface markers. The most important of these surface markers is α-galactose-1,3-galactose (α-gal), a carbohydrate present in the cell membrane of most mammalian species excepting human beings and old world primates. Recognition of this structure leads to hyperacute rejection of the transplanted organ, which is defined as the destruction of the donor organ within 24 h after transplantation via antibody-mediated complement activation, injury of endothelial tissue, followed by thrombosis and finally interstitial haemorrhage. If hyperacute rejection is successfully controlled, further hurdles are the development of an adaptive immune response and thrombotic micro-angiopathies which result from incompatibilities between the porcine and human coagulation cascades, or even the presence of a constant low-level inflammation leading to chronic rejection. Genetic engineering of pigs has offered many possibilities: for example in α-1,3-galactosyltransferase-knockout pigs hyperacute rejection is successfully controlled leading to far improved lengths of survival, but consistent graft function has still been difficult to achieve even with islets from multi-transgenic pigs. (Bottino et al., 2014; Cooper et al., 2016; Rosales & Colvin, 2019)

Pertaining to islet-xenotransplantation, promising research has been published for the survival and function of adult and neonatal porcine islets in different primate species for several months. However, to date, it was not possible to show consistent graft function and survival. Furthermore, even with genetically altered donor animals heavy immunosuppression remains a necessity to prevent graft rejection. (Cardona et al., 2006; Hering et al., 2006; Thompson et al., 2011; Shin et al., 2015; Cooper et al., 2016)

The use of adult animals is mandatory for whole organ transplantations due to organ sizes, and neonates are not a viable option. On the other hand, this is not a consideration pertaining to isolated pancreatic islets, where other factors become more important such as the high fragility and comparably low survival of adult islets *in vitro*. Taken together with the danger of viral transmission and the fact that the quality of islets strongly depends on the conditions in which the animals were reared along with their age and health, this complicates clinical application of adult porcine islets. (Clayton et al., 1996; Korbutt et al., 1996; MacKenzie et al., 2003)

In contrast to this, neonatal porcine islet-like cluster (NICC) are easy to isolate in reproducibly good quality with clinical-grade purity and remain stable and show higher vitality *in vitro* (Emamaullee et al., 2006). In addition, NICC display an increased resistance towards hypoxia-induced apoptosis (Emamaullee et al., 2006; He et al., 2018) and to the human pro-inflammatory cytokines IL-1β, TNF-α, and IFN-γ (interleukin 1β, tumour necrosis factor α, interferon γ) which are known to be cytotoxic to human islets (Harb et al., 2007) making them promising candidates for islet transplantation. As is common for neonatal pancreatic islets compared to adult islets, NICC contain a comparably low number of β-cells, and need to mature for 6-8 weeks either *in vitro* or *in vivo* before showing an adequate metabolic reaction and normalising blood-glucose levels (MacKenzie et al., 2003; Emamaullee et al., 2006; Elliott et al., 2007; Köllmer et al., 2016; He et al., 2018; Li et al., 2019). Isolated NICC mature into fully functional islets, but show slightly different cellular composition than isolated adult islets. Matured NICC contain only 6 % non-β-cells, whereas this ratio is approximately 20 % in isolated adult porcine islets (Yoon et al., 1999). The main advantage of adult porcine islets over NICC is that they barely express α-gal, whereas NICC show very high levels of the antigenic carbohydrate (Van Der Windt et al., 2007; Cooper et al., 2016;) which heightens the need for intense immunosuppression.

2.2.3 Encapsulation of islets

To avoid the complications associated with immunosuppression, prevent allo- or xeno-rejection and heighten the availability of islet transplantation for a broader range of patients, the encapsulation of islets is an attractive and heavily researched strategy. Encapsulation approaches can be divided into two main strategies, micro- and macroencapsulation (Figure 5). Common to all approaches is that they are based on semi-permeable materials that are permissive for small molecules such as oxygen, nutrients and insulin, but form a barrier for immune cells and preferably also for antibodies and inflammatory cytokines (De Vos & Marchetti, 2002; Calafiore et al., 2006; Farney et al., 2016).

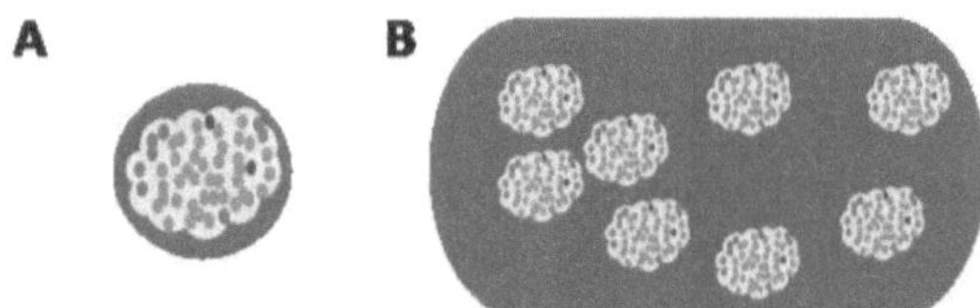

Figure 5: Schematic depiction of encapsulation approaches. A) Microencapsulation: Each individual islet is covered by a thin layer of hydrogel. B) Macroencapsulation: A large number of islets is collectively encased in a macroscopic hydrogel-based device.

2.2.3.1 Alginate as encapsulation material

The majority of approaches for islet encapsulation is based on a protective layer of alginate which is a linear anionic polysaccharide found in brown algae comprised of (1,4)-linked β-D-mannuronate (M) and α-L-guluronate (G) residues arranged in varying M, G, or MG blocks (Figure 6 A). Alginates for research are usually available as water-soluble alginic acid sodium salts in varying grades of molecular weight (Mw). Alginate can easily be crosslinked at room temperature and neutral pH by a number of different multivalent cations resulting in different gel characteristics, although only Ca^{2+}, Sr^{2+}, and low concentrations of Ba^{2+} are not toxic to cells at low concentrations (Smidsrød & Skjåk-Braek, 1990). While there is evidence that Ba^{2+} can also bind M residues, the divalent cations mainly bind to blocks of G residues, and crosslinking of alginate chains results in a characteristic "egg-box" structure of reversibly interconnected molecules (Figure 6 B). Strength of crosslinking increases from Ca^{2+} via Sr^{2+} to Ba^{2+}, but naturally also with the amount of G-residues. Due to their high capacity for binding water, high biocompatibility, permeability for oxygen and nutrients, and gelation under mild crosslinking conditions, alginate hydrogels are suitable for cell encapsulation and have been successfully used with a range of different cell types including hepatocytes, mesenchymal stem cells (MSC), and pancreatic islets. Furthermore, important in regards to clinical applicability, alginate has been approved for medical use by the U.S. Food and Drug Administration e.g. as wound covering. (Martinsen et al., 1989; Smidsrød & Skjåk-Braek, 1990; Gombotz & Wee, 1998; Kuo & Ma, 2008; Hunt et al., 2009; Lee & Mooney, 2012)

For soft tissue engineering (TE) applications, alginate hydrogels are ideally suited not only because of their cell compatibility, but also to a large part because mammalian species lack enzymes to cleave the alginate chains and thereby degrade the gels (Lee & Mooney, 2012). Especially relevant for TE applications is the immunogenicity of a given material and while alginate has been shown to be biocompatible in a myriad of studies over the years, there has often been a lack of reproducibility in biocompatibility studies with highly differing amounts of immune reaction and fibrotic overgrowth which strongly impacts diffusion through the membrane and thereby cell survival (Dusseault et al., 2006). This has in parts been attributed to the use of M-rich alginates which might leak and provoke an immune response, but more likely is a result of impurities in the alginate preparations (De Vos et al., 1997a; Ertesvåg & Valla, 1998; Orive et al., 2002; Draget & Taylor, 2011). Since alginates are isolated from algae, many commercially available preparations contain various impurities (Klöck et al., 1994), and in the past a large focus of research has been on the development of purification protocols. The contaminants can leak out from the crosslinked hydrogels and elicit an immune response through their sole presence, but could also affect the morphology and biocompatibility of alginate coatings by reducing the intrinsic wettability of the gel and interfere with the interaction between single chains during crosslinking (Tam et al., 2006). Proper purification of the alginate preparations has been shown to greatly reduce fibrotic overgrowth (De Vos et al., 1997b; Mallett & Korbutt, 2009), influence survival of pancreatic islets *in vitro* (Langlois et al., 2009) or even to completely prevent an immune response (Rokstad et al., 2011; Lee & Mooney, 2012).

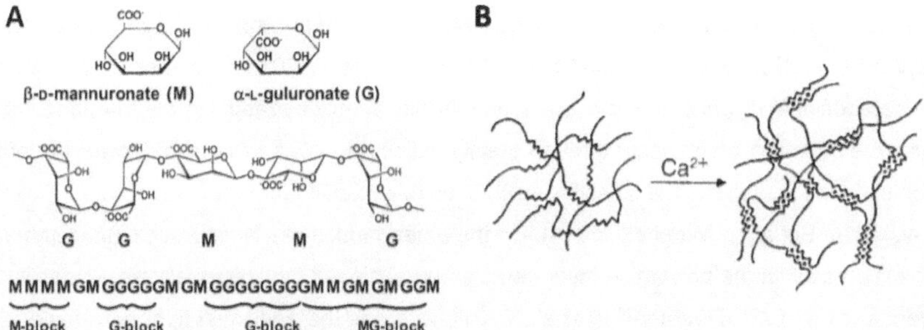

Figure 6: Alginate. A) Structure of alginate with β-D-mannuronate (M) and α-L-guluronate (G) in the top row, linked molecules in the middle and a schematic depiction of M, G and MG block in the bottom row (Draget & Taylor, 2011). B) Crosslinking of alginate with divalent cations binding to the G residues resulting in a characteristic "egg-box" structure (Smidsrød & Skjåk-Braek, 1990).

2.2.3.2 Alginate-based islet encapsulation approaches

The general feasibility of encapsulating pancreatic islets of different species in either micro- or macrocapsules while retaining their functionality has been described in a number of preclinical but also clinical studies in different species over the years. The main difference between the approaches is that in microencapsulation each capsule only contains a single islet encased in a thin protective layer of hydrogel, whereas in macroencapsulation the device can hold the entire transplant volume (De Vos & Marchetti, 2002; Dimitrioglou et al., 2019). For both, micro- and macroencapsulation of islets, alginate has been shown to be a promising candidate as it creates a barrier which is impermeable for cells of the immune system, yet barely impacts the diffusion of glucose and insulin whereby the functional response of islets can be retained (Rayat et al., 2000; Omer et al., 2003; Bochenek et al., 2019).

<u>Microencapsulation</u> of islets (Figure 5 A) is usually achieved by suspending the islets in a low-viscosity hydrogel solution such as alginate and generating small droplets by air-flow or electro-static forces which are dropped into crosslinking solution, generally resulting in bead sizes between 200 and 800 µm in diameter (Van Schilfgaarde & De Vos, 1999; Gasperini et al., 2014; Scharp & Marchetti, 2014; Salg et al., 2019).

The main advantage of microencapsulation is the minimal diffusion distance improving the supply with oxygen and nutrients as well as the reaction time to glucose stimulation while still retaining the immunoprotective barrier function. While alginate acts as a barrier to all cells of the immune system, small molecules such as antibodies and cytokines can diffuse through the membrane, and, especially for microencapsulation, large efforts have been undertaken in the past to reduce the permissiveness of the capsules for all components of the immune system. This can be accomplished by encasing the droplets in an additional layer, this one a polyamine layer such as poly-lysine. Polyamines are immune-reactive though, especially if the binding to the alginate layer is incomplete which happens with the use of high-G alginates, necessitating a further layer of alginate, which in turn increases the diffusion distance. (Uludag et al., 2000; De Vos et al., 2003; Scharp & Marchetti, 2014; Köllmer et al., 2016; Strand et al., 2017)

These additional layers can improve biocompatibility simply by reducing the frequency of in-complete capsules which occur through gravity pulling the islets towards the lower rim of the droplet during the fall into the crosslinking solution (Van Schilfgaarde & De Vos, 1999; Rokstad et al., 2014; Scharp & Marchetti, 2014). On the other hand, a similar improvement in immuno-protection as with the polyamine layer can also be achieved by using a stronger crosslinking agent such as Ba^{2+} (Duvivier-Kali et al., 2001), whereas the additional tight polyamine layer reduces islet survival by promoting the accumulation of metabolic waste products within the capsule (De Vos et al., 2003) and has been shown to negatively impact insulin release (De Haan et al., 2003). Furthermore, the use of additional polyamine layers seems to reduce the function of xenogeneic islets (Köllmer et al., 2016).

Microencapsulation approaches have the advantage of short diffusion distances through a favourable surface-to-volume ratio (Salg et al., 2019), but if the individual islet capsules are in close vicinity they tend to clump, resulting in necrotic centres (Bochenek et al., 2019). Furthermore they are almost impossible to retrieve in case of graft failure, and to achieve normoglycaemia in human beings 5,000-10,000 islet equivalents (IEQ, the standardised estimation between islet number and volume) per kg body weight are required (McCall & Shapiro, 2012; Ludwig et al., 2013). Even with optimised protocols for microencapsulation the size of each islet increases by 2-10-fold (300-1000 µm in diameter), resulting in a far greater overall transplant volume than with non-encapsulated islets, which limits the choice of suitable transplantation sites (Zhu et al., 2018). On the other hand, a study from 2015 indicated that the size of microcapsules impacts their immunogenicity with a higher degree of fibrotic capsular overgrowth on capsules of 0.5 than of 1.5 mm in diameter (Veiseh et al., 2015) indicating that to reduce the immune response the transplant volume would need to increase even further.

<u>Macroencapsulation</u> of islets (Figure 5 B) is based on collectively encasing a large number of islets, which is practical for extrahepatic transplantation sites and provides the possibility of achieving a high density of islets in a relatively compact device, so that only a low number of devices is needed to reach a curative dose of islets. On the other hand, macroencapsulation reduces the surface-to-volume ratio by far. Despite the possibility of high islet densities, a large capsule size is necessary to achieve the required IEQ resulting in a further increase in diffusion distances which in turn impacts the function of transplanted islets. (Chicheportiche & Reach, 1988; Korsgren, 2017; Buchwald et al., 2018; Hwa & Weir, 2018)

Physiologically, pancreatic islets are highly vascularized and supplied with a large amount of oxygen, whereas encapsulated islets rely mainly on supply through diffusion. With larger diffusion distances the likelihood of hypoxia within the transplant increases, which has been shown to lead to a loss of function in pancreatic islets (Lehmann et al., 2007; Colton, 2014). In light of the impact of diffusion distance on oxygenation of islets and insulin release, the main foci of macroencapsulation research have been the maximisation of the surface-to-volume ratio, enhanced vascularisation, or an external supply of oxygen. Examples for alginate-based macroencapsulation approaches which combine a high surface-to volume ratio with sufficient stability are the TRAFFIC device, an alginate covered nylon fibre presented by An *et al.* (An et al., 2017), or an alginate-filled honeycomb structure developed by Marchioli *et al.* (Marchioli et al., 2015). A successfully applied approach for an external supply with oxygen is the "beta-Air" device that has also been shown to provide full immunoprotection (Barkai et al., 2013; Ludwig et al., 2013; Carlsson et al., 2018). In contrast to microencapsulation approaches, macroscopic devices have already been commercialized in some cases, such as the "beta-Air" and the so-called "islet sheet" (Lamb et al., 2011) which are both alginate-based, but also others such as the "TheraCyte" (Kumagai-Braesch et al., 2013) and the "Cellpouch" device (Pepper et al., 2015), the exact compositions of which are confidential. Even with thin planar devices with a large surface-to-volume ratio, the upscaling to curative doses of islets remains challenging though (Hwa & Weir, 2018).

2.2.3.3 Transplantation of encapsulated islets

For both, micro- and macroencapsulation, a number of pre-clinical but also preliminary clinical studies have been undertaken with varying results over the years. The species chosen as donors and recipients were mice, rats, pigs, primates and humans in most cases, while studies with bovine and canine islets remain a minority.

For alginate-based microencapsulation, many promising studies in rodents have been conducted showing biocompatibility and stability of the capsule materials *in vivo* as well as survival and function of the transplanted islets for extended periods of time. Both, alginate-polycation (De Vos et al., 2003) and simple alginate (Duvivier-Kali et al., 2001; Schneider et al., 2005; Veiseh et al., 2015) capsules were shown to be immunoprotective and containing functional islets for more than 6 months. Furthermore, the xenogeneic transplantation of encapsulated human islets into immune-competent mice led to a normalisation of the blood-glucose regulation for up to 9 months (Schneider et al., 2005). Overall, these remarkable results from small animals have been difficult to transfer to primates however (Tuch et al., 2009; Scharp & Marchetti, 2014; Carlsson et al., 2018): With allogeneic transplantation of encapsulated islets from human donors it was possible to achieve sufficient immunoprotection for up to 3 years, but while a reduction in the requirement of exogenous insulin and circulating C-peptide could be observed (Tuch et al., 2009; Basta et al., 2011), none of the patients reached insulin-independence. It could be possible to improve these results with chemically modified alginates which have shown promise in nonhuman primates (NHP), but long-term studies on these alginates *in vivo* have yet to be published (Bochenek et al., 2019). For the xenogeneic transplantation of porcine islets, a striking first success was achieved by Sun *et al.* with alginate-polylysine-alginate encapsulated porcine islets transplanted into nonhuman primates without immunosuppression. Out of the 9 NHP used in that study seven became insulin-independent initially, and one remained so for more than 2 years (Sun et al., 1996). To date, it has not been possible to replicate this accomplishment in NHP (Elliott et al., 2005; Dufrane et al., 2006), or human patients (Elliott et al., 2000; Matsumoto et al., 2014; Matsumoto et al., 2016) though, with neither adult nor neonatal porcine islets being able to reverse the diabetic condition. On the other hand, xenotransplantation studies of adult porcine islets into rodents led to a normalisation of blood glucose (Cappai et al., 1995; Duvivier-Kali et al., 2004) and encapsulated NICC were shown to mature *in vivo* followed by a normalisation of blood-glucose levels (Omer et al., 2003).

Comparable to microencapsulation, different macroencapsulation devices, some of them alginate-based, have shown remarkable promise in rodents with full reversal for up to 6 months after syngeneic (Lacy et al., 1991; Pileggi et al., 2006) and allogeneic transplantation without immunosuppression (Barkai et al., 2013; An et al., 2017). As the transplantation of rodent islets into larger beings such as humans is not feasible due to the high number of islets required, studies with NHP or human patients concentrated on the use of human or porcine islets. While it was possible to achieve complete immunoprotection resulting in the survival of porcine islets transplanted xenogeneically between several months and 10 years (Elliott et al., 2007; Dufrane et al., 2010; Vériter et al., 2014; Ludwig et al., 2017), functionality was lost over time. Overall, none of the macroencapsulation strategies tested in pre-clinical and clinical trials could show clear evidence for fully functional encapsulation strategy, since especially the normalisation of blood-glucose levels could only be achieved in a small number of patients for a finite amount of time in each case (Hwa & Weir, 2018; Zhu et al., 2018; Dimitrioglou et al., 2019).

2.3 3D bioprinting in medical research

In general, macroencapsulation approaches have a number of advantages for the transplantation of pancreatic islets, yet the upscaling to clinically relevant sizes and especially to clinically relevant islet densities remains a major challenge, mainly due to increasing diffusion distances (Hwa & Weir, 2018; Bochenek et al., 2019). The development of macrocapsules with defined macropores to increase the surface-to-volume ratio therefore seems to be a promising strategy, which can be realised by employing 3D printing.

Over the last 30 years, 3D bioprinting, or computer-aided additive manufacturing, developed into a broad research field with a variety of technologies for different medical applications, such as the generation of patient-specific implants supportive structures, or patient-individual models for the planning of surgeries and prosthetics (Bauermeister et al., 2016; Tack et al., 2016; Yan et al., 2018). Another field of application is TE research, i.e. the generation of patient-individual tissue constructs containing live cells which can also be supplied with bioactive drugs or proteins such as for the induction of vascularization or the prevention of inflammation (Billiet et al., 2012). If live cells are to be used, the material characteristics are a viscosity which does not impair cell survival through shear stress but allows for shape fidelity until crosslinking under physiological conditions. Further requirements are cytocompatibility, the support of cellular functions, and, depending on the application, either biodegradability or stability *in vivo* (Badwaik, 2019).

2.3.1 Extrusion-based 3D bioprinting

Additive manufacturing techniques in general are used to create layered structures. The most promising of these for the generation of volumetric cell-containing constructs is extrusion-based 3D printing (Figure 7 A), in this case termed 3D bioprinting (in the present book referred to as bioplotting or plotting), whereby the layers are deposited strand by strand. This technique enables the generation of macroporous constructs (scaffolds) in clinically relevant sizes and a variety of shapes (Figure 7 B) from highly-viscous materials with high cell densities. Further-more, with multichannel plotting, different materials and cell types can be used simultaneously and with precise spatial distribution within a scaffold (Figure 7 C). Plotting has so far been used successfully with a variety of different cell types such as fibroblasts, chondrocytes, hepatocytes, and MSC as stated in recent reviews (Badwaik, 2019; Matai et al., 2020).

Apart from a wide variety of cell types, a multitude of materials have been investigated for the plotting of cells, but to date alginate remains one of the most commonly used biopolymers and, as mentioned, is also often employed for islet encapsulation. At low concentrations, the matrix-forming alginate supports the survival of different cell types, however, as reviewed by Malda *et al.* alginate solutions with a low polymer content have a very low viscosity whereas successful plotting requires a highly viscous shear-thinning hydrogel (blend) to achieve shape-fidelity during the plotting process (Malda et al., 2013). Increasing the viscosity of alginate can be achieved by creating a blend with other biopolymers such as methylcellulose (MC), which is known for its use as a thickening agent in food industry (Coffey et al., 2006). The addition of MC to an alginate solution creates a highly viscous hydrogel blend ideal for plotting which to the best of the author's knowledge was first published by Schütz *et al.* from our group (Schütz et al., 2017, published online 2015). With the increased viscosity of this blend it was possible to create scaffolds with up to 50 layers with lasting shape fidelity during the plotting process prior to crosslinking (Figure 7 B).

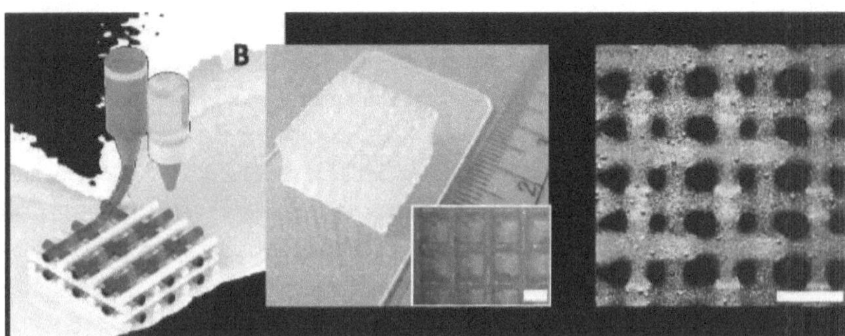

Figure 7: 3D bioplotting. A) Schematic depiction of extrusion-based plotting using two different materials. B) Plotted 3D scaffold consisting of 3 % alginate & 9 % methylcellulose (Alg/MC). Scale bar = 1 mm. (Schütz et al., 2017) C) Scaffold created by multichannel plotting with alternating strands of Alg/MC containing algae (*Chlamydomonas reinhardtii*) in green, and strands of Alg/MC containing SaOS-2, cells from a human bone osteosarcoma cell line, in blue. Scale bar = 3 mm. (Lode et al., 2015)

Furthermore, the blend supported survival and differentiation of MSC. The same blend was later used by Li *et al.* in 2017 for plotting of mouse fibroblasts, who did not incorporate the cells into the blend prior to plotting though but plotted material and cell layers alternatingly (Li et al., 2017). In a following study by our group performed in collaboration with this author, the blend consisting of 3 % alginate and 9 % methylcellulose (Alg/MC) was further characterised in terms of the influence of different sterilisation methods on MC. In a comparison between autoclaving, supercritical CO_2 ($scCO_2$) treatment, γ-irradiation, and ultraviolet (UV) irradiation, especially the highly energetic γ-irradiation was shown to impact the Mw of MC and thereby the plottability of the blend, whereas use of $scCO_2$ negatively influenced cytocompatibility (Hodder et al., 2019). Within the blend MC provides stability during the plotting process and increases the shear-thinning properties, thereby enabling the fabrication of macroporous scaffolds. Furthermore the simple presence of non-crosslinked MC within, but likely also its release from the crosslinked alginate network creates microporosity within the scaffold strands (Schütz et al., 2017; Hodder et al., 2019). It has also been shown that this microporosity can at least partially be tailored by the amount of MC used and could influence cell viability (Gonzalez-Fernandez et al., 2019).

2.3.2 Bioplotting of islets

With the use of plotting for the encapsulation of pancreatic islets, it could be possible to combine the advantages of micro- and macroencapsulation, that is encase a large number of islets together in a single scaffold for extra-hepatic transplantation and easy retrieval while retaining short diffusion distances. Furthermore, pancreatic islets could be plotted together with supportive cell types such as MSC with complete control over the spatial distribution of both cell types (Yue et al., 2016).

Despite the advantages so far only few studies on applying 3D printing techniques for diabetes therapies have been published, and of these the majority describe 3D printed matrices which are retrospectively filled with islets, not bioplotted constructs. 3D printed matrices usually consist of poly-lactic acid or poly(lactic-co-glycolic acid). Such matrices were shown to improve culture time when filled with extracellular matrix (ECM)-based gels (Daoud et al., 2011), or to support stem cell (SC)-derived insulin-producing cells, human islets, and pancreatic organoids when filled with fibrin, platelet lysate, and collagen / Matrigel respectively (Farina et al., 2017; Song & Millman, 2017; Soltanian et al., 2019). All of these gels are biodegradable in the human body though, and do not provide long-term protection from the immune system. On the other hand, 3D printing was recently also employed to generate a stable microporous surrounding structure for an alginate sheet containing cells of the insulin producing cell line INS-1 (Espona-Noguera et al., 2019).

Plotting of islets is a more complex issue, as in addition to the requirements for normal encapsulation, i.e. immune protection and support of functionality, it is also required that the hydrogels are viscous enough to remain stable until crosslinking, which often interferes with the diffusion of glucose and insulin. The first publication reporting on bioplotted islets was by Marchioli *et al.* who used a hydrogel blend consisting of 4 % alginate and 5 % gelatine, and could show a high viability but no functionality. As the human islets recovered functionality after removal from the bioplotted constructs and the diffusion of glucose was shown to be slower than in plain alginate, it is likely that the dense meshwork of the scaffold interfered with the functionality through impaired diffusion of glucose and insulin (Marchioli et al., 2015). Improved functionality of human and murine islets and SC-derived insulin producing cells in porcine ECM-based gels were shown in a study by Kim *et al.* who reported functionality of islets in the blend but did not explicitly show functionality in plotted scaffolds (Kim et al., 2019). Furthermore, the ECM-based material is likely to lack immunoprotective properties due to its fast biodegradability. Probable immunoprotection through the use of 2 % alginate with 7.5 % methacrylated gelatine and the co-plotting of a second cell type was presented by Liu *et al.* (Liu et al., 2019). They employed the so-called core-shell technique to plot murine islets in the protected core surrounded by a shell containing endothelial progenitor cells. However, in this study it was again possible to show high islet survival but no functional response to glucose stimulation.

In summary, to date it was possible to show viability but no satisfactory functionality of 3D bioplotted human and murine islets embedded in different materials.

3 Materials & Methods

3.1 Cell culture

3.1.1 Cell lines

Human telomerase reverse transcriptase immortalized mesenchymal stem cells (hTERT-MSC) (Böker et al., 2008) were kindly provided by Prof. Matthias Schieker (Laboratory of Experimental Surgery and Regenerative Medicine, Ludwig Maximilian University, Munich, Germany). hTERT-MSC were stored in freezing medium (Cryo-SFM; PromoCell, Germany) in liquid N_2 and were cultured in α-MEM (Biochrom, Germany) supplemented with 10 % (v/v) fetal bovine serum (FBS; Gibco® by ThermoScientific, USA), 100 U/ml Penicillin / 100 µg/ml Streptomycin (Life Technologies, USA) and 1 % (v/v) L-glutamine (Life Technologies). Medium was changed every 3-4 days. For cell expansion, 1×10^6 hTERT-MSC were plated per T175 flask and sub-cultivated once a week at approximately 80 % confluency.

Rat insulinoma derived INS-1 cells were a kind donation from Prof. Emeritus Claes B. Wollheim (MD Department of Cell Physiology and Metabolism University Medical Center 1, Geneva, Switzerland). INS-1 were stored in Cryo-SFM at -80°C and cultured in RPMI 1640 (Gibco) supplemented with 10 % (v/v) heat-inactivated FBS (HI-FBS), 20 mM HEPES pH 7.4 (Roth, Germany), 100 U/ml Penicillin / 100 µg/ml Streptomycin, 1 mM sodium pyruvate (AppliChem, Germany), 2 mM L-glutamine, and 50 µM 2-Mercaptoethanol (Sigma, USA). Medium was changed every 2-3 days. For expansion of cells, INS-1 were plated at a density of 1×10^7 per T175 flask and sub-cultivated twice a week at approximately 70 % confluency.

Adherent cell lines were cultured at 37°C and 5 % CO_2. For sub-cultivation or use in experiments, adherent cell lines were detached from culture flasks with Trypsin/EDTA (0.05 % Trypsin, 0.02 % EDTA; Biochrom) and cell count was determined after trypan blue (Sigma) staining by use of a Neubauer counting chamber.

3.1.2 Primary islets from rat

All islet isolations from rat were performed according to guidelines established by the "Technische Universität Dresden" Institutional Animal Care and Use Committee. Pancreata were obtained from 10-12 week old wild type female Wistar rats and digested with collagenase as described by Barkai et al. (Barkai et al., 2013) with slight modifications. For each of the twelve isolations performed within this work, islets from 10 rats were pooled. Briefly, the pancreata were infused with 10 ml of glucose-free RPMI 1640 medium without supplements (Gibco) containing 1 mg/ml collagenase (Sigma) and 0.1 mg/ml DNase (Roche, Switzerland) during the dissection and kept on ice until digestion at 37°C for 13 min. Digestion was stopped by addition of ice-cold wash buffer consisting of RPMI 1640 with 5.5 mM glucose and supplemented with 10 % HI-FBS. The tissue was homogenized, and islets were purified by centrifugation using a discontinuous Ficoll-gradient (densities 1.125/1.096g/1.08g/1.069g/cm^3 in Euro Collins Solution; Sigma) for 15 min at 1590 g and 4°C. Purified islets were washed twice and kept in culture medium consisting of RPMI 1640 with 5.5 mM glucose, supplemented with 10 % HI-FBS, 20 mM HEPES pH 7.4, and 100 U/ml Penicillin / 100 µg/ml Streptomycin overnight under cell culture conditions. Exocrine debris was then removed manually, islet equivalents (IEQ) were determined using dithizone staining (chapter 3.3.2.2, page 33), and islets were cultured at 37°C and 5 % CO_2 in suspension culture or in plotted scaffolds for up to 14 days. Medium was changed every other day.

3.1.3 Neonatal porcine islet-like cell clusters

NICC were isolated at the Gene Center Munich and transferred to Dresden via courier on day 3 after isolation. Pancreata were obtained from neonatal wild-type pigs < 8 days of age and pieces were digested with collagenase at 37°C as described by Korbutt *et al.* (Korbutt et al., 1996). Thereafter, the digest was filtered and washed repeatedly with Hank's Balanced Salt Solution (HBSS). NICC were cultured for 3 days in recovery medium consisting of Ham's F12/M199 with protease inhibitors, antioxidants and additional nutrients at the Gene Center. After arrival in Dresden, medium was changed to maturation medium consisting of Ham's F-10 (Sigma) supplemented with 0.5 % (w/v) bovine serum albumin (BSA, Roth), 10 mM glucose (Sigma), 50 µM 3-Isobutyl-1-methylxanthin (IBMX, Sigma), 100 U/ml Penicillin / 100 µg/ml Streptomycin, 2 mM L-glutamine, 10 mM Nicotinamide (Sigma), and 1.6 mM $CaCl_2$ (Merck Millipore, Germany) as described by Korbutt *et al.* (Korbutt et al., 1996). Culture conditions for NICC were equivalent to those for primary islets from rat. For each isolation, NICC from 1-3 neonatal pigs were pooled.

3.2 <u>Material preparation and characterisation</u>

3.2.1 Hydrogel preparation

The hydrogel blend used for plotting, which had previously been established in this laboratory (Schütz et al., 2017), consisted of 3 % (w/v) alginate and 9 % (w/v) methylcellulose (MC; Sigma; Mw = 88 kDa) with a degree of substitution of 1.5-1.9 for maximum water solubility. Research-grade alginate, routinely used in the laboratory for the preparation of this blend, had been purchased from Sigma (viscosity 5-40 mPa*s), whereas clinical-grade alginate, chosen in regard to its use in islet transplantation studies (Barkai et al., 2013), was from NovaMatrix (Norway; Pronova Up MVM, viscosity > 200 mPa*s). Alginate was dissolved in phosphate buffered saline (PBS; Gibco) overnight while stirring. Sterilization of the dissolved alginate and the methylcellulose powder was achieved via autoclaving for 20 min at 120°C in a table-top autoclave (D-23; Systec, Germany). On the day of plotting, the Alg/MC blend was prepared through vigorous stirring of the appropriate amount of powdered sterile MC into the sterile alginate solution at room temperature and left to swell for 1.5 h.

3.2.2 3D plotting of cell-free hydrogels for material characterisation

The system used for 3D plotting was the BioScaffolder 3.1 from GeSiM mbH (Radeberg, Germany) operated under sterile conditions. The Alg/MC blend was carefully transferred into a sterile cartridge and dispensed through a dosing needle (Nordson GmbH, Germany), with an inner diameter of 610 µm, at a pressure of 70-80 kPa. 3D scaffolds were constructed through layer-by-layer strand deposition, at 10 mm/sec with a 90° change of orientation after each layer. Scaffold dimensions were 9 mm side length with 3 mm strand distance and 4 layers, each layer comprised of a single connected strand (Figure 8). After plotting, the constructs were crosslinked in 1 ml of 70 mM strontium chloride (SrCl$_2$; Roth) for 10 min, washed in 1 ml culture medium to remove residual SrCl$_2$ and kept at 37°C and 5 % CO$_2$ for up to 14 days. The media used for storage of cell-free hydrogels were DMEM (DMEM GlutaMAX™; Gibco) supplemented with 10 % (v/v) FBS and 100 U/ml Penicillin / 100 µg/ml Streptomycin; and RPMI 1640 supplemented with 10 % (v/v) HI-FBS, 20 mM HEPES pH 7.4, 100 U/ml Penicillin / 100 µg/ml Streptomycin, 1 mM sodium pyruvate, 2 mM L-glutamine and 50 µM 2-mercaptoethanol.

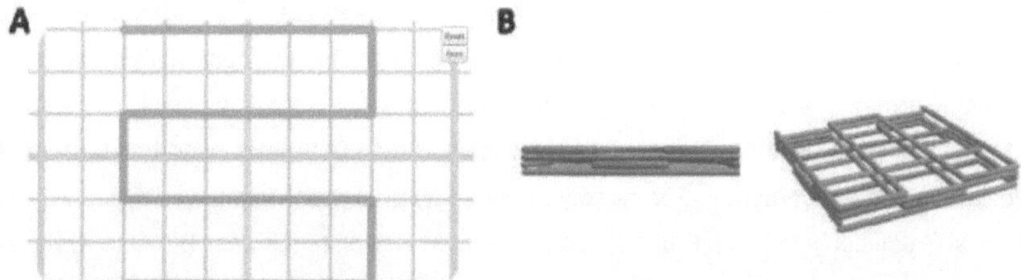

Figure 8: Schematic depiction of scaffold geometry. A) One scaffold layer comprised of a single connected strand shown in green colour. B) A complete scaffold with 4 layers.

3.2.3 Rheological characterisation

Rheological measurements were performed using a plate rheometer (Rheotest RN 4; Rheotest, Medingen, Germany).

The viscosities of Alg/MC pastes were determined at room temperature using a plate diameter of 50 mm, and a plate-plate distance of 0.5 mm. Shear thinning was tested for Alg/MC pastes prepared with research-grade and clinical-grade alginate by constantly increasing rotational shear rate from 0 to 100 s^{-1} (increment 0.08 s^{-1}). Before measurement, the pastes were left to swell for 1.5 h analogous to pastes used for cell culture experiments.

For the determination of crosslinking density, first the viscoelastic region of plotted and cross-linked Alg/MC scaffolds, prepared as described above, was determined with an initial amplitude sweep test. Based on that oscillatory frequency sweep tests (f = 0.01–10 s^{-1}) were performed at 40 Pa.

3.2.4 Quantification of ion release

The Fluitest CA CPC assay method (Analyticon® Biotechnologies AG, Germany), which detects divalent ions, was used to measure the Ca^{2+}- or Sr^{2+}-concentration of the culture supernatants at progressive intervals during scaffold incubation. Cell-free scaffolds of similar size and structure as used for cell plotting were incubated for 21 days under cell culture conditions in 1 ml DMEM or RPMI 1640 supplemented as described in chapter 3.1.1 (page 26). The supernatant was collected every 3-4 days and 1 ml of fresh medium was added. The Fluitest assay was performed as per the manufacturer's instructions and absorbance was measured on a microplate reader (Infinite M200 Pro; Tecan, Switzerland) at 570 nm.

3.2.5 Determination of methylcellulose content

For quantitative analysis of MC release, a quantitative Mykoval™-based assay was used. Alg/MC scaffolds were incubated for 21 days under cell culture conditions in 1 ml DMEM or RPMI 1640 supplemented as described in chapter 3.1.1 (page 26). The supernatant was collected every 3-5 days and 1 ml of fresh medium was added. The fluorophore Mykoval™ (Hund Wetzlar, Germany), a fluorescence marker primarily applied for detection of cellulose and chitin in fungal cell walls (Koch & Pimsler, 1987; Rasconi et al., 2009), was used to determine MC released into the supernatant. For measurements, 180 µl of supernatant was mixed with 20 µl Mykoval™ solution in a black F-bottom polystyrene 96 well plate (Greiner Bio-One, Germany). The samples were incubated for 5 min protected from light and measured using a microplate reader, excitation and emission wavelengths used were 400 and 450 nm, respectively. The assay was calibrated with a concentration range of 0.003-0.375 % MC via detected fluorescence signal and regression analysis to obtain sample concentration was performed via non-linear regression (Model: one-site saturation) using GraphPad Prism 8 for Windows (GraphPad Software, USA).

3.2.6 Preparation of cell-free hydrogel discs

In order to analyse permeability of the hydrogel, the Alg/MC was compared to plain alginate samples, both prepared as hydrogel discs of similar size and surface, since 3 % plain alginate cannot be plotted into macroporous constructs with any shape-fidelity.

To obtain uniform samples with even surfaces for uptake and release experiments (chapter 3.2.7.1, page 30 f.), metal rings with an inner diameter of 12 mm and a height of 0.9 mm were placed on a Teflon membrane wetted with 70 mM $SrCl_2$. The rings were filled with either 3 % (w/v) alginate or 3 % / 9 % (w/v) Alg/MC, covered with a second wetted Teflon membrane and incubated in 70 mM $SrCl_2$ for 30 min for complete crosslinking. To create an approximation of macroporosity, a biopsy punch with an inner diameter of 2 mm (pfm medical, Germany) was used to punch holes into each disc (Figure 9).

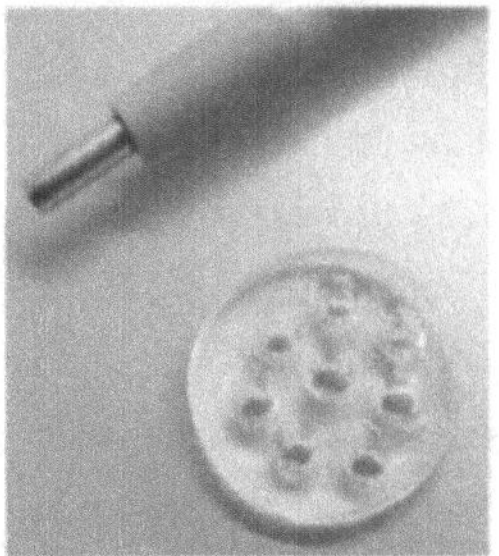

Figure 9: Representative image of a crosslinked alginate hydrogel disc punctured with a biopsy punch. Disc diameter 15 mm, height 2.5 mm.

To obtain samples for measurements in a diffusion chamber system (chapter 3.2.7.2), Alg/MC as well as plain alginate discs were prepared within stainless steel washers (Toolcraft, Germany) of 40 mm inner diameter and a height of 0.5 or 1 mm. Gels within washers were manufactured between 2 filter papers (smooth medium fast filtration papers MN 616, 0.2 mm height and 70 cm diameter; Macherey-Nagel, Germany) wetted with 70 mM $SrCl_2$, flattened, and incubated in 70 mM $SrCl_2$ for 15 min for complete crosslinking.

3.2.7 Permeability measurements

3.2.7.1 Uptake and release experiments

Glucose: Hydrogel discs of plain alginate and Alg/MC, or plotted Alg/MC scaffolds, were prepared as described and saturated with 3 g/L glucose (Sigma) in cell culture conditions for up to 7 days with medium changes every 2 days. The solution used for saturation was HBSS (Thermo Fisher, USA) for comparison of the materials (alginate vs Alg/MC), and RPMI 1640 without supplements for comparison of the alginates (research-grade vs clinical-grade). Release experiments were performed on day 1, 4, and 7 of saturation. For release, the hydrogels were transferred into 1 ml glucose-free HBSS or culture medium and further incubated under cell culture conditions. After 30 min, a sample of 100 µl was taken, after 2 h the remaining 900 µl were removed and the hydrogels were dissolved in 2 ml of 100 mM sodium citrate (Merck Millipore) for 3 h at room temperature. All samples were stored at 4°C until quantification of glucose which was done with the Glucose Assay Kit I (Eton Bioscience, USA) as to the manufacturer's instructions and fluorescence was measured at 490 nm using a microplate reader. For calculation of release in percent, the glucose measured from the supernatant was compared to the total amount of glucose, i.e. the amount measured from the supernatant added to the amount measured from the dissolved scaffold.

Insulin: To keep the concentration of insulin constant, i.e. to keep the timeframe for the experiment as short as possible only uptake was measured. Alginate discs and plotted Alg/MC scaffolds were prepared as described above and kept in RPMI 1640 under cell culture conditions for up to 7 days. On day 1, 4, and 7, triplicates were incubated in 1 ml medium each with 10 ng/ml human recombinant insulin (Sigma). After 2 h, supernatants were collected and stored at -20°C until measurement, hydrogels were dissolved in 3 ml of 100 mM sodium citrate at 4°C. Insulin in the supernatants and dissolved scaffolds was quantified using human insulin enzyme-linked immunosorbent assay (ELISA) kits (Mercodia, Sweden) according to the manufacturer's instructions and assayed on a microplate reader at an absorbance of 450 nm. For normalization, the insulin content was calculated as ng insulin per 100 mg material based on the wet weight of the corresponding hydrogel samples.

3.2.7.2   Diffusion chamber system

The final system chosen for diffusion chamber measurements was the "Osmosis and Electrochemistry-Chamber, DURAN®" (PHYWE, Germany).

Gels for measurements in this system were prepared as described briefly in chapter 3.2.6 (page 29) and in more detail in chapter 4.1.3.2 (page 46), and inserted between the chamber halves during chamber assembly. Chamber halves were filled with 58 ml. To align the filling level in both halves, ceramic beads (Precellys 2.8 mm zirconium oxide beads; Bertin Technologies, France) were added on one side.

For diffusion of glucose, chambers were filled with 10 mM $SrCl_2$ solution, with a concentration of 0 or 5 g/L glucose in either half. For diffusion of insulin, chambers were filled with Krebs Ringer bicarbonate buffer (137 mM NaCl, 4.7 mM KCl, 1.2 mM KH_2PO_4, 1.2 mM $MgSO_4$*$7H_2O$, 2.5 mM $CaCl_2$*$2H_2O$, 25 mM $NaHCO_3$ (all from Merck Millipore), 0.25 % (w/v) BSA), with a concentration of 0 or 250 ng/ml insulin in either half. Prior to insulin diffusion experiments, the chamber system was incubated with Krebs Ringer bicarbonate buffer with 0.25 % BSA for coating to reduce the binding of insulin to the glass.

The assembled chamber system was kept at 37°C on a magnetic stirrer for diffusion measurements; 200 µl sample volume were taken from each chamber half in regular intervals of at least 30 min for a minimum of 3 h.

For an exact measurement of the mean height of hydrogel discs each disc was carefully measured at 10 different positions with callipers after removal from the chamber system and values were averaged. Callipers were judged to result in sufficiently precise measurements after verification with quantitative analysis of cross-sections imaged microscopically.

To assess glucose or insulin accumulating in the hydrogel discs, the discs were dissolved in 10 ml of 1 M sodium hydrogen carbonate (Merck Millipore) after measurement of height. Glucose was measured via quantification of reducing sugars with the 3,5-dinitrosalicylic acid assay (DNS-assay), which can be used to detect much higher concentrations of glucose than the Glucose Assay Kit I. The DNS reagent consisted of 8.5 mM potassium sodium tartrate (stock solution 42.5 mM in 2 M NaOH) and 48 mM DNS (stock solution 96 mM in distilled water; all reagents from Merck Millipore). For the actual measurement, equal volumes of sample and DNS reagent were mixed, heated to 99°C for 10 min in a Thermocell mixing block (Bionova, Italy), and quickly cooled down to 4°C. The reaction mix was diluted 1:5 with cold distilled water and absorbance at 540 nm was measured on a microplate reader. Insulin was quantified applying the human insulin ELISA kit (Mercodia) according to the manufacturer's instructions and assayed on a microplate reader at an absorbance of 450 nm.

3.3 <u>Plotting and characterisation of cell-laden constructs</u>

3.3.1 Incorporation of cells & scaffold preparation

For the printing of cell lines, the adherent cells were detached and 5×10^6 hTERT-MSC or 3×10^7 INS-1 per gram Alg/MC were suspended in 100 µl culture medium per gram and mixed with the material.

In case of islet plotting, islets were centrifuged under gentle conditions (1 min at 200 g, decreased acceleration and deceleration) and 3,000-6,000 rat IEQ or 10,000-45,000 porcine IEQ per gram Alg/MC were suspended in 100 µl culture medium per gram Alg/MC and mixed with the material. Murine islets were used one day after isolation, while neonatal porcine islet-like cluster were kept in culture for up to 10 days after isolation before plotting.

For incorporation into the material, single cells or islets were resuspended in the appropriate amount of medium and gently mixed (folded) into the Alg/MC-blend with a spatula.

3D plotted scaffolds (chapter 3.2.2, page 28) were prepared analogous to cell-free scaffolds. Needle diameters were 610 or 840 µm, and the pressures used were 70-80 kPa for experiments with cell lines and 40-50 kPa for islet experiments. All scaffolds were crosslinked in 1 ml of 70 mM $SrCl_2$ for 10 min, and incubated in the respective medium (chapter 3.1, page 26 f.) under cell culture conditions for up to 14 days.

3.3.2 Staining methods for the characterisation of (embedded) cells

3.3.2.1 MTT staining

For a visual assessment of metabolic activity, samples were incubated in 0.5 mg/ml thiazolyl blue tetrazolium bromide (MTT, Sigma) in culture medium under cell culture conditions for 2 h. Images were taken using a stereo light microscope (Leica M205 C).

3.3.2.2 Dithizone (DTZ) staining

For a visual assessment of presence of insulin, free control and plotted islets were briefly incubated in 2 mg/ml DTZ (Sigma) dissolved in 20 % Dimethyl sulfoxide (DMSO; Sigma) in PBS. Images were taken using a stereo light microscope.

3.3.2.3 Live/dead staining

Cell viability was determined using a live/dead viability/cytotoxicity kit (Molecular Probes, USA). The stainings for live and dead cells, calcein AM and ethidium homodimer-1, were diluted in culture medium to 2 and 4 µM, respectively, and plotted scaffolds containing cell lines or islets, as well as free control islets were incubated in the staining solution for 30 min before confocal laser scanning microscopy was performed using a Leica TCS SP5.

For a quantitative assessment of cell viability of INS-1, area of live and dead cells was analysed using the particle analyser of Image J V1.44p (National Institutes of Health, USA). Size of image sections was approximately 900x700x180 µm.

For a semi-quantitative assessment of islet viability, plotted and free control islets were imaged and visually sorted into viability categories (0, 25, 50, 75, 100 % viable) before % viability was calculated as described in Karaoz et al. (Karaoz et al., 2010).

For semi-quantitative assessment of spherical morphology, islets plotted with an inner needle diameter of 610 or 840 µm were imaged and visually sorted into the categories "impacted" and "not impacted", before percent spherical morphology was calculated from the percentage of "not impacted" islets from the total counted.

3.3.2.4 Immunofluorescence

Plotted scaffolds containing islets as well as control islets in suspension culture were fixed overnight in formaldehyde (Merck Millipore) diluted to 4 % (v/v) in HBSS at 4°C. During the following day, the fixed samples were washed with HBSS while shaking gently, with changes of HBSS every 2-3 h. All samples were embedded in Tissue-Tek O.C.T (Sakura Finetek, USA) and cryosections were prepared using a Microm HM 560 Cryostat (Thermo Fisher).

For immunostaining, the cryosections were incubated in PBS at 70°C for 20 min, permeabilized with 0.2 % (v/v) Triton X-100 (Serva, Germany) in PBS and incubated with background sniper (BS966L; Biocare medical, USA) for 11 min at room temperature to block unspecific antibody binding sites.

Primary antibodies used for murine islets were guinea pig polyclonal anti-insulin antibody (1:100, ab7842; Abcam, UK) and mouse monoclonal anti-glucagon antibody (1:2000, G2654; Sigma) incubated overnight at 4°C. Secondary antibodies used were goat anti-guinea pig Alexa Fluor 488 (1:1000, A11073; Life Technologies) and goat anti-mouse Alexa Fluor 568

(1:750, A11031; Life Technologies) applied for 1 h at room temperature. 4',6-Diamidin-2-phenylindol (DAPI, 5 µg/ml; Roche) was applied for 1 h for cell nucleus-specific staining. Primary antibodies used for NICC were mouse monoclonal anti-insulin antibody (clone K36AC10, 1:1000, I2018; Sigma), rabbit polyclonal anti-glucagon antibody (1:200, 2760S; Cell Signaling Technology, USA), and rat monoclonal anti-somatostatin antibody (clone YC7, 1:100, MAB354; Merck), whereby anti-insulin and anti-glucagon were applied overnight at 4°C, and anti-somatostatin for 2 h at RT. Secondary antibodies used were goat anti-mouse Alexa Fluor 488 (1:500, A11001; Life Technologies), goat anti-rabbit Alexa Fluor 568 (1:1000, A11011; Life Technologies), and goat anti-rat Alexa Fluor 647 (1:500, A-21247; Thermo Fisher) applied for 30 min at room temperature. DAPI (5 µg/ml) was applied for 1 h for cell nucleus-specific staining.

All antibodies were diluted in blocking buffer consisting of 0.2 % (v/v) Triton X-100, 2 % (w/v) BSA and 2 % (v/v) goat serum (Gibco) in PBS. Between each staining step, samples were washed at least once with 0.1 % PBS-Tween (Serva).

Cryosections stained for insulin, glucagon, somatostatin, and nuclei were imaged on a Leica TCS SP5.

3.3.2.5 Nuclear apoptosis staining

For the staining of apoptotic nuclei, the In Situ Cell Death Detection Kit TMR red (Sigma), which detects TdT-mediated dUTP-X nick end labelling (TUNEL), was used according to the manufacturer's instructions. Apoptosis in islets was quantitatively assessed by counting nuclei of 25 islets of varying sizes and calculating % nuclei stained for TUNEL compared to all nuclei stained by DAPI.

Cryosections stained for apoptotic nuclei and nuclei were imaged on a Leica TCS SP5.

3.3.3 Functional analysis of islets: Glucose stimulated insulin release (GSIR)

Analysis of islet reaction to stimulation with glucose was done via GSIR assay. For the plotted islets, whole scaffolds were used as single samples, while for the control islets, either 20 rat islets or 50 NICC of varying sizes were picked manually for each sample. On day 1, 4, 7, 11 & 14 after plotting, scaffolds and free control islets were treated with low (3.3 mM) or high (16.4 mM) glucose in Krebs Ringer bicarbonate buffer and secreted insulin was quantified. First, all samples were exposed to 3.3 mM glucose for 2 h (resting conditions); for stimulation, samples were divided in two groups: one was treated with 3.3 mM glucose and the other with 16.4 mM glucose for 3 h. In addition, for murine islets one experiment was performed where all samples were first rested for 1.5 h then stimulated in low-high-low glucose for 2.5 h each. During high-glucose stimulation, NICC were additionally exposed to 100 nM of the GLP-1 analogue liraglutide (Victoza®; Novo Nordisk A/S, Denmark) per ml medium.

Insulin was measured from supernatants stored at -20°C until quantification via high-range rat insulin or porcine insulin ELISA kits (Mercodia) performed to the manufacturer's instructions and assayed on a microplate reader at an absorbance of 450 nm. For normalization, insulin content was calculated in relation to 100 ng DNA. To determine the DNA-content, samples were frozen at -80°C. To dissolve the scaffolds all samples were thawed and incubated in 3 ml of 100 mM sodium citrate on a shaker until complete dissolution. Free control islets were incubated in only 1 ml of 100 mM sodium citrate but otherwise treated identically. Cells were lysed overnight in a 60°C water bath followed by 10 min ultrasonication in an ice-cold water bath. Samples were frozen again until measurement of DNA-content which was performed using the QuantiFluor dsDNA system (Promega, USA) as per the manufacturer's instructions and measured on a microplate reader. Excitation and emission wavelengths were 485 and 535 nm, respectively.

For calculation of the stimulation index (SI) the released insulin was first normalized to the DNA-content of each sample as described. This was followed by dividing the amount of insulin released in high glucose stimulation by the amount released in low glucose. For each condition (plotted vs free control islets, low vs high glucose), at least nine samples over the course of up to seven different experiments were analysed for experiments performed with murine islets and clinical-grade alginate for the timepoints day 1, 4, and 7. For NICC, stimulation with glucose was performed on five isolations whereby liraglutide was used in two of them.

3.4 <u>Statistics</u>

Sample size is denoted by "n =" and expresses number of replicates within one experiment for the majority of data depicted. In case of stimulation indices of islets, n denotes number of replicate isolations.

Data were tested for statistically significant differences ($p < 0.05$) using a 95 % confidence interval. For 2 sample groups at a single timepoint 2-tailed t-tests were used for comparison. Two sample groups over multiple timepoints were compared via 1-way ANOVA, multiple sample groups over multiple timepoints with 2-way ANOVA, each with post-hoc Tukey. All statistical analyses were performed using GraphPad Prism 8 for windows.

4 Results

The present book consists of four parts. Among these, the first part deals with the characterisation of the cell-free plotting material investigating key features of the hydrogel, and the second part with the incorporation of cells into the material as prerequisite for bioplotting. The third part describes 3D plotting of primary adult islets from rats as a proof-of-concept for the feasibility of the envisaged method, and in part four preliminary data for the plotting of the more clinically relevant neonatal porcine islet-like cluster is provided.

4.1 <u>Adaptation & characterisation of cell-free Alg/MC</u>

The basic material chosen for the plotting of islets was an alginate/methylcellulose hydrogel blend which had previously been established in this lab by using alginate for research purposes ("research-grade" alginate) and $CaCl_2$ for crosslinking (Schütz et al., 2017). In the present work, the blend was adapted for preparation with endotoxin-free alginate ("clinical-grade" alginate) used in clinical trials for the encapsulation of pancreatic islets (Ludwig et al., 2013), and for crosslinking with $SrCl_2$ to achieve compatibility with the islet-specific culture medium. The different compositions of the hydrogel blend were characterized in terms of viscosity, stability of the crosslinked scaffolds over time, crosslinking density and MC content, as well as permeability for glucose and insulin with uptake and release assays in addition to analyses with a diffusion chamber system.

In all cases the hydrogel consisted of either 3 % alginate or 3 % / 9 % Alg/MC, and crosslinking was achieved with either 100 mM $CaCl_2$ (Schütz et al., 2017) or 70 mM $SrCl_2$ (Ludwig et al., 2012). Except if stated otherwise in the respective subsection, all samples were incubated under cell culture conditions in DMEM supplemented with FBS and antibiotics (in the following referred to as DMEM[+]) or RPMI 1640 supplemented with HI-FBS, antibiotics, HEPES, sodium pyruvate, L-glutamine and 2-Mercaptoethanol (in the following referred to as RPMI[+]) as described in detail in chapter 3.1 (page 26 f.).

4.1.1 Paste viscosity and scaffold stability

The use of research-grade and clinical-grade alginate resulted in pastes which demonstrated shear thinning behaviour with a decrease in viscosity under shear strain (Figure 10). Comparison between pastes at a shear rate of 1-100 s^{-1} revealed a significantly lower viscosity for the paste prepared with research-grade alginate. All pastes were plottable by using pressures between 40 and 80 kPa, and both scaffold types could be crosslinked with Ca^{2+} and Sr^{2+} ions.

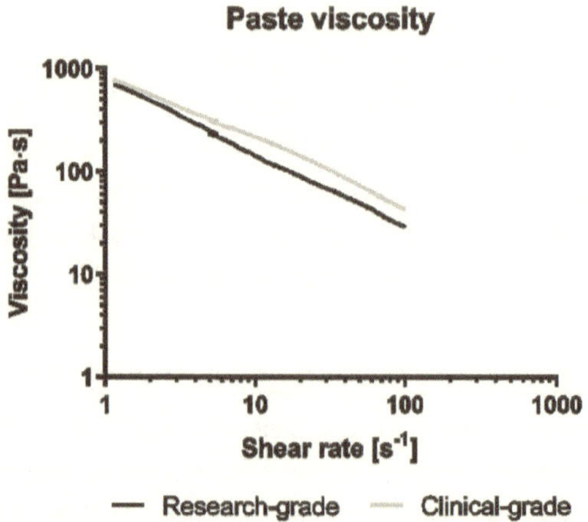

Figure 10: Paste viscosity. Viscosity over shear rate of Alg/MC pastes prepared with research-grade or clinical-grade alginate. Mean, n = 4.

The hydrogel blend had previously been used for culture of cells in DMEM- or α-MEM-based media, the medium used for the culture of murine islets *in vitro* is RPMI-based though. Preliminary experiments revealed a lack of stability of scaffolds crosslinked with $CaCl_2$ and stored in RPMI⁺ medium, which led to a disintegration within the first day (Figure 11 A). When crosslinking was achieved via $SrCl_2$ instead, plotted macroporous scaffolds maintained stability and high shape-fidelity over a duration of 21 days in culture independent of the alginate used (Figure 11 A&B). The crosslinking of both types of alginate in plotted Alg/MC scaffolds with $SrCl_2$ was verified with rheological measurements of scaffolds one day after plotting (Figure 11 C). Scaffolds prepared with the two different alginates showed almost constant storage moduli over the whole range of angular velocities measured, with a higher storage modulus apparent in the scaffolds prepared with research-grade alginate though, indicating a higher crosslinking density.

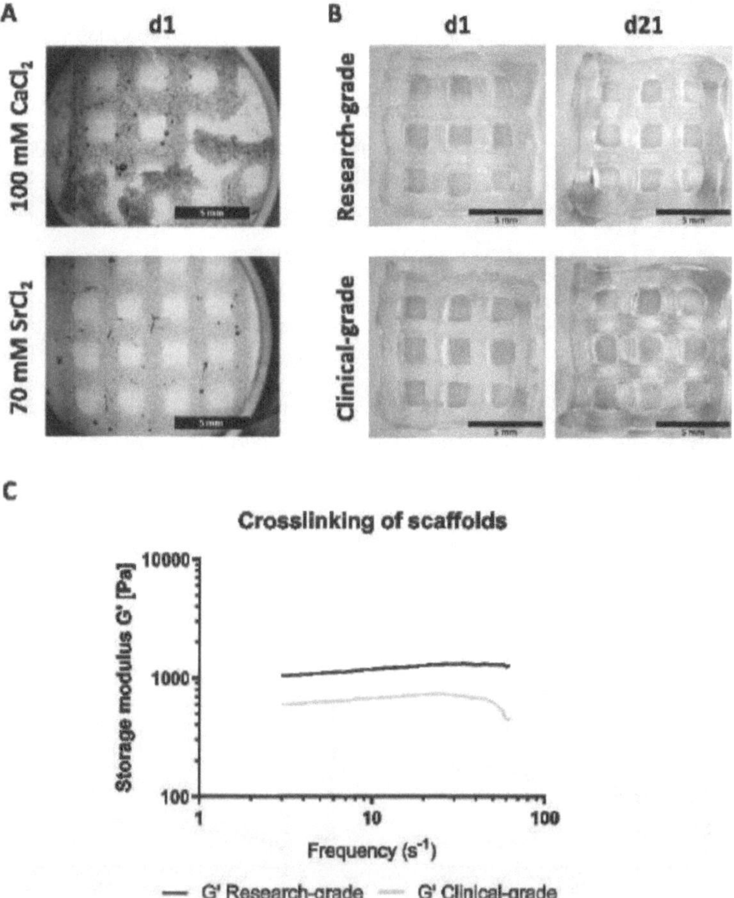

Figure 11: Shape fidelity and crosslinking density of cell-free plotted Alg/MC scaffolds. A) Representative images of plotted and Ca^{2+}- (top) or Sr^{2+}- (bottom) crosslinked research-grade Alg/MC scaffolds on day 1 after plotting. Scale bars = 5 mm. B) Representative images of plotted and Sr^{2+}-crosslinked Alg/MC scaffolds over 21 days in culture, indicating high shape fidelity and stability. Scale bars = 5 mm. C) Storage modulus of plotted scaffolds crosslinked with 70 mM $SrCl_2$ on day 1 after plotting, which indicates complete crosslinking and a higher crosslinking density for research-grade alginate. Mean, n = 4.

4.1.2 Scaffold composition during incubation under cell culture conditions

The hydrogels used for this study are composed of alginate, methylcellulose and $CaCl_2$ or $SrCl_2$. Ca^{2+} and Sr^{2+} ions crosslink alginate molecules reversibly (Lee & Mooney, 2012), while the MC remains non-crosslinked. Therefore, even though the scaffolds remain stable over time in culture, the overall composition of the material changes when ions and MC are released from the scaffolds into the supernatant.

Release of ions

Having observed a lack of stability in Ca^{2+}- but not Sr^{2+}-crosslinked scaffolds stored in RPMI[+] while they remain stable in DMEM[+] (Schütz et al., 2017), plotted and crosslinked Alg/MC scaffolds prepared from both alginates were systematically tested for the release of crosslinking ions over 21 days of culture. Owing to the mentioned lack of stability, release of ions from scaffolds crosslinked with $CaCl_2$ and $SrCl_2$ was observed for culture in DMEM[+] (Figure 12 A), whereas for culture in RPMI[+] only $SrCl_2$-crosslinked scaffolds could be used (Figure 12 B).

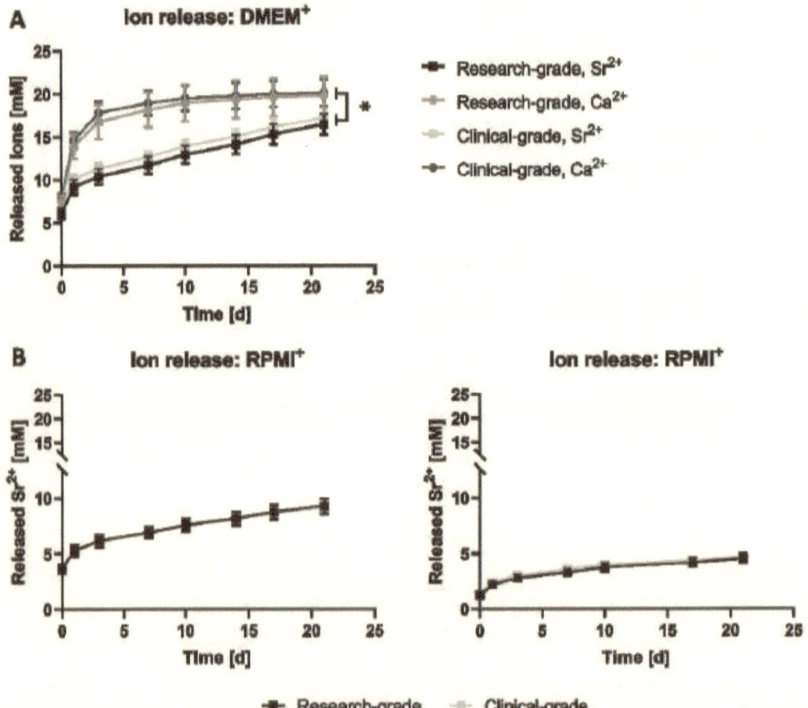

Figure 12: Release of crosslinking ions in different cell culture media. Cumulative release of ions from plotted scaffolds crosslinked with 70 mM $SrCl_2$ or 100 mM $CaCl_2$ prepared with research-grade and clinical-grade alginate over 21 days of culture. A) Release of Ca^{2+} & Sr^{2+} ions into DMEM[+]. Mean ± SD, n = 6, significances indicate *$p<0.05$. B) Release of Sr^{2+} ions into RPMI[+] displayed for two repeat experiments in the left and right graph whereby the data points are nearly identical in the left graph, so that the two curves cannot been seen clearly. Mean ± SD, n = 6 for each.

For all scaffolds, a burst release of ions shortly after crosslinking could be observed and release of ions was independent of the alginate type (Figure 12). For scaffolds stored in DMEM[+] (Figure 12 A), a distinct difference between the release of Ca^{2+} and Sr^{2+} ions was visible, with the former being released to a much higher degree at early timepoints but plateauing after day 10. In contrast to that, after the initial burst Sr^{2+} ions were released in a linear fashion over the whole time of observation. Cumulatively, significantly more Ca^{2+} and Sr^{2+} ions had been released into $DMEM^+$ until day 21. For scaffolds stored in $RPMI^+$ (Figure 12 B), the concentration of Sr^{2+} ions detected in the supernatant was 2-3 times lower than in $DMEM^+$ overall, but differed strongly between the three repeat experiments. This difference between the repeat experiments is depicted in Figure 12 B (left and right), for the third repetition which closely resembled Figure 12 B (right) please refer to Figure 61, addendum. Manner of release also varied between the experiments with a continuous increase in released ions over 21 days in the first, and a plateau after day 10 in the following two experiments.

As mentioned, the overall release of Sr^{2+} ions measured was lower in $RPMI^+$ than in $DMEM^+$ although the observation that scaffolds crosslinked with Ca^{2+} remain stable during incubation in $DMEM^+$ but not in $RPMI^+$ medium indicated a rapid and stronger loss of crosslinking ions in $RPMI^+$. This is likely caused by the formation of precipitates in the media (Figure 62, addendum), leading to a reduced concentration of the soluble ions which are detected in the assay used.

<u>Release of methylcellulose</u>
Apart from the loss of crosslinking ions, the release of MC over time also changes scaffold properties. On the one hand, the MC fibres themselves could have a reinforcing effect on scaffold stability (Schütz et al., 2017), on the other hand, the removal of MC fibres over time could possibly influence diffusion characteristics of the scaffolds. MC is a derivative of cellulose and can be detected by similar methods such as staining with Mykoval™ (Hodder et al., 2019). Figure 13 depicts the release of MC from different scaffolds analysed quantitatively with Mykoval™ in two repeat experiments (Figure 13 A&B; for better visibility of data points in Figure 13 A without standard deviation refer to Figure 63, addendum). Analogous to the experiments performed for ion release, plotted Alg/MC scaffolds prepared from both alginates were systematically tested for the release of MC over 21 days of culture under cell culture conditions in $DMEM^+$ and $RPMI^+$ but additionally in 10 mM $SrCl_2$ (low molar crosslinking solution) which is used in later permeability experiments (chapter 4.1.3.3, page 50 ff.). Both quantitative repeat experiments were executed with the same general setup, i.e. substances, concentrations and incubation times both for scaffold preparation and analysis were similar, but conducted one year apart and with different batches of material.

A similarity observed in all experiments was a burst release within the first day (specifically during crosslinking and washing at room temperature and the first 24 h of incubation at 37°C), which plateaued after day 3 at the earliest (Figure 13 B) and day 10 at the latest (Figure 13 A). For the first experiment (Figure 13 A), where scaffolds crosslinked with $CaCl_2$ or $SrCl_2$ were incubated in $DMEM^+$, and scaffolds crosslinked with $SrCl_2$ were incubated in $RPMI^+$, overall release of MC ranged between 60-80 %. Standard deviations in this experiment were very high in all conditions and no significant differences between either the crosslinking ions or the alginate types could be detected.

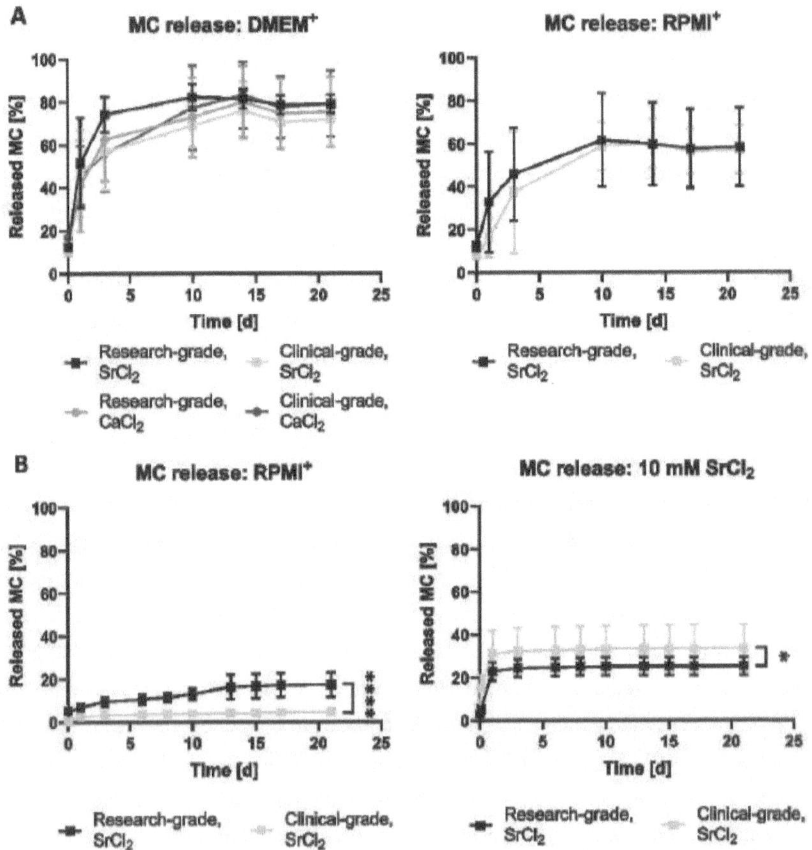

Figure 13: Release of MC in different media. Cumulative release of MC from plotted and crosslinked Alg/MC scaffolds prepared with research-grade or clinical-grade alginate over 21 days of culture. A) Release of MC from scaffolds crosslinked with 70 mM SrCl₂ or 100 mM CaCl₂ and incubated in DMEM⁺ (left), and release from scaffolds crosslinked with 70 mM SrCl₂ and incubated in RPMI⁺ (right). Mean ± SD, n = 6 for each. B) Release of MC from scaffolds crosslinked with SrCl₂ and incubated in RPMI⁺ (left) or 10 mM SrCl₂ (right). Mean ± SD, n = 10 for each, significances indicate *$p<0.05$, ****$p<0.0001$.

For the second experiment (Figure 13 B), only SrCl₂ was used as a crosslinking ion and scaffolds were incubated in either RPMI⁺ or 10 mM SrCl₂. In this experiment, the overall amount of released MC lay between 5 and 30 %, and standard deviations were much lower or even marginal in case of clinical-grade alginate incubated in RPMI⁺.

Release was higher after incubation in 10 mM $SrCl_2$. In a comparison between the alginates, the amount of MC released from research-grade Alg/MC scaffolds surpassed the release from clinical-grade scaffolds in a highly significant manner when incubated in RPMI[+], but was significantly lower when scaffolds were incubated in 10 mM $SrCl_2$. In a comparison between the repeat experiments, scaffolds crosslinked with $SrCl_2$ and incubated in RPMI[+] showed a striking difference in the overall amount of release (60 % vs 20 % in case of research-grade and 60 % vs 5 % in case of clinical-grade alginate).

4.1.3 Permeability for glucose & insulin

An important characteristic of any hydrogel used for the encapsulation of pancreatic islets is the permeability for relevant molecules, specifically for glucose and insulin. Alginate encapsulation has been shown to have a negligible impact on the insulin response of pancreatic islets when small diffusion distances were used (Fritschy et al., 1991; Buchwald et al., 2018), but as mentioned, the addition of MC to the gel influences its characteristics and could alter the permeability of the blend compared to plain alginate. Furthermore, due to variations in the M:G content and the chain lengths of different alginate preparations resulting in different pore sizes, the choice of alginate type could have an influence on permeability as well.

Permeability testing was therefore performed for plain alginate and Alg/MC hydrogels prepared with research-grade and clinical-grade alginate, all crosslinked with 70 mM $SrCl_2$, and analysed with two different setups: For an insight into the behaviour of macroporous plotted scaffolds, uptake & release studies were performed for said scaffolds with hydrogel discs as a bulk material control. To further characterise the gel properties independent of geometry, diffusion of glucose and insulin was also investigated in a diffusion chamber setup which has been established within this work.

4.1.3.1 Uptake and release

<u>Glucose</u>

To gain insight into whether the presence of MC affects release of glucose, a direct comparison of research-grade alginate or Alg/MC gels was conducted on bulk samples with retroactively added macropores (Figure 9, page 30) as plain alginate, due to its low viscosity, does not lend itself to plotting. For this material comparison, hydrogels were stored under cell culture conditions in HBSS containing 3 g/L glucose overnight to deliver glucose into the gels, before being transferred to HBSS without glucose to measure the release after 30 min and 2 h (Figure 14). Overall uptake of glucose was approximately 70 mg for alginate and 120 mg for Alg/MC gels. Within 30 min of incubation in glucose-free HBSS, almost the entirety of the glucose was released into the supernatant and the release did not increase further within the additional 1.5 h of incubation. No difference in the ratio of glucose release could be observed between the materials, indicating that the addition of MC into the alginate does not impact permeability for glucose. A direct comparison to alginate was therefore omitted for further glucose uptake and release experiments.

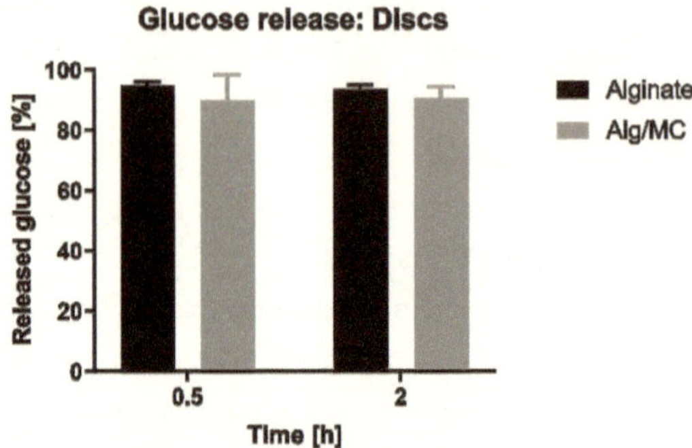

Figure 14: Glucose release from alginate and Alg/MC gel discs. Macroporous gel discs were prepared with research-grade alginate, crosslinked with 70 mM $SrCl_2$, and incubated in HBSS with 3 g/L glucose for 24 h for glucose uptake. Release is depicted after 30 min and 2 h in HBSS w.o. glucose. Mean ± SD, n=3.

To investigate the glucose permeability of plotted Alg/MC scaffolds, that is of the specific geometry also used in later cell culture experiments, the hydrogel blend was prepared with research-grade and clinical-grade alginate and the samples were stored in RPMI 1640 with 3 g/L glucose for uptake and without glucose for release. As investigated in chapter 4.1.2 (page 38 ff.), the scaffold composition changes during prolonged incubation under cell culture conditions and the declining crosslinking density and loss of fibres could influence the permeability characteristics. Uptake and release of glucose was therefore investigated for scaffolds incubated under cell culture conditions for up to 7 days as schematically depicted in Figure 15 A.

Overall uptake of glucose, compared to the amount of material in the respective scaffolds, increased between day 1 and 7 of incubation for both alginate types used. A significant difference between the alginate types could only be detected at the first timepoint, with a lower uptake by scaffolds prepared with clinical-grade alginate (Figure 15 B). Percentage of released glucose (Figure 15 C&D) was calculated from the overall glucose inside the gel. In general, throughout the whole observation period of 7 days, the plotted scaffolds did not undergo a significant change in terms of glucose permeability and the percentage of released glucose was significantly lower from scaffolds prepared with research-grade than from those with clinical-grade alginate. The only exception to this is the release of glucose from research-grade Alg/MC scaffolds after 2 h on day 1 after plotting, which showed a much higher release than at any other timepoint.

In contrast to release experiments performed in HBSS for the comparison between alginate and Alg/MC (Figure 14), where almost all of the glucose contained in the samples originally could be detected in the supernatant after only 30 min, percentage of release was lower from plotted scaffolds in RPMI, with a maximum of 80 % detected in the supernatant after 2 h (Figure 15 D).

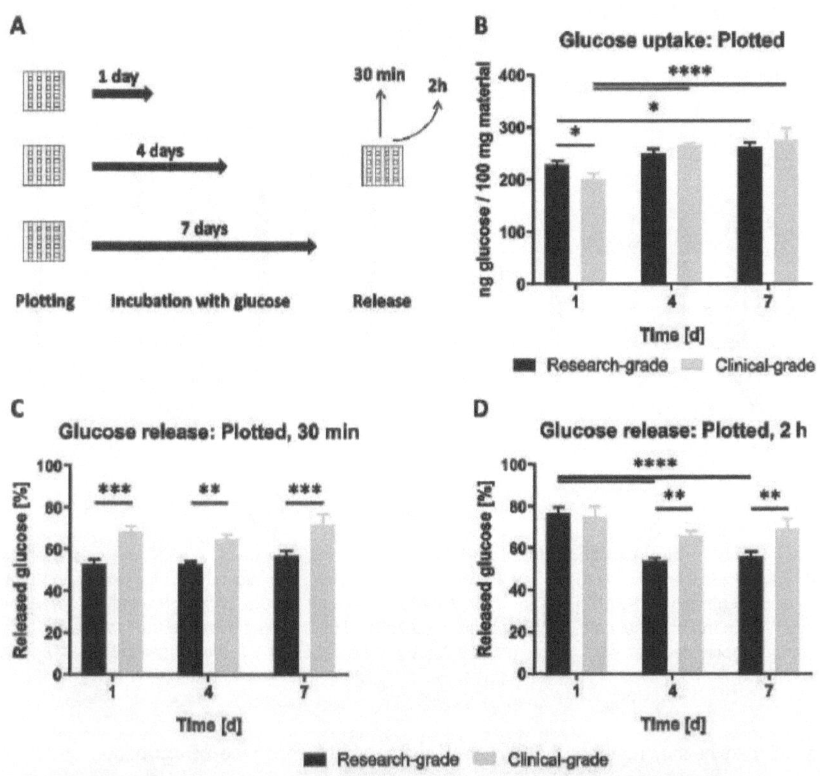

Figure 15: Glucose uptake into and release from plotted Alg/MC scaffolds. Scaffolds were prepared with research-grade or clinical-grade alginate, crosslinked with 70 mM $SrCl_2$, and incubated in RPMI 1640 with 3 g/L glucose for up to 7 days under cell culture conditions before being transferred to glucose-free RPMI 1640. A) Schematic depiction of the glucose release experiment from plotted scaffolds. Released glucose was quantified after 30 min and 2 h. B) Uptake of glucose into scaffolds treated as described in A, quantification from dissolved scaffolds. C&D) Release of glucose from scaffolds treated as described in A. Release is depicted after 30 min (C) and 2 h (D). Mean ± SD, n=3. Significances in all graphs indicate *$p<0.05$, **$p<0.01$, ***$p<0.001$, ****$p<0.0001$.

<u>Insulin</u>

Preliminary experiments indicated a time-dependent reduction in the concentration of insulin measured in RPMI 1640 at 37°C, with a first drop in concentration after only 5 h, and a loss of approximately 20 % after 24 h as measured by ELISA (data not shown).

For this reason, permeability for insulin was assayed not as release from but as uptake into the hydrogel after 30 min and 2 h. Samples analysed were macroporous alginate and Alg/MC discs, as well as plotted Alg/MC scaffolds, all prepared with both, research-grade and clinical-grade alginate and crosslinked with 70 mM $SrCl_2$. Scaffolds were incubated under cell culture conditions for 1 or 7 days prior to uptake experiments and the medium used for the entire experiment was RPMI 1640.

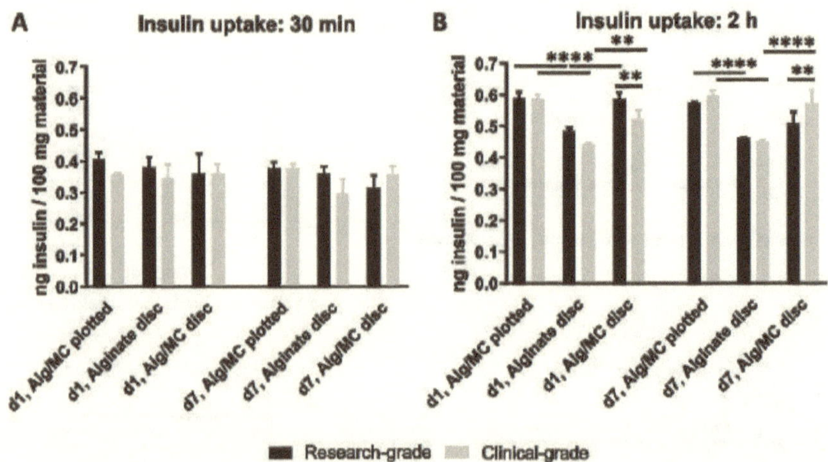

Figure 16: Insulin uptake into alginate and Alg/MC gels. Alginate discs, Alg/MC discs, and plotted Alg/MC scaffolds were prepared with research-grade or clinical-grade alginate, crosslinked with 70 mM $SrCl_2$ and incubated in RPMI 1640 for 1 or 7 days under cell culture conditions. Ingress of insulin (10 ng/ml) into the material calculated as absolute uptake of insulin normalized to the wet weight of the hydrogel samples depicted after 30 min (A) and 2 h (B). Mean ± SD, n=3, significances indicate **$p<0.01$, ****$p<0.0001$.

After 30 min neither material composition, nor geometry, nor time of incubation under cell culture conditions showed any influence on insulin uptake (Figure 16 A). Geometry of Alg/MC samples and time of prior incubation did not influence uptake after 2 h either. However, at the 2 h timepoint (Figure 16 B) a distinct difference between plain alginate and Alg/MC samples could be observed, with the Alg/MC samples taking up more insulin overall. Between the alginate types, a significant difference could only be detected for Alg/MC discs but not for plotted Alg/MC scaffolds nor for the plain alginate discs at the 2 h timepoint. To be able to give a rough estimate on the percentage of insulin taken up per scaffold, it would be necessary to regard the density of the hydrogel scaffolds as equal to that of the supernatant. In this case, 0.4 ng insulin per 100 mg material would equal 40 % and 0.6 ng per 100 mg material would correspond to 60 %.

4.1.3.2 Development of a reliable diffusion chamber system

To be able to characterize diffusion of relevant molecules through the hydrogels used independent of geometry, it was necessary to establish a workflow for the use of a diffusion chamber. Requirements for the chamber system were foremost a protocol for the reproducible preparation of hydrogel discs, the possibility to gently but firmly fix the hydrogel discs between the chamber halves and the possibility to tightly seal the chamber system, both between the chamber halves and towards the outside to avoid leakage but also evaporation. To mimic the conditions in the plotted scaffolds as closely as possible, the gel discs needed a large surface-to-volume ratio. To prevent the formation of a concentration gradient within one chamber half, the contents of each chamber half needed to be stirred continuously necessitating the addition of stir bars and the use of magnetic stirrers. Further requirements were a horizontal setup to eliminate the influence of gravity, a large internal volume to minimise the effect of sampling, and reusability of the chamber.

<u>Osmosis chamber</u>

The final chamber system chosen was the "Osmosis and Electrochemistry-Chamber, DURAN®" (for previous models investigated as diffusion chambers see Figure 64, addendum), which has a large inner volume, a large inner diameter, and is marketed for the use of semi-permeable membranes of any kind while being easy to assemble and to clean. The chamber itself (Figure 17) consists of two halves of borosilicate glass (DURAN®), each 9 cm in length with an inner diameter of 3 cm, a filling volume of approximately 65 ml, and can be closed by a screw cap. To assemble the system, at least one rubber seal ring has to be placed between the chamber halves before the whole chamber is placed within the provided plastic fixture and tightened with screws. For a tightly sealed system, the semi-permeable membrane or hydrogel disc must either be prepared within one rubber seal ring or be placed between two rings before chamber assembly. The sealing of the chamber with a hydrogel disc between the halves occurs solely by pressure from the 10 mm broad flange on the central side of each half.

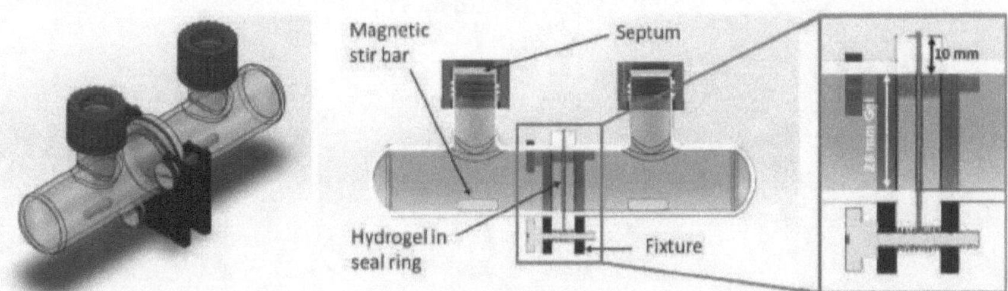

Figure 17: Schematic depiction of the osmosis chamber. From left to right: 3D view, 2D view with labelled components, and magnification of the interface between the chamber halves. The total diameter of the gel is 48 mm, with an exposed surface 28 mm in diameter and an outer rim of 10 mm where the gel is pressed between the chamber halves for a tight fit.

Preparation of hydrogel discs for the osmosis chamber

The requirement for large flat hydrogel discs of reproducible size and firmly connected to seal rings necessitated the development of a protocol for their preparation. In initial tests, the gel discs were prepared within one rubber seal ring, however this reduces the rim of the hydrogel disc which is exposed to pressure between the flanges (Figure 17, right) from 10 to 4 mm. Therefore, gel disc preparation was changed to use stainless steel seal rings with an inner diameter of 4 cm, equal to the diameter of the flanges.

The final protocol for gel disc preparation and chamber assembly was comprised of the following steps and is illustrated in Figure 18: Filter papers were wetted with 70 mM $SrCl_2$ before one seal ring was placed on each and the gels were filled into the cavity while taking care that both, top and bottom side of the seal ring were covered with hydrogel. Subsequently, another $SrCl_2$-wetted filter paper was placed on top of the gel and the gels were rolled out and flattened down to the height of the seal ring (Figure 18 A) by using a large stir bar. The rationale behind using filter papers during gel preparation was to enable crosslinking from top and bottom while keeping the gels on a flat surface and to have a smooth but bendable surface for easy removal of the gels after crosslinking. Wetting the filter papers with $SrCl_2$ and thereby starting the crosslinking process immediately after the gels came in contact with the filter paper was necessary to avoid diffusion of fluid gel parts into the dry filter paper which results in gel and filter forming an inseparable unit during crosslinking.

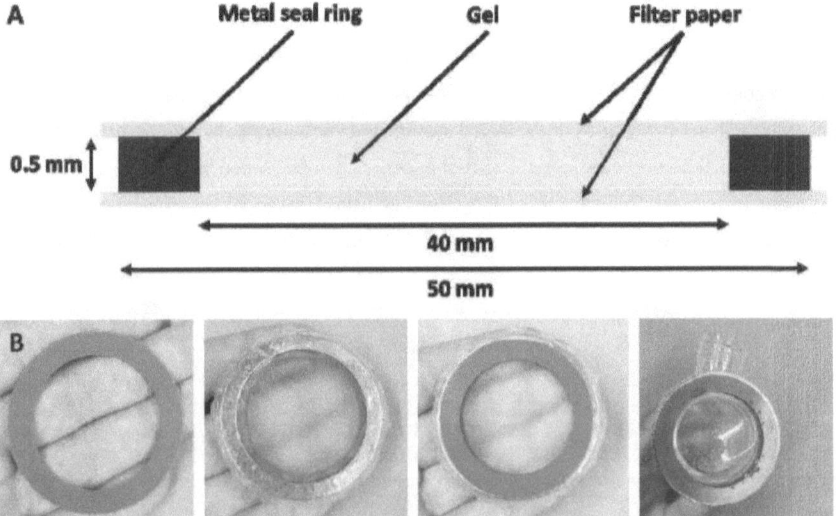

Figure 18: Preparation of hydrogel discs for the osmosis chamber. A) Schematic depiction of the preparation of hydrogel discs in seal rings between filter papers wetted with 70 mM $SrCl_2$. B) Sequence of steps for placing a gel disc between the chamber halves. From left to right: rubber seal ring, gel disc within metal seal ring, second rubber seal ring, and placement of the stack on the opening of one chamber half.

After flattening, the gels were crosslinked in 70 mM $SrCl_2$ for 15 min, overhangs were trimmed and gels were stored in 10 mM $SrCl_2$ for up to 7 days, according to the experimental setup, before chamber assembly. For assembly (Figure 18 B), excess liquid was carefully blotted away and the hydrogel discs were placed between two rubber seal rings, which were then placed between the chamber halves.

To mimic cell culture conditions as closely as possible, cell culture medium was used for storage of gel discs and as chamber content in initial experiments. However, under these conditions, fluid accumulated within the discs after insertion into the chamber, leading to large swellings in both alginate and Alg/MC gels (Figure 19 A&B). As depicted in Figure 19 C, the inner area of the gel discs stored in cell culture medium is often not uniform but comprised of unconnected parts. Storage in different buffer solutions such as HBSS or the incorporation of stiff meshes into the gel discs for additional stability could not prevent the formation of swellings. With respect to structural unity 10 mM $SrCl_2$ were therefore used for storage of gel discs and chamber filling in the majority of diffusion chamber experiments.

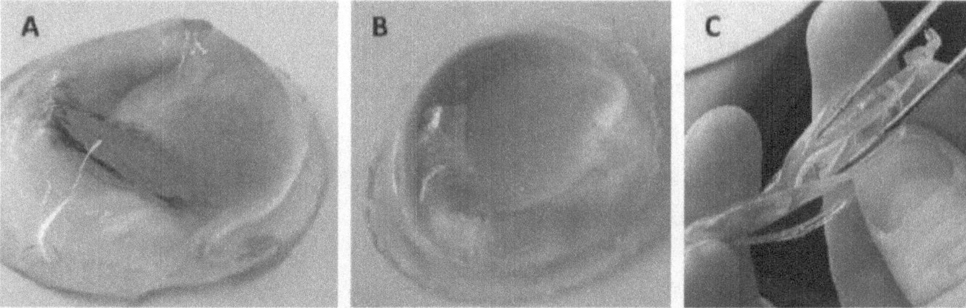

Figure 19: Optimisation of the storage conditions for stable hydrogel discs. A&B) Gel storage and chamber content RPMI 1640: Alginate (A) and Alg/MC (B) gel discs filled with fluid after removal from the osmosis chamber. C) Exemplary depiction of a gel disc stored in RPMI 1640 with unconnected gel parts.

Ex-factory, each chamber half has a maximal filling volume of 65 ml, not accounting for stir bars, but the halves are not entirely identical in inner volume. If both halves are separated by a (semi-permeable) layer and filled with the same volume of liquid, the filling level on both sides is not equal (Figure 20 A). To avoid the possibility of different pressures on both sides influencing diffusion, adjustment of the filling level was realised by the use of stir bars of different sizes and the addition of ceramic beads (Figure 20 B). The beads did not interfere with the movement of the stir bars, nor did they damage the gels.

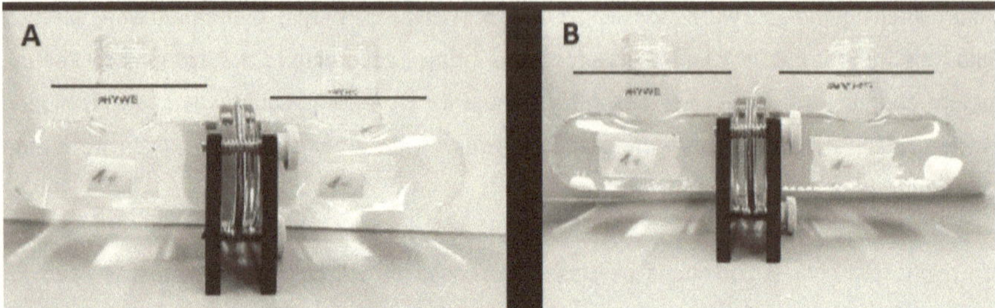

Figure 20: Adjustment of the filling level. Representative depiction of the filling level in a fully assembled osmosis chamber, each chamber half containing 58 ml of 10 mM $SrCl_2$. A) Uneven filling level due to slight differences in chamber volume. B) Adjustment of the filling level with stir bars in different sizes and ceramic beads.

As mentioned above, sealing of the chamber towards the outside to prevent leakage from the system, as well as sealing between the halves to prevent the movement of molecules by any way other than diffusion through the gel, is realised solely by pressure applied to seal rings and the gel. While the seal rings are inherently stable, there was a possibility that the gel discs themselves could get torn at the rim by the application of too much pressure. For proof-of-concept experiments, the chamber was assembled with both, alginate and Alg/MC discs (depicted for Alg/MC in Figure 21), filled with 10 mM $SrCl_2$ and phenol red in one half. With phenol red for a visual assessment it is evident that the insertion into the chamber did not damage the gel and the halves were indeed separated by a semipermeable membrane through which the phenol red molecules diffused over the course of 24 h.

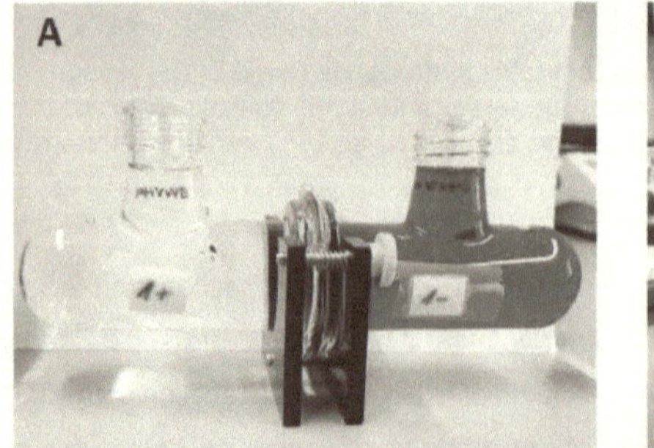
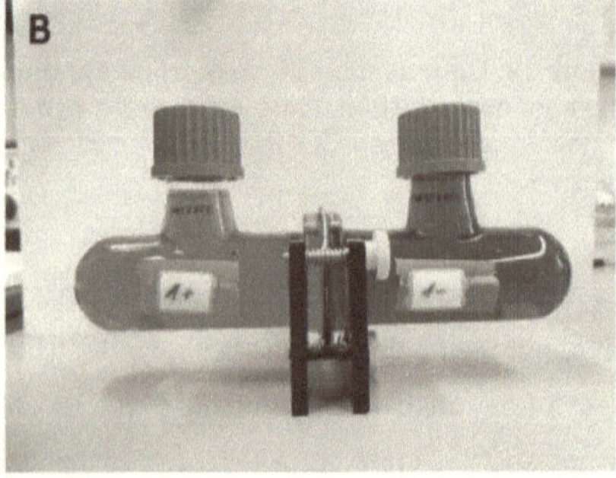

Figure 21: Proof-of-concept of chamber tightness and function with phenol red. A) Newly assembled chamber with an Alg/MC gel disc separating the halves and 10 mM $SrCl_2$ with and without phenol red in the right and left half respectively. B) Diffusion of phenol red from right to left after 24 h at 37°C.

4.1.3.3 Permeability measurements in a diffusion chamber system

As for the uptake and release experiments, the main intent behind using the diffusion chamber setup was to compare the Alg/MC blend with an alginate control, to compare gel discs prepared with research-grade or with clinical-grade alginate, and to compare gel discs of either composition after storage for 1, 4, and 7 days under cell culture conditions. Comparisons in terms of permeability were performed for the main molecules relevant for the function of pancreatic islets, i.e. glucose and insulin, but due to the ease of analysis, the main focus was on permeability for glucose which was also used for parameter optimisation. Experiments for parameter optimisation concerned the time until near equilibrium as well as the impact of gel height, of crosslinking ions, and of solution used for chamber filling on the rate of glucose diffusion.

All gels were prepared as described in the previous section (page 47 f.), crosslinked with 70 mM $SrCl_2$, and stored in 10 mM $SrCl_2$ for up to 7 days before chamber assembly except if specifically stated otherwise. The molecules were always added to one chamber half, the donor compartment, from where they diffused into the other half, the acceptor compartment.

<u>Glucose</u>

Concentration of glucose was 5 g/L in the donor and 0 g/L in the acceptor compartment in all conducted experiments and 10 mM $SrCl_2$ were used as chamber filling except if stated otherwise.

To be able to estimate a time frame during which diffusion progressed linearly, in an initial experiment glucose diffusion through research-grade alginate and Alg/MC gels was monitored over a period of 30 h until near equilibrium (Figure 22 A). After a lag-phase of 30 min, glucose could be measured in the acceptor compartment and diffusion progressed linearly from 2 h onwards independent of gel composition. After approximately 14 h the concentration curve entered the stationary phase and approached the saturation point (equilibrium). In this initial experiment, a slight difference between diffusion through the alginate and the Alg/MC gel discs was visible, which could not be detected in any of the following analyses though. To investigate whether this difference could be due to a different amount of glucose being retained within the alginate and Alg/MC gels, the glucose content in gel discs of both types was analysed after chamber runs but no trend could be detected (data not shown). For the observation until equilibrium, glucose content is displayed for the donor and acceptor compartment to illustrate the decrease in glucose concentration in the donor compartment in proportion to a rise in concentration in the acceptor compartment as a proof-of-concept. For all further diffusion measurements presented in this work, only the concentration in the acceptor compartment is shown.

Despite optimisation of the protocol for gel preparation and the use of pressure to flatten hydrogel discs to a uniform height, slight differences between the individual gels remain, therefore it was necessary to investigate the influence of gel height on permeability. Alginate gels were prepared in metal seal rings of either 1 mm or 0.5 mm height and diffusion was observed over the course of 3 h (Figure 22 B). An increased height of the gel disc led to a longer lag-phase until glucose could first be measured in the acceptor compartment (1 h vs 30 min for the 1 mm gel and the 0.5 mm gel, respectively), a later begin of the linear phase, a more shallow slope of the linear increase (0.13 vs 0.27), and a much lower concentration of glucose in the acceptor compartment after 3 h incubation time (300 mg/L vs 700 mg/L). This highlighted the necessity to precisely measure the height of each gel after the run.

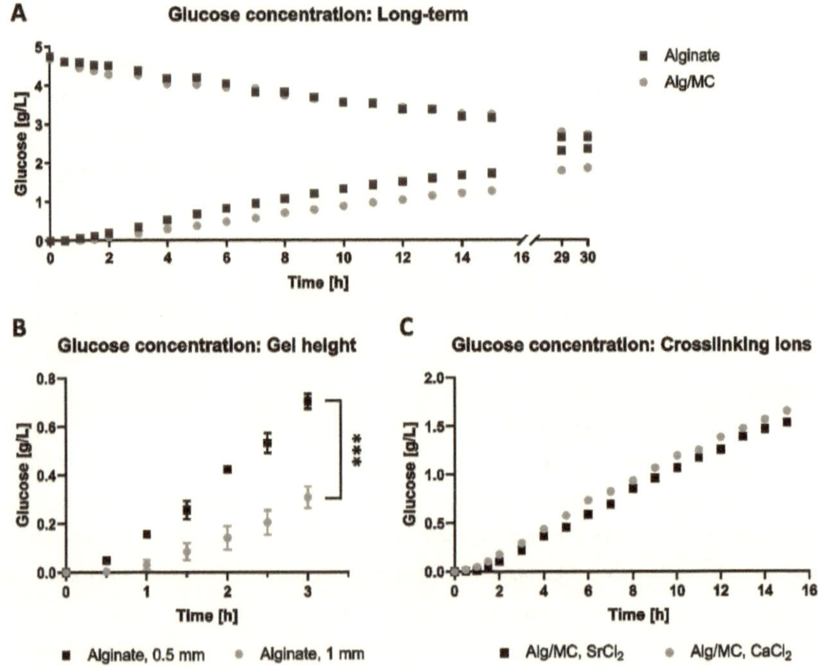

Figure 22: Parameters for glucose diffusion. Alginate and Alg/MC gel discs prepared with research-grade alginate. A) Alginate and Alg/MC gels were crosslinked with 70 mM SrCl$_2$ and incubated in 10 mM SrCl$_2$ under cell culture conditions for 1 day. Glucose concentration over a timeframe of 32 h until near equilibrium between the chamber halves. The declining and the increasing data set depict the concentration in the donor and receptor chamber respectively. n = 1, data were not adjusted for gel height. B) Alginate gel discs were crosslinked with 70 mM SrCl$_2$ and incubated in 10 mM SrCl$_2$ under cell culture conditions for 1 day. Glucose concentration in the acceptor compartment in dependence of the diffusion distance, i.e. the height of the hydrogel discs. Discs prepared in 1 and 0.5 mm seal rings with an effective gel height of 1.7 and 0.9 mm respectively. Mean ± SD, n = 3, significances indicate ***$p<0.001$, data were not adjusted for gel height. C) Alg/MC gel discs were crosslinked with 100 mM CaCl$_2$ or 70 mM SrCl$_2$ and incubated in 20 mM CaCl$_2$ or 10 mM SrCl$_2$ under cell culture conditions for 1 day. Glucose concentration in the acceptor compartment in dependence of the ions used for crosslinking. n = 1, data were adjusted for gel height.

According to Fick's law, the speed of diffusion is inversely proportional to the diffusion distance (Helmich, 2018). The comparison between gel heights presented here also showed an approximately proportional relationship between concentration in the acceptor compartment and gel height, therefore in all further experiments the precise height was multiplied with the glucose concentration in the acceptor compartment to eliminate the factor of height differences between gels.

To investigate the influence of different crosslinking ions which can result in different pore sizes, Alg/MC gel discs were crosslinked with either 100 mM $CaCl_2$ or 70 mM $SrCl_2$ and diffusion was observed over 16 h. The use of different crosslinking ions did not influence lag-time, slope, or overall glucose concentration in the acceptor compartment (Figure 22 C) and was therefore determined to have no influence on glucose diffusion.

In light of these results and the fact that a maximum surface-to-volume ratio was desired, all further experiments were conducted with gels prepared in 0.5 mm seal rings, crosslinked with 70 mM $SrCl_2$ and the time frame selected for further glucose diffusion chamber experiments was 0-4 h with sampling every 30 min.

For comparison between alginates, gel compositions and gel ages analogous to analysis time-points in cell culture experiments, glucose diffusion was analysed for alginate and Alg/MC gel prepared with research-grade and clinical-grade alginate and stored for up to 7 days. Figure 23 gives an overview over the comparison between alginate and Alg/MC gels at the different time-points, Figure 24 depicts a comparison between research-grade and clinical-grade alginate.

For all gels tested, the initial lag-phase lasted 30 min and glucose diffusion progressed into the linear phase after 1 h. When corresponding alginate and Alg/MC gels are compared, the amount of glucose measured in the acceptor compartment after 4 h was not significantly different between the gel compositions (Figure 23). The only visible but not significant trend was observed between research-grade alginate and Alg/MC gels incubated for 1 day, with a slightly higher rate of diffusion through the plain alginate gel (Figure 23 A). This was not visible for gels aged 4 and 7 days at which timepoints diffusion of glucose through research-grade Alg/MC increased slightly compared to day 1. Save this slight trend, no difference between differently aged gels could be detected (for a visual comparison between differently aged gels refer to Figure 65, addendum).

In a comparison between gels prepared with research-grade and clinical-grade alginate, statistical analyses did not detect any significant differences between gels either, but there is a distinct trend towards quicker diffusion of glucose through plain alginate gels prepared with research-grade alginate independent of gel age (Figure 24 A, C, E). This trend was not visible for Alg/MC gels (Figure 24 B, D, F).

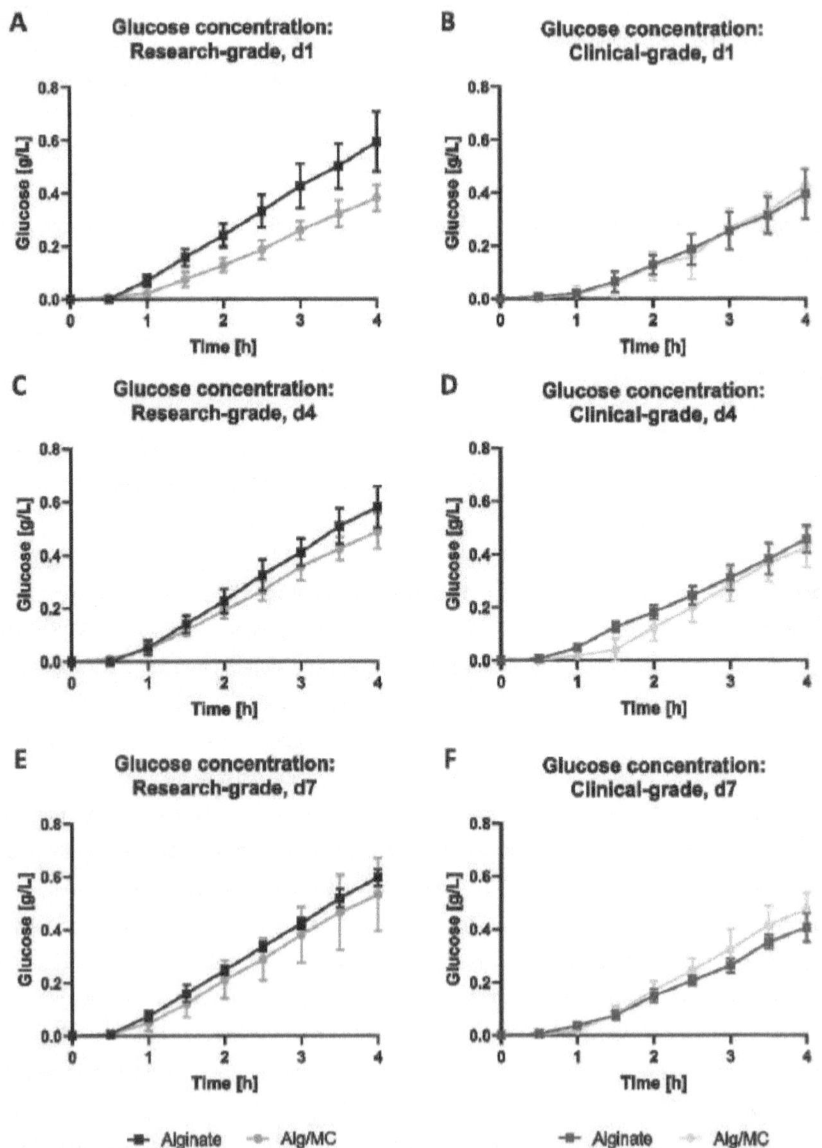

Figure 23: Glucose concentration compared by gel composition. Glucose concentration is depicted for the acceptor compartment. Alginate and Alg/MC gel discs were prepared with research-grade (left) or clinical-grade (right) alginate and crosslinked with 70 mM $SrCl_2$. Incubation of discs in 10 mM $SrCl_2$ under cell culture conditions for 1 day (A, B), 4 days (C, D), or 7 days (E, F) before mounting in the chamber filled with 10 mM $SrCl_2$. Samples of 200 µl were taken from both compartments every 30 min during a period of 4 h. Mean ± SD, n = 3, data were adjusted for gel height.

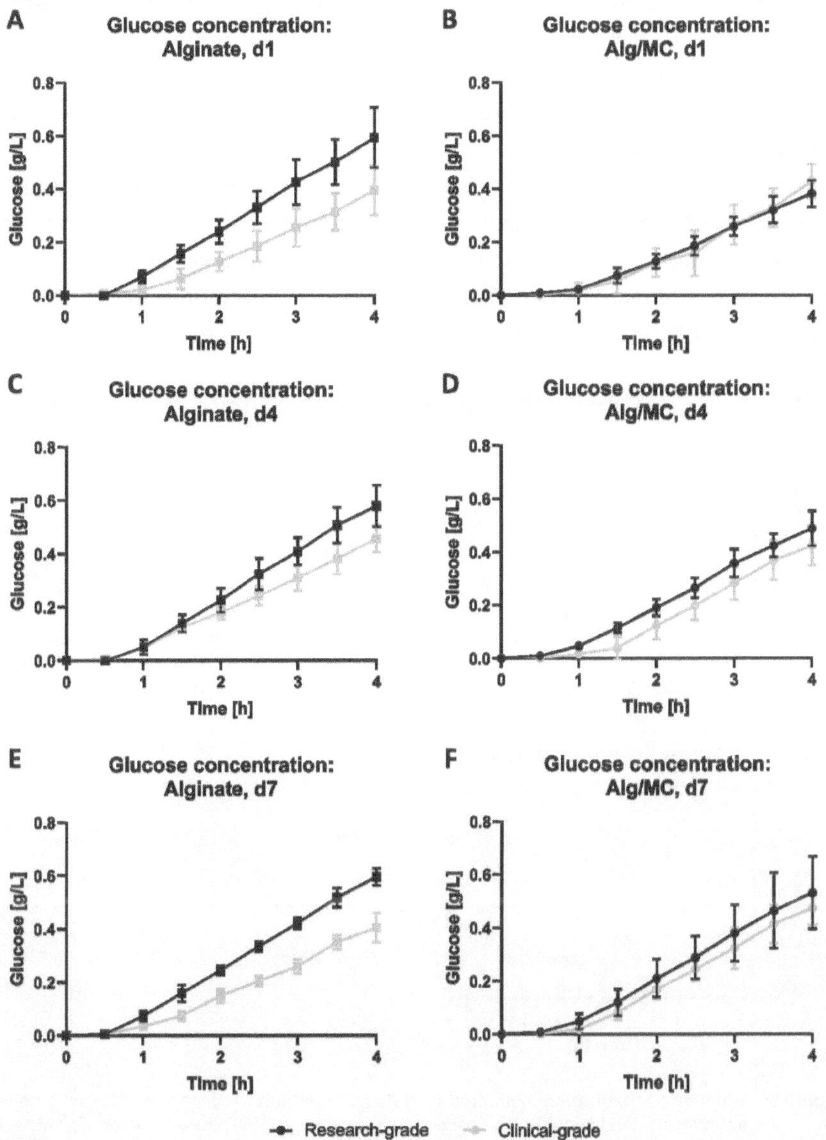

Figure 24: Glucose concentration compared by type of alginate. Glucose concentration is depicted for the acceptor compartment. Alginate (left) and Alg/MC (right) gel discs were prepared with research-grade or clinical-grade alginate and crosslinked with 70 mM SrCl$_2$. Incubation of discs in 10 mM SrCl$_2$ under cell culture conditions for 1 day (A, B), 4 days (C, D), or 7 days (E, F) before mounting in the chamber filled with 10 mM SrCl$_2$. Samples of 200 µl were taken from both compartments every 30 min during a period of 4 h. Mean ± SD, n = 3, data were adjusted for gel height.

In the interest of gel stability, 10 mM $SrCl_2$ was used for storage of gel discs and for chamber content for glucose measurements in these experiments. However, as stimulation of islets, as performed for this book, is done in Krebs Ringer bicarbonate buffer, an additional experiment concerning a possible influence of solvents was performed for research-grade Alg/MC gel discs (Figure 25).

Overall speed of diffusion was slightly lower than in the previous experiments with gels of the same makeup (Figure 23 A, C, E) and the lag-phase lasted longer. In a comparison between different chamber fillings (Figure 25) and differently aged gels (for a visual comparison between differently aged gels refer to Figure 66, addendum), the rate of diffusion was comparable between all conditions tested.

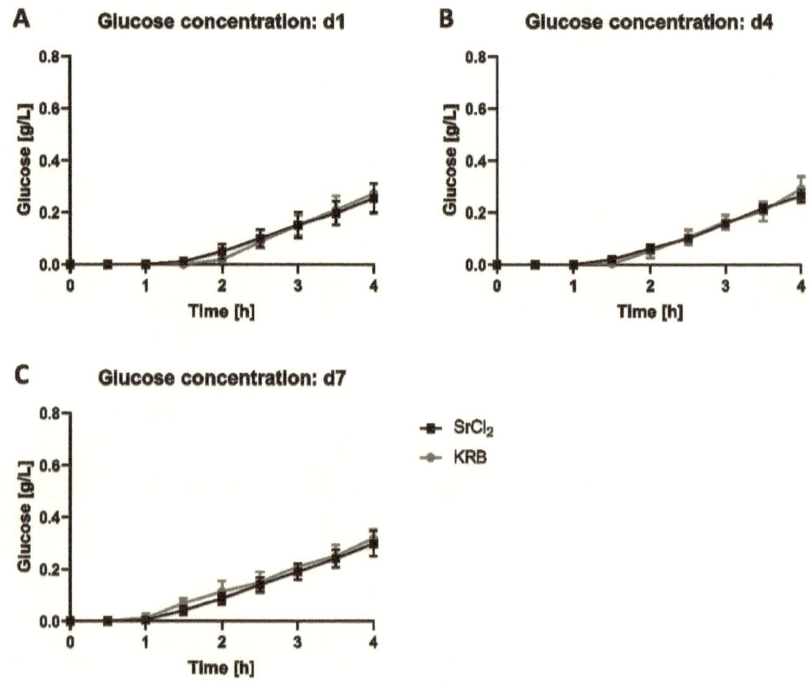

Figure 25: Glucose concentration compared by diffusion medium. Glucose concentration is depicted for the acceptor compartment. Alg/MC gel discs were prepared with research-grade alginate and crosslinked with 70 mM $SrCl_2$. Incubation of discs in 10 mM $SrCl_2$ or Krebs-Ringer buffer for 1 day (A), 4 days (B), or 7 days (C) before mounting in the chamber filled with 10 mM $SrCl_2$ or Krebs-Ringer buffer. Samples of 200 µl were taken from both compartments every 30 min during a period of 4 h. Mean ± SD, n = 3, data were adjusted for gel height.

Insulin

Concentration of insulin was 250 ng/L in the donor and 0 ng/L in the acceptor compartment and Krebs-Ringer buffer was used as chamber filling in all conducted experiments to mimic the conditions used for islet stimulation as closely as possible. As insulin is a larger molecule than glucose and diffusion might therefore be slower, time of observation was extended to 6 h and sampling was conducted every 30 min for the first hour followed by sampling every hour. The three gel types tested for a preliminary insight into the diffusion of insulin were research-grade plain alginate, research-grade Alg/MC, and clinical-grade Alg/MC.

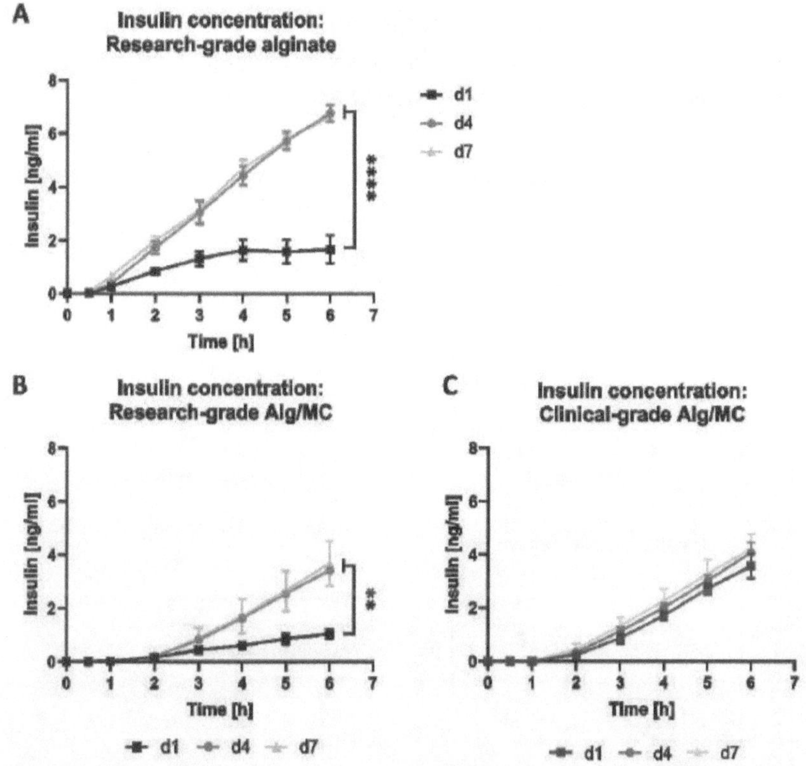

Figure 26: Insulin concentration compared by incubation time. Insulin concentration is depicted for the acceptor compartment. Gel discs were prepared with research-grade alginate (A), research-grade Alg/MC (B), and clinical-grade Alg/MC (C). All discs were crosslinked with 70 mM $SrCl_2$. Incubation of discs in KRB under cell culture conditions for 1, 4, or 7 days before mounting in the chamber filled with KRB. Samples of 200 µl were taken from both compartments every 30 min for the first hour and every 60 min during a further period of 5 h. Mean ± SD, n = 3, significances in all graphs indicate **$p<0.01$, ****$p<0.0001$.

Overall, the lag-time was slightly longer than for glucose but all conditions entered the linear phase after a maximum of 2 h. In a comparison between differently aged gels, the rate of diffusion changed significantly between day 1 and later timepoints for both alginate and Alg/MC gels prepared with research-grade alginate (Figure 26 A&B). For Alg/MC gels prepared with clinical-grade alginate on the other hand, rate of diffusion remained constant independent of gel age (Figure 26 C).

In a comparison between gel types at different timepoints after gel preparation, diffusion of insulin at day 1 through research-grade alginate and Alg/MC gels was comparable, but significantly higher through clinical-grade Alg/MC gels (Figure 27 A). For gels aged 4 and 7 days on the other hand, diffusion though plain alginate was significantly higher than diffusion through Alg/MC gels independent of alginate type (Figure 27 B&C).

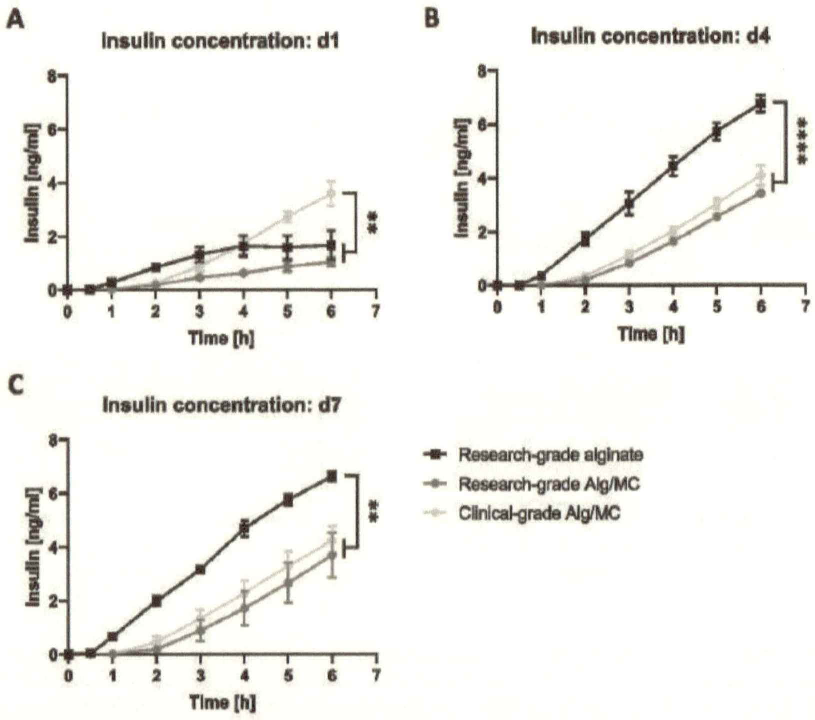

Figure 27: Insulin concentration compared by gel composition. Insulin concentration is depicted for the acceptor compartment. Alginate gel discs (A) were prepared with research-grade alginate, Alg/MC gel discs with research-grade (B) or clinical-grade (C) alginate. All discs were crosslinked with 70 mM $SrCl_2$. Incubation of discs in KRB under cell culture conditions for 1, 4, or 7 days before mounting in the chamber filled with KRB. Samples of 200 µl were taken from both compartments every 30 min for the first hour and every 60 min during a further period of 5 h. Mean ± SD, n = 3, significances in all graphs indicate **$p<0.01$, ****$p<0.0001$.

4.2 Adaptation & characterisation of islet cell incorporation into the Alg/MC blend

The Alg/MC blend had been developed and previously been shown to be suitable for the plotting of mammalian single cells of mesenchymal origin (Schütz et al., 2017). In previous studies using this blend it became apparent that the sterilisation of MC not only influences the material and plotting properties but also the survival and behaviour of embedded cells, chondrocytes in that case (Hodder et al., 2019). In general, different cell types react differently towards materials and since none of the cell types used in the previous studies were endocrine cells, the blend was analysed for cytocompatibility with the insulin producing INS-1 as a model cell line preliminary to islet plotting experiments. In addition to being crucial with respect to clinical application, the sterilisation of the material components influences the viscosity of the blend, which is an important parameter with respect to islet plotting. The majority of encapsulation approaches concerning these sensitive cell clusters is based on soft alginate-based gels (chapter 2.2.3, page 17 ff.) to minimise shear stress. With respect to the sizable difference between the viscosity of plain alginate and of Alg/MC, it was imperative to appraise methods for the careful incorporation of islets into the blend and investigate the effect of shear stress applied to cells during the plotting itself. To reduce this shear stress, plotting needles with a large inner diameter of 610 and 840 µm were chosen and compared concerning their influence on islet morphology.

For islets and especially islet plotting, it is highly important to measure the cell number as precisely as possible since the functional analysis depends on the ratio of released insulin compared to the number of cells. Furthermore, a precise measurement of cell count between scaffolds was required since a completely homogeneous distribution of islets over all scaffolds of a batch cannot be guaranteed even with the optimised incorporation methods discussed later. For the precise determination of cellular content from plotted scaffolds, a protocol for complete dissolution of scaffolds and complete lysis of cells was developed (Figure 67, addendum).

4.2.1 Sterilisation of MC: influence on β-cell survival and behaviour

The sterilisation of alginate solutions by autoclaving is well established (Jeong et al., 2012; Kundu et al., 2015; Park et al., 2017), influence of sterilisation methods on MC on the other hand has been shown to be a crucial factor for plottability of the Alg/MC blend and the viability of cells encapsulated therein (Hodder et al., 2019). To test the influence of sterilisation methods applied to MC prior to paste preparation as well as the influence of the material blend itself on endocrine cells, INS-1, cells from a rat insulinoma β-cell-line, were plotted in research-grade Alg/MC pastes. The alginate solution was autoclaved, sterilisation methods used on dry MC were autoclaving, supercritical CO_2 ($scCO_2$) treatment or ultraviolet (UV) irradiation.

The cell-containing scaffolds were crosslinked with 70 mM SrCl₂ and incubated for up to 21 days. Viability was characterised in terms of metabolic activity via MTT staining, live/dead staining, cluster formation over time and measurement of DNA-content (Figure 28 & Figure 29; for a depiction of live and dead images separately refer to Figure 68-Figure 70, addendum).

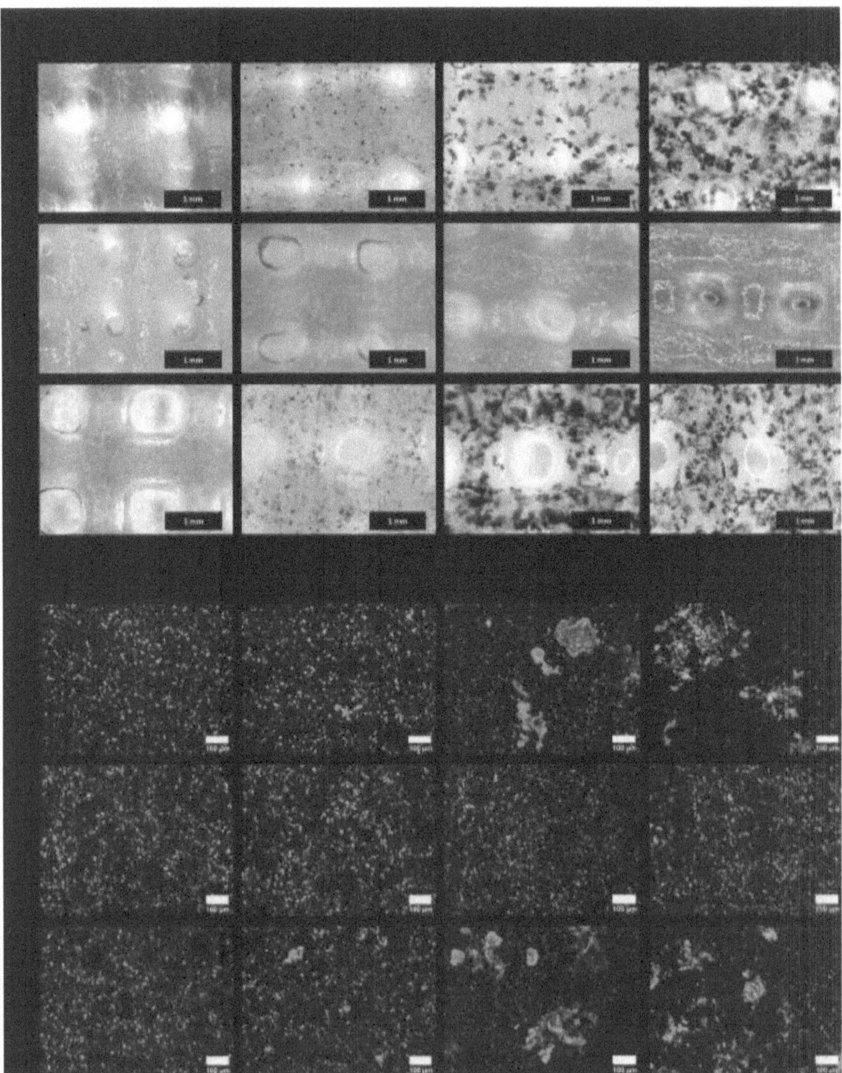

Figure 28: Qualitative depiction of the influence of different sterilisation methods applied to MC on the viability of INS-1 cells. INS-1 cells in plotted research-grade Alg/MC scaffolds crosslinked with 70 mM SrCl₂ and incubated in RPMI⁺ under cell culture conditions for up to 21 days. A) Representative images of INS-1 stained with MTT for metabolic activity. Scale bars = 1 mm. B) Representative images of INS-1 stained for live (green) and dead (red) cells. Separate live and dead images are presented in Figure 68-Figure 70, addendum. Scale bars = 100 μm.

One day after plotting, no metabolically active INS-1 cells could be detected in either of the scaffolds. In scaffolds prepared with autoclaved or UV-irradiated MC, metabolically active cells were first detected on day 7 and the amount of MTT-positive cells increased strongly over time (Figure 28 A). The highest amount of cells was detected after 21 days in scaffolds prepared with autoclaved MC, but already on day 14 in scaffolds prepared with UV-irradiated MC. In scaffolds of both variants, the cells, naturally prone to cluster growth (Lee et al., 2011), formed large metabolically active clusters over time. In scaffolds prepared with $scCO_2$-sterilised MC on the other hand, no metabolically active cells could be detected over the whole time of observation.

Live/dead staining (Figure 28 B) qualitatively displayed an approximately even amount of live and dead single cells on day 1 after plotting, independent of the sterilisation method. Analogous to MTT staining (Figure 28 A), INS-1 cells in scaffolds that had been prepared with either autoclaved or UV-irradiated MC formed large clusters of live cells over time. Cluster formation first appeared on day 7 after plotting, number and size of clusters increased until day 14 and remained mostly constant until day 21, at which point the borders of the clusters appeared less clearly defined though. Number of dead cells is reduced over time, especially between day 14 and day 21 after plotting with no difference visible between the two sterilisation methods. In contrast to that, when scaffolds were prepared with $scCO_2$-sterilised MC live cells were present throughout the whole time of incubation, but no cluster formation could be detected (Figure 28 B).

For quantitative analysis of live/dead staining, area of live and dead cells was calculated and is presented as ratio of live / total cells (% viability) as well as absolute overgrown area of the analysed images (Figure 29 A&B). Number of cells is reflected in the DNA-content of scaffolds over time (Figure 29 C). Ratio of cell survival (Figure 29 A) showed a highly significant increase from day 1 to day 7 without further increase towards day 21 when UV- and $scCO_2$-sterilised MC had been used. In samples prepared with autoclaved MC, increase of viability was not significant between day 1 and day 7, but highly significant between day 7 and day 14 of culture. Absolute area of live cells (Figure 29 B) and DNA content (Figure 29 C) confirmed the qualitative results from MTT and live/dead images in Figure 28. Both parameters showed an increase over time when MC had been sterilised with wet heat or UV-irradiation and a decrease in the $scCO_2$-samples. As had become evident in the MTT-staining, number and area of cells were highest on day 21 for autoclaved but already on day 14 for UV-treated MC samples. Area in autoclaved samples increased significantly between day 7, 14 and 21 of culture, whereas in UV-treated samples increase was only significant between day 1 and day 7. For DNA-content, differences between the groups were not tested for significance due to a low number of samples. Interestingly, despite a lack of visibly metabolically active cells from $scCO_2$ samples, a much higher DNA content could be measured and both, DNA and area of live cells increased slightly between day 1 and 7. After that, DNA content dropped sharply while the area remained constant. From day 14 on, overall rate of survival and absolute area of living cells were significantly lower in $scCO_2$-sterilised samples compared to autoclaved and UV-irradiated samples. While both, autoclaved and UV-irradiated MC supported survival of INS-1, autoclaving was chosen for islet experiments with respect to its approval as a clinically applicable sterilisation method.

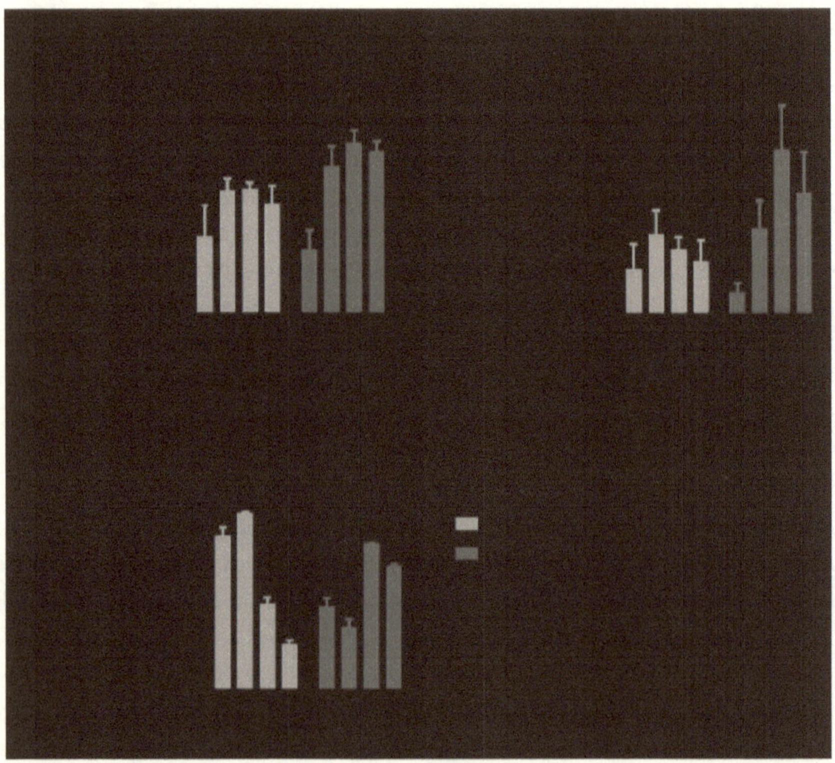

Figure 29: Quantitative analysis of the influence of different sterilisation methods applied to MC on the viability of INS-1 cells. INS-1 cells in plotted research-grade Alg/MC scaffolds crosslinked with 70 mM $SrCl_2$ and incubated in $RPMI^+$ under cell culture conditions for up to 21 days. A) Percent viability calculated from the area of live cells. Mean ± SD, n = 3 scaffolds, 5 images each. B) Absolute area of live cells. Mean ± SD, n = 3 scaffolds, 5 images each. C) DNA-content per scaffold. Mean ± SD, n = 2 scaffolds.

4.2.2 Incorporation of pancreatic islets into the highly viscous Alg/MC blend

The high viscosity of the Alg/MC blend can lead to strong shear stress during cell incorporation. Especially the pancreatic islets, which are large but relatively sensitive cell clusters, have to be incorporated carefully to retain their overall morphology. At the same time, a sufficiently homogeneous distribution of islets in the paste is required to ensure a sufficiently homogenous distribution of islets in the scaffolds. In preliminary experiments, a very low number of islets (approximately 2000 IEQ per gram material) had been incorporated with an incorporation method derived from that used for single cells. This resulted in a very uneven distribution of islets between scaffolds of the same batch ranging from zero to five metabolically active islets per scaffold and a loss of round-shaped islet morphology (data not shown).

Following this, different methods for the thorough but gentle incorporation of sensitive cell constructs were investigated to achieve a homogeneous cell-material mixture (Figure 30 A). The method derived from the incorporation of single cells ("stirring"), consisted of the deposition of a defined amount of material into a falcon tube, centrifugation, addition of the cell suspension on top, and incorporation via stirring with a spatula. For a slight modification of this protocol ("gentle folding in") the centrifugation step was omitted and a defined amount of material was distributed on the side of the tube after which the cell suspension was distributed along the entire material and gently folded in with a spatula. Further methods tested were blending of material and cell suspension via two connected syringes starting out with the material in one, and the cell suspension in the other syringe, and a gentle pressure to move the entire content between the syringes ("syringe"), and the use of the so called "Cellmixer" from CELLINK. With the Cellmixer, the material and cell suspension are also deposited in different connected syringes, but blending takes place via a single move through a screw thread. These methods were first compared concerning their effect on spheroids of hTERT-MSC as a model for cell clusters, however spheroids created from single cells of a cell line are more fragile than even primary islets and only a small number remained intact during either incorporation method preventing the use (data not shown). Use of the cell mixer was restricted by a fast clogging of the narrow screw thread and therefore discontinued.

The methods "stirring", "gentle folding in" and "syringe" were qualitatively compared based on their influence of islet morphology and survival of murine islets in plotted scaffolds. Islets folded in but unplotted, and free islets were used as controls. Two representative examples of each variant are shown in Figure 30 B. The majority of islets remained alive in all cases, a trend towards a higher number of dead cells with a loss of islet morphology was indicated though. Islet morphology was preserved in a majority of islets when the cell suspension was gently folded in, with a far greater number of intact islets than when the methods "stirring" or "syringe" were used. Even with gentle incorporation some islets were frayed at the edges though. As no difference between unplotted islets, and plotted islets which had been folded in could be observed, this was attributed to the shear stress during the process of incorporation and not during the plotting. Due to its low impact on islet morphology the method "gentle folding in" was chosen for incorporation of islets into the material for all further experiments.

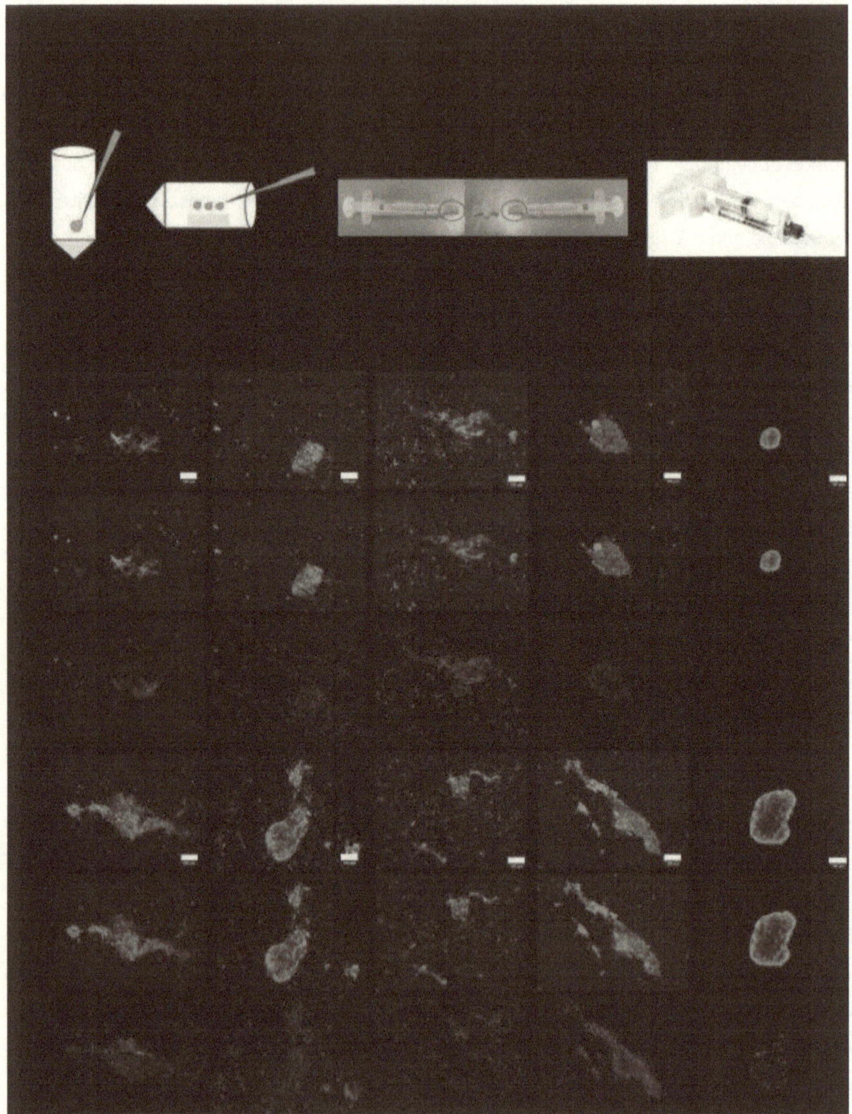

Figure 30: Incorporation of murine islets into the Alg/MC blend. A) Schematic depiction of methods used to incorporate cells into the material. Islets were pipetted onto the material and incorporated with a spatula (I&II), or the material and the islets were deposited in separate containers and incorporation was achieved with pressure (III&IV (CELLINK, 2020)). B) From top to bottom: Representative images of survival & morphology of islets stained for live (green) and dead (red) cells. Islets were incorporated into research-grade Alg/MC with the methods I-III depicted in A. Scaffolds were plotted with an inner needle diameter of 610 µm, crosslinked with 70 mM $SrCl_2$ and incubated in $RPMI^+$ under cell culture conditions for up to 7 days. Islets folded in in but unplotted, and free islets in suspension culture served as controls. Scale bars = 100 µm.

4.2.3 Needle diameter for the plotting of pancreatic islets

Apart from shear stress during incorporation, islets are additionally exposed to shear stress during extrusion through plotting needles which is higher with smaller outlet diameters (Emmermacher et al., 2020). Since islet sizes naturally range lies from 50 to 350 µm in average diameter, conical plotting needles with an inner diameter of either 610 or 840 µm were compared as to their influence on cell survival and islet morphology, both qualitatively (Figure 31) and quantitatively (Figure 32).

Chosen for the qualitative assessment in this work is an array of six images for each needle type which illustrates the cell survival and percentage of undamaged islets in a representative fashion. In qualitative image analysis, a slight correlation between impaired islet morphology and number of dead cells was visible, with both being higher after use of the 610 µm needle (Figure 31).

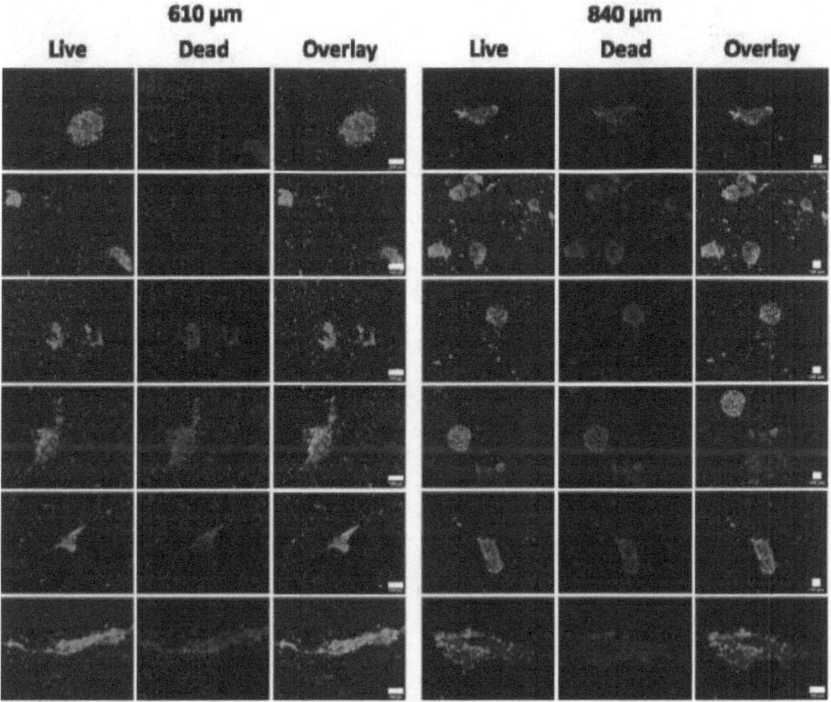

Figure 31: Qualitative viability and morphology of murine islets depending on the inner diameter of the plotting needle. Plotted islets in research-grade Alg/MC scaffolds crosslinked with 70 mM $SrCl_2$ and incubated in RPMI+ under cell culture conditions for up to 14 days. Representative images of islets stained for live (green) and dead (red) cells. Scaffolds were plotted with a needle of 610 µm (left) or 840 µm (right) inner diameter. Scale bars = 100 µm.

Quantitative analysis on the other hand only partially confirmed the impression from the qualitative analysis, with needle diameter significantly impacting morphology (Figure 32 B), but not viability (Figure 32 A).

With a larger needle, a higher number of islets showed spherical morphology, therefore a needle diameter of 840 μm was chosen for further islet plotting experiments.

Figure 32: Quantitative viability and morphology of murine islets depending on the inner diameter of the plotting needle. Plotted islets in research-grade Alg/MC scaffolds crosslinked with 70 mM SrCl$_2$ and incubated in RPMI$^+$ under cell culture conditions for up to 14 days. A) Semi-quantitative assessment of islet viability on the basis of live/dead stainings as shown in Figure 31. Mean ± SD, n = 1 isolation for 610 μm on day 1, n = 3 isolations for all other conditions, each 10-101 islets. B) Semi-quantitative assessment of islet morphology on the basis of live/dead stainings as shown in Figure 31. Each islet was visually assessed for impaired spherical morphology. Mean ± SD, n = 3 isolations, each 8-93 islets.

4.3 Plotting of adult murine pancreatic islets

In previous chapters, the basic suitability of the adapted Alg/MC blend concerning plottability and stability of the gel as well as optimised methods for incorporation and analysis of cell clusters were ascertained. In the following, a detailed analysis of islets embedded within plotted and crosslinked clinical-grade Alg/MC scaffolds by using primary adult islets from rat as a model for proof-of-concept plotting experiments is presented.

In accordance with the results concerning material characterisation and islet incorporation, the basic parameters chosen for islet plotting were the Alg/MC blend with autoclaved MC, gentle folding in, plotting with a needle diameter of 840 µm, and crosslinking with 70 mM $SrCl_2$. All gels were prepared with clinical-grade alginate, except if specifically stated otherwise. Islet containing scaffolds as well as control islets in suspension culture were incubated in $RPMI^+$ under cell culture conditions for up to 7 days.

To assess the overall impact of 3D plotting on murine islets, parameters chosen for analysis were metabolic activity, the presence of insulin within islets, size distribution, viability, and presence of apoptotic nuclei compared to control islets. In a second step a thorough examination of islet functionality via presence of pancreatic hormones and stimulation with glucose was performed.

4.3.1 Distribution, morphology and viability of bioplotted murine islets

Islet-containing scaffolds were stained with MTT and DTZ to get a visual overview over distribution of insulin-containing metabolically active cell clusters within the hydrogel strands (Figure 33 A&B). In all analysed scaffolds, a sufficiently homogeneous distribution of islets could be detected, the islets were metabolically active throughout the time of incubation (Figure 33 A), and presence of insulin could be detected via dithizone until at least day 7 after plotting (Figure 33 B).

Plotted and free control islets were also analysed for size distribution as ascertained by means of counting nuclei in immunofluorescently stained cryosections (Figure 33 C). While islets substantially vary in size by nature, it could be observed throughout the whole time of observation, that free control islets tended to be larger on average than plotted islets. Furthermore, from day 4 to day 7 of culture a slight, but not significant, trend in size reduction could be observed in both groups.

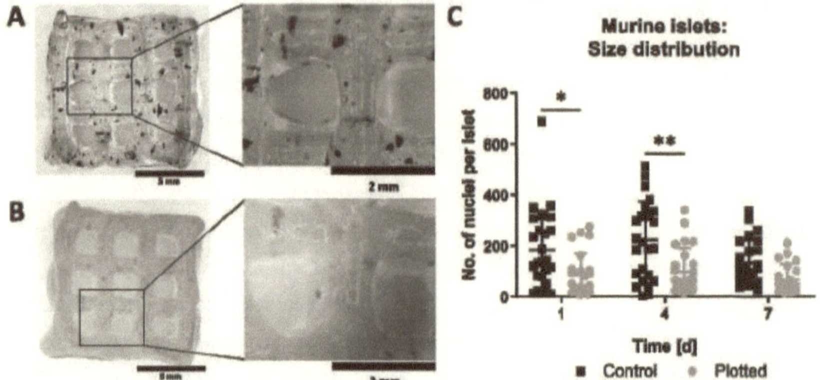

Figure 33: Placement and size distribution of murine islets. Plotted islets in clinical-grade Alg/MC scaffolds crosslinked with 70 mM $SrCl_2$ and control islets in suspension culture incubated in RPMI[+] under cell culture conditions for up to 7 days. A) Representative images of islets stained for metabolic activity with MTT, day 1 after plotting. B) Representative images of islets stained for presence of insulin with DTZ, day 7 after plotting. Scale bars = 5 mm (left) and 2 mm (right). C) Size of islets determined by counting of nuclei in DAPI stained 2D cross-sections. Mean ± SD, n=1 isolation, 25 islets, *$p<0.05$, **$p<0.01$.

In-depth examination of survival of plotted islets was done through the staining of live vs dead cells (Figure 34-Figure 36), and the staining of nuclei for DNA and DNA fragmentation (Figure 38). Main focus lay on survival for up to seven days (Figure 34 & Figure 35), which is the timeframe reported for preservation of islet functionality *in vitro*. However, in light of the fact that islet-containing scaffolds eventually need to preserve survival and function of islets over a long period of time for medical application, survival of plotted islets was also observed up to day 14 as a first indicator for long-term survival (Figure 36).

As previously observed in the experiments conducted for optimisation of incorporation (chapter 4.2.2, page 61 ff.) and needle diameter (chapter 4.2.3, page 64 ff.), live/dead staining revealed that the complete surface area visible in the images of the islets showed green staining indicating live cells at all timepoints and in both sample types, control and plotted. Additionally however, nearly all islets also showed red signal in the periphery, but in most cases the number of dead cells per islet was very low (Figure 34). The semi-quantitative evaluation of the stainings (Figure 35) demonstrated a slightly higher rate of survival in the control than the plotted scaffolds, with the disparity being highest on day 4 but overall negligible. Interestingly, while the percentage of live cells increased from day 1 to day 4 in the control, it only did so from day 4 to day 7 in the plotted scaffolds. Semi-quantitative assessment was mainly done on islets from one experiment for a direct comparison between all timepoints of control and plotted islets from the same isolation. Selective control stainings for plotted islets in 10 of the 14 performed isolations showed the same overall effect in qualitative analysis though (data not shown).

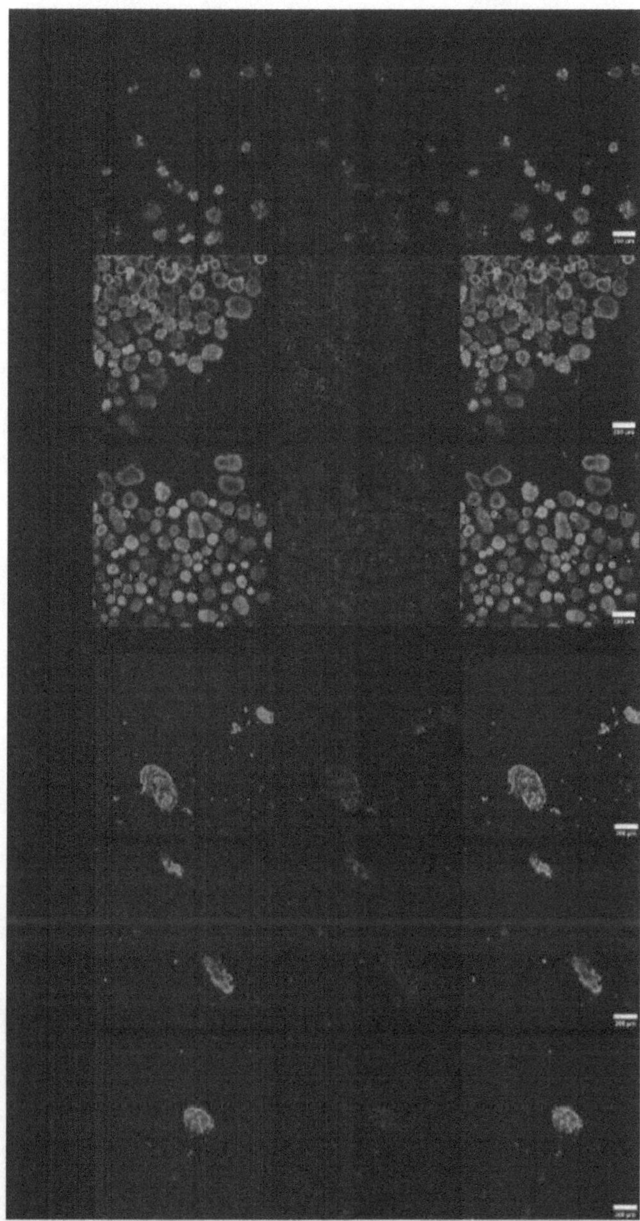

Figure 34: Qualitative viability of murine islets. Plotted islets in clinical-grade Alg/MC scaffolds cross-linked with 70 mM $SrCl_2$ and control islets in suspension culture incubated in RPMI⁺ under cell culture conditions for up to 7 days. Representative images of islets stained for live (green) and dead (red) cells. A) Free control islets. B) Islets in plotted Alg/MC scaffolds. Scale bars = 200 µm for all.

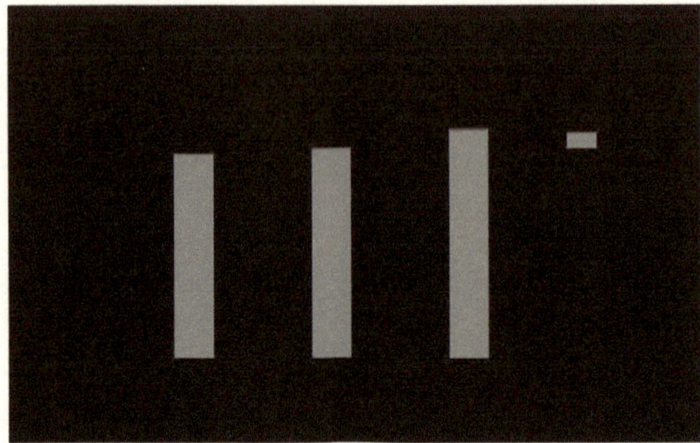

Figure 35: Quantitative viability of murine islets. Plotted islets in clinical-grade Alg/MC scaffolds crosslinked with 70 mM SrCl$_2$ and control islets in suspension culture incubated in RPMI⁺ under cell culture conditions for up to 7 days. Semi-quantitative assessment of islet viability on the basis of live/dead stainings as shown in Figure 34. Mean ± SD, n = 1 isolation, 62-177 islets.

When survival of plotted islets was observed over a longer timeframe (Figure 36 & Figure 37), the overall trend was similar to short-term observations with only minor changes in percentage of survival over the whole time but a slight increase in live cells between day 1 and day 7 after plotting. Over the course of the next week of incubation, this increase receded again, so that survival after 14 days of incubation under cell culture conditions was comparable to survival immediately after plotting (Figure 37). In accordance with the presence of dead cells throughout the time of observation, cell number as measured by DNA content in general decreased over time (Table 1).

Table 1: DNA content of plotted Alg/MC scaffolds containing adult murine islets. DNA content was normalised to the DNA content measured on day 1 after plotting. Clinical-grade Alg/MC scaffolds were crosslinked with 70 mM SrCl$_2$ and incubated under cell culture conditions for up to 21 days. Plot 1-8 denote different islet isolations. Mean, n corresponds to number of samples in GSIR denoted in Table 3-Table 10, addendum.

	d1	d4	d7	d11	d14	d21
Plot 1	100	42.1	15.4	20.9	13.1	18.5
Plot 2	100	54.5	42.1	29.1	20.3	18.7
Plot 3	100	94.2	127.7	72.4		
Plot 4	100	68.3	60.5	41.1	49.1	32.6
Plot 5	100	77.1	65.4	48.5	33.4	
Plot 6	100	63.9	72.7	68.2	85.7	
Plot 7	100	86.7	53.9	31.2		
Plot 8	100	80.9	55.9			

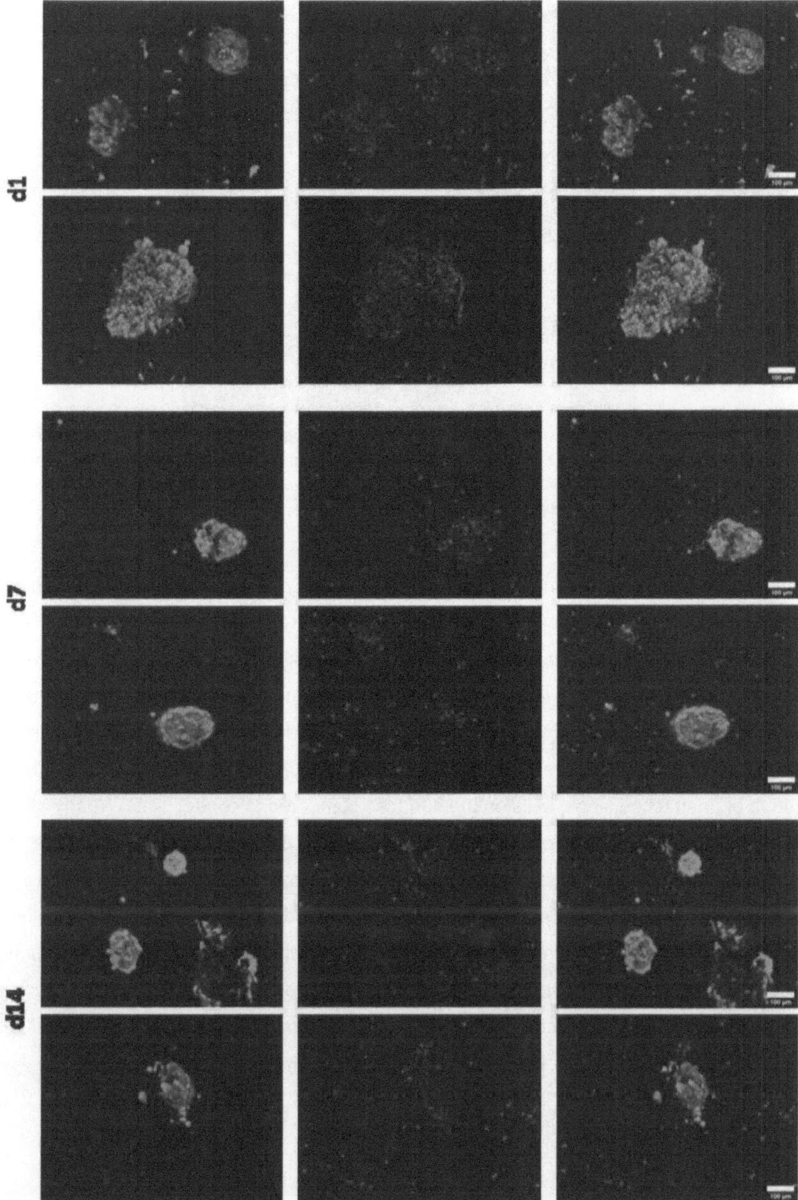

Figure 36: Qualitative viability of murine islets over 14 days. Plotted islets in clinical-grade Alg/MC scaffolds crosslinked with 70 mM SrCl$_2$ incubated in RPMI$^+$ under cell culture conditions for up to 14 days. A) Representative images of islets stained for live (green) and dead (red) cells. Scale bars = 100 μm.

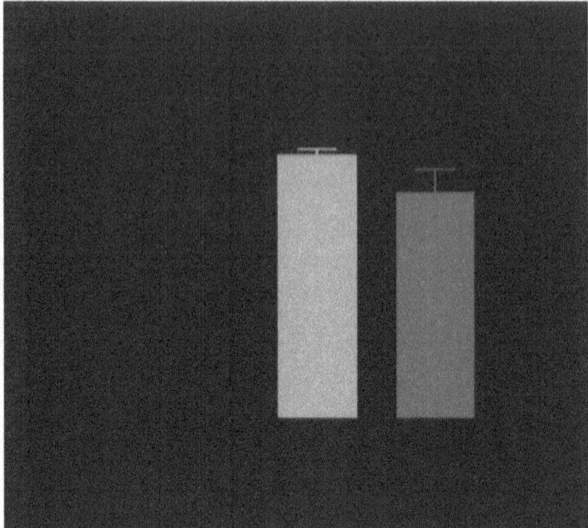

Figure 37: Quantitative viability of murine islets over 14 days. Plotted islets in clinical-grade Alg/MC scaffolds crosslinked with 70 mM $SrCl_2$ incubated in $RPMI^+$ under cell culture conditions for up to 14 days. Semi-quantitative assessment of islet viability on the basis of live/dead stainings as shown in Figure 36. Mean ± SD, n = 3 isolations, each 24-70 islets.

TUNEL-staining for apoptotic nuclei observed for up to 7 days (Figure 38 & Figure 39) showed the same trend as staining for live vs dead cells, but in a more pronounced manner. Qualitative analysis of TUNEL and DAPI stained islets (Figure 38) revealed that most islets in both groups, control and plotted, were approximately spherical in shape, but that there was a higher number of larger islets in the control group, which is also revealed in quantitative depiction of size in Figure 33 C (page 67). Despite their largely comparable shapes plotted islets had a higher likelihood of unattached single cells on the surfaces compared to control islets. Nearly all analysed samples of both groups contained apoptotic cells in different amounts. In plotted scaffolds apoptotic nuclei were predominantly located in the outer areas or areas where a tear likely had happened. In free control islets on the other hand, especially in a number of larger islets apoptotic nuclei were mainly located in the centre, or where the centre of the islets seems to be missing entirely. In quantitative analysis of overall percentage of live cells, a trend towards higher survival of free control islets was observed, especially for day 4 and day 7 after plotting; this difference was not significant in statistical analysis though (Figure 39).

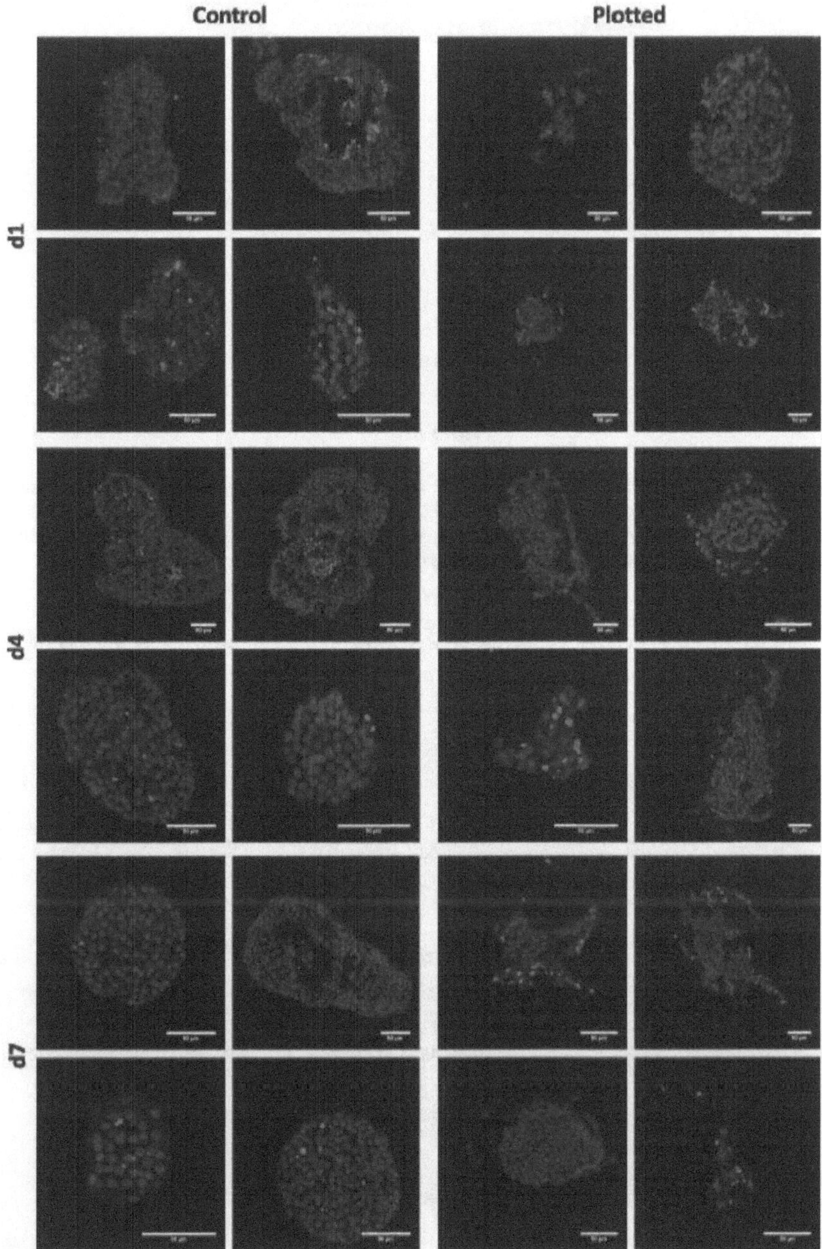

Figure 38: Qualitative depiction of intact and apoptotic nuclei in murine islets. Plotted islets in clinical-grade Alg/MC scaffolds crosslinked with 70 mM $SrCl_2$ and control islets in suspension culture incubated in RPMI⁺ under cell culture conditions for up to 7 days. Representative images of TUNEL and DAPI stained cryosections. Scale bars = 50 μm.

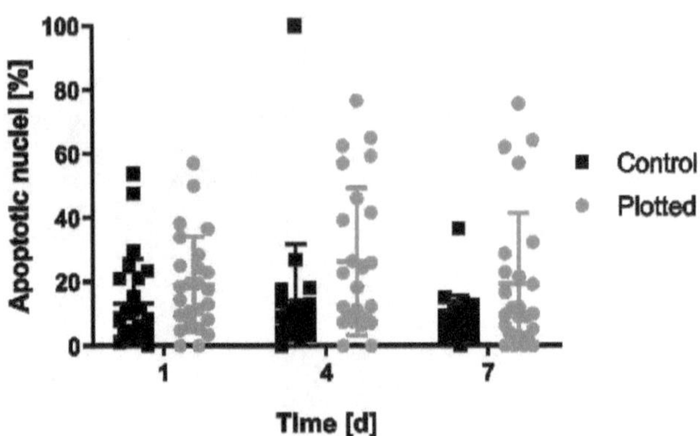

Figure 39: Quantitative depiction of intact and apoptotic nuclei in murine islets. Plotted islets in clinical-grade Alg/MC scaffolds crosslinked with 70 mM $SrCl_2$ and control islets in suspension culture incubated in RPMI+ under cell culture conditions for up to 7 days. Percent apoptotic nuclei per islet calculated from TUNEL and DAPI stained cryosections. Mean ± SD, n=1 isolation, 25 islets.

In the free control group, some islets appeared to fuse which is shown exemplarily in Figure 38, control, d4, upper right image, and depicted more thoroughly in Figure 40. The islets this pertains to are still distinctly recognizable as two separate islets, which are connected in one place via a cellular bridging. This bridging neither influenced overall islet morphology, nor number of apoptotic cells. While the phenomenon was independent of size or time in culture, it seemed to be restricted mainly to free control islets where the fusion was observed in approximately 10 % of islets. In a survey of all images of plotted murine islets, such a fusion was only detected one single time.

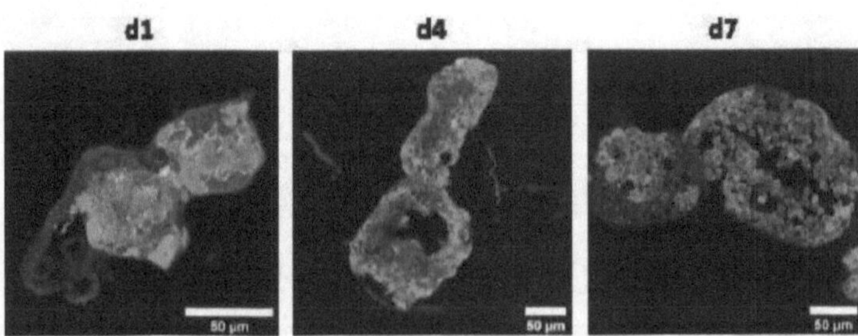

Figure 40: Aggregation of individual murine control islets. Control islets in suspension culture incubated in RPMI+ under cell culture conditions for up to 7 days. Exemplary images of aggregated islets immunofluorescently stained for insulin (green) and glucagon (red). Nuclei (blue) were stained with DAPI. Scale bars = 50 µm.

4.3.2 Functionality of bioplotted murine islets

The functionality of islets was assessed by analysing the production and localisation of insulin and glucagon inside the islet, and ultimately the release of insulin in response to glucose stimulation.

Cryosections of control and plotted islets fixed on day 1, 4, and 7 after plotting were immuno-histochemically stained for nuclei, insulin and glucagon (Figure 41). Both, insulin and glucagon were detected in the majority of islets in all investigated conditions and throughout the whole time of observation. Insulin was located nearly throughout the whole islet, whereas glucagon could only be found in the outer areas in a far smaller subset of cells than insulin. Both hormones did not appear in the same cells. This was for the most part independent of islet size or shape, even large or slightly frayed islets still contained both hormones on day 7, although it has to be noted that in some larger islets, insulin was not as prevalent in the centre as towards the outer areas. As has been stated when referring to DAPI/TUNEL stained islets, insulin/glucagon stainings again showed that overall control islets are larger and more often rounded in shape, but tend to contain empty areas (Figure 41 A). Plotted islets had a higher likelihood of unattached single cells on the edges, which did not impair production or localisation of either hormone though (Figure 41 B, day 1).

Functionality of islets was investigated via glucose-stimulated insulin release whereby islets were exposed to either low (3.3 mM) or high (16.4 mM) glucose. Functional analysis was performed on free control islets (denoted as "ctrl") and on islets embedded in plotted scaffolds (denoted as "plot"), whereby the numbering indicates different islet isolations. Plotted scaffolds were prepared with either research-grade (Figure 42) or clinical-grade alginate (Figure 43 & Figure 44). For analysis, the released insulin was normalized to DNA followed by calculation of the stimulation index (SI), the ratio of insulin released under high-glucose to insulin released under low-glucose stimulation. For functional murine islets, the SI is defined as ≥ 2 (Carter et al., 2009).

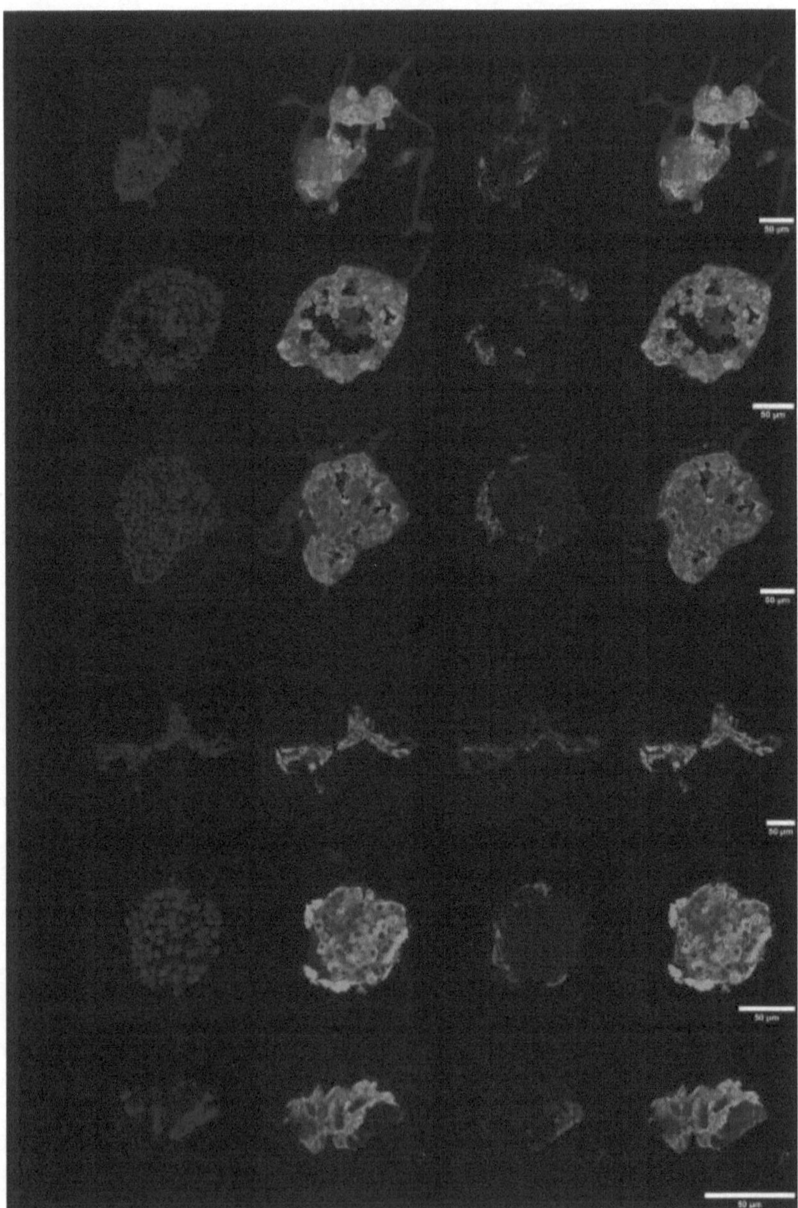

Figure 41: Presence of pancreatic hormones in murine islets. Plotted islets in clinical-grade Alg/MC scaffolds crosslinked with 70 mM $SrCl_2$, and control islets in suspension culture incubated in RPMI$^+$ under cell culture conditions for up to 7 days. Representative images of islets immunofluorescently stained for insulin (green) and glucagon (red). Nuclei (blue) were stained with DAPI. A) Free control islets. B) Islets in plotted Alg/MC scaffolds. Scale bars = 50 µm for all.

Stimulation of islets plotted in research-grade Alg/MC was performed for up to five isolations and is depicted as single data points representing different isolations; free islets served as control (Figure 42). The majority of control islets showed functionality at all timepoints although SI on day 4 was unexpectedly high (Figure 42 A). For plotted islets on the other hand, in none of the five performed isolations a functional response with an SI > 2 could be detected. At each timepoint, at least two isolations resulted in an SI > 2 though, i.e. they released a slightly higher amount of insulin in response to high than in response to low glucose (Figure 42 B).

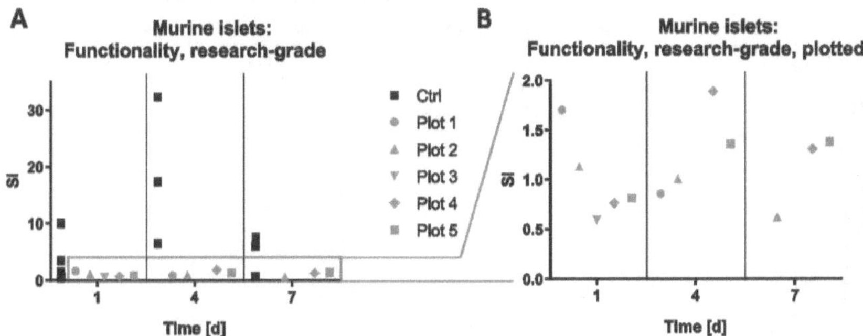

Figure 42: GSIR of murine islets in research-grade Alg/MC. Plotted islets in research-grade Alg/MC scaffolds crosslinked with 70 mM $SrCl_2$ and control islets in suspension culture incubated in RPMI$^+$ under cell culture conditions for up to 7 days. SI of up to 5 different islet isolations. A) SI of control and plotted samples. B) SI of only plotted samples from A for better visibility.

For scaffolds prepared with clinical-grade alginate, the functional response is depicted as the absolute amount of released insulin normalised to the DNA content to illustrate the scale of release, as well as the SI to illustrate the ratio between low and high glucose. The amount of released insulin from free control and plotted islets over a cultivation time of up to 14 days is exemplarily depicted for 3 out of 7 different isolations (Figure 43, for a complete overview over all isolations in graphical depiction and numerically refer to Figure 71 & Figure 72, addendum, and Table 3-Table 9, addendum, respectively). Overall, the amount of insulin varied strongly between isolations but also between replicates within isolations, which was much stronger in the free control though. Especially at early timepoints, control islets released disproportionately higher amounts of insulin in response to high glucose in the majority of the isolations. Release from control islets generally decreased strongly towards later timepoints.

The SI calculated from the released insulin is depicted in Figure 44 with the single isolations differentiated by colour. The SI of control islets varied strongly between isolations, especially on day 1 and 4 after plotting but in general decreased until day 7.

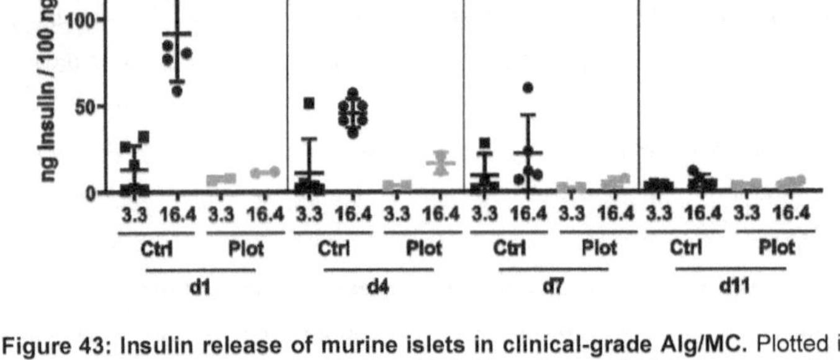

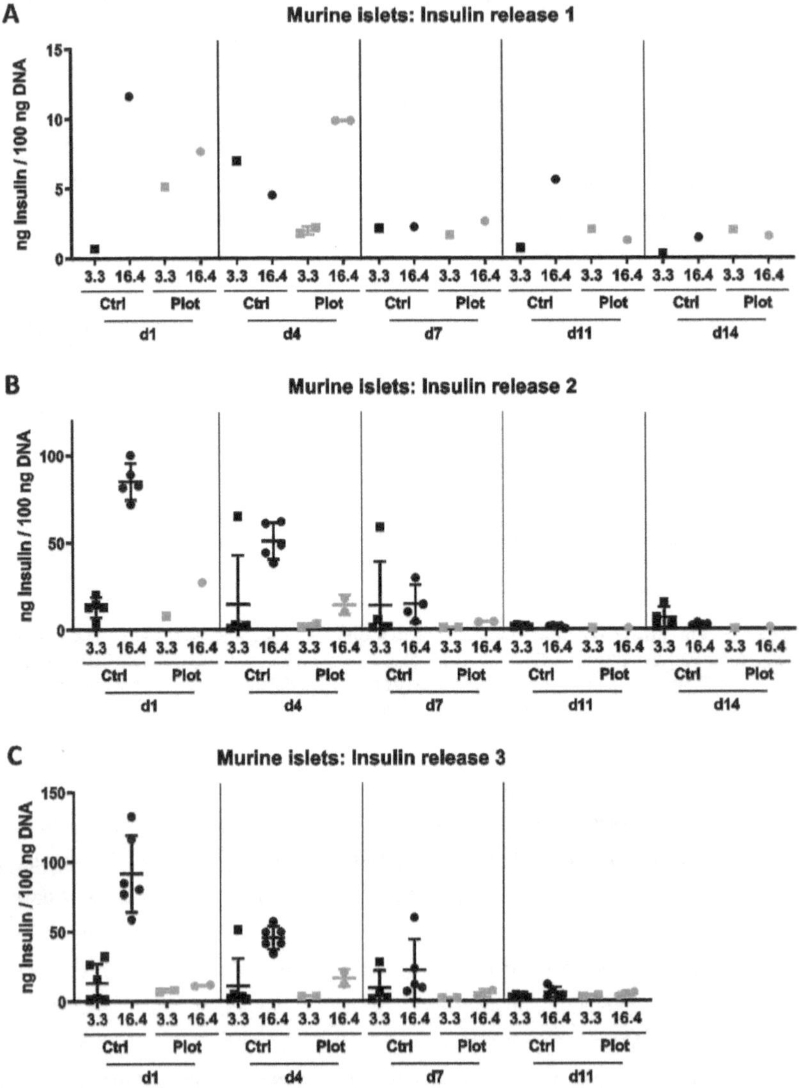

Figure 43: Insulin release of murine islets in clinical-grade Alg/MC. Plotted islets in clinical-grade Alg/MC scaffolds crosslinked with 70 mM $SrCl_2$ and control islets in suspension culture incubated in $RPMI^+$ under cell culture conditions for up to 7 days. Single values of ng insulin released in response to either low (3.3 mM) or high (16.4 mM) glucose stimulation normalised to 100 ng DNA. Stimulation over a cultivation time of 14 days exemplarily depicted for 3 out of 7 isolations. Data points for each isolation depict replicate samples. For an overview over the calculated values refer to Table 3-Table 5, addendum.

Plotted islets on the other hand, were non-functional on day 1 after plotting, but the functionality was on par with the control on day 4 and 7. In an average of the isolations, the SI of the free control decreases from 9.2 on day 1 via 4.8 on day 4 to 1.8 on day 7 whereas the SI of plotted islets is 1.8 on the first day and increases to 4.5 on day 4 before decreasing again to 2.4 on day 7. On day 4 and day 7 of incubation, control and plotted islets from the majority of the isolations reacted similarly with either both or none giving an SI $\geq$ 2. An SI < 1 on the other hand, was rarely detected, and between day 1 and day 7 of incubation only present in control but never in plotted samples. After 11 days of culture, the majority of isolations was non-functional. Interestingly, in a preliminary insight into functionality of islets after 14 days of culture, control and plotted islets from the same isolation reacted very differently. Functionality testing on day 14 was performed for only two isolations with a low number of replicates though. No significances were detected.

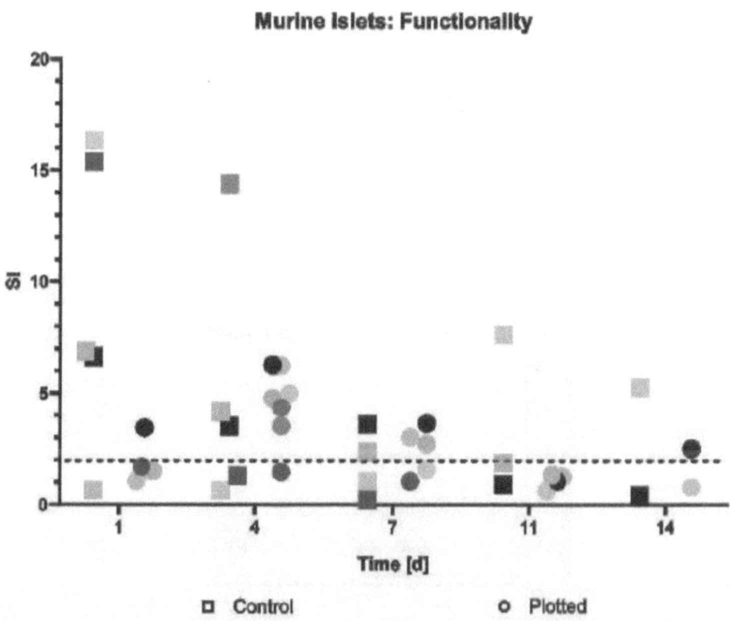

Figure 44: GSIR of murine islets in clinical-grade Alg/MC. Plotted islets in clinical-grade Alg/MC scaffolds crosslinked with 70 mM SrCl$_2$ and control islets in suspension culture incubated in RPMI$^+$ under cell culture conditions for up to 7 days. SI of insulin released in response to either low (3.3 mM) or high (16.4 mM) glucose stimulation of up to 7 isolations over a cultivation time of 14 days. Different isolations are differentiated by colour. SI was calculated on the basis of insulin release as depicted in Figure 43 and in Table 3-Table 9, addendum.

In vivo, pancreatic islets need to react to glucose stimulation by an increase in insulin release, followed by a decrease concomitant to a decrease in blood-glucose levels. For a preliminary insight into the ability to repeatedly react to changes in glucose concentration, murine islets were additionally exposed to successive low-high-low stimulation on day 1 and day 4 after plotting (Figure 45). In accordance with the results presented for functionality of murine islets presented on previous pages, for low-high-low stimulation the overall amount of released insulin varied strongly between control and plotted islets with plotted islets releasing less insulin, but also varied within the control. Independent of timepoint it could be shown for all sample groups that the amount of released insulin corresponded to the glucose settings, with a low release in low glucose, followed by a high release in high glucose and then going back to a low release when low glucose was applied once more.

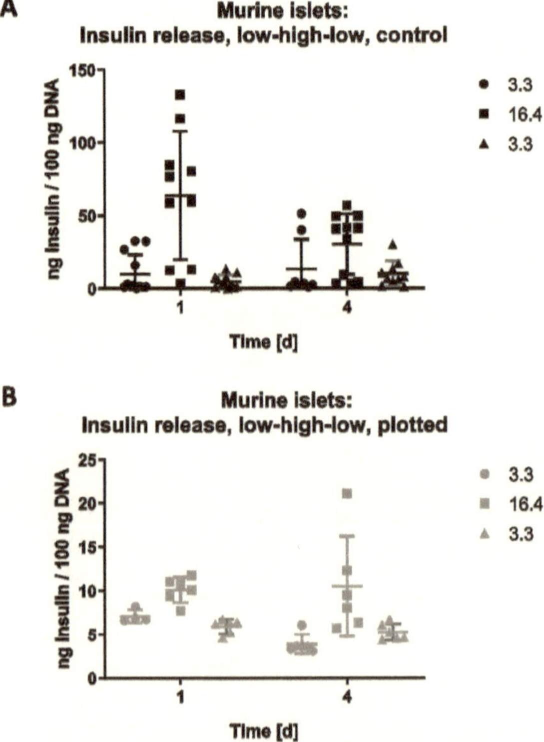

Figure 45: Insulin release of murine islets in clinical-grade Alg/MC in response to successive exposure to low-high-low glucose. Plotted islets in clinical-grade Alg/MC scaffolds crosslinked with 70 mM $SrCl_2$ and control islets in suspension culture incubated in RPMI+ under cell culture conditions for up to 4 days. Single values of ng insulin released in response to consecutive low-high-low (3.3 mM – 16.4 mM – 3.3 mM) glucose stimulation normalized to 100 ng DNA. A) Free control islets. B) Islets in plotted Alg/MC scaffolds. n = 1 isolation, data points depict replicate samples.

4.4 Plotting of neonatal porcine islet-like cell clusters (NICC)

Murine islets are a suitable system for a proof-of-concept of the survival and function of plotted islets but lack clinical applicability. Neonatal porcine islet-like cell clusters on the other hand, are clinically relevant as a promising candidate for the xenotransplantation of islets for patients with Diabetes mellitus type 1 (Korbutt et al., 1996; Cooper et al., 2015).

Out of the much broader topic of xenotransplantation of NICC in plotted scaffolds, this work aimed at investigating the general compatibility of the Alg/MC blend and plotting process with NICC. This first foray is meant to provide information on the general feasibility of the concept while disregarding other aspects relevant for transplantation of NICC, such as maturation within the scaffolds and sufficient immunoprotection, for the moment. These extensive topics will be the focus of future studies.

Analogous to adult murine islets, first considerations involved the analysis of morphology and survival after incorporation into the material and plotting, followed by a preliminary examination of functionality via detection of presence of pancreatic hormones and reaction to glucose stimulation. All experiments were performed according to the optimised protocol for murine islets with clinical-grade alginate, careful folding in, a needle diameter of 840 µm, and crosslinking with 70 mM SrCl$_2$.

4.4.1 Distribution, morphology and viability of bioplotted NICC

To investigate to what extent NICC tolerate the incorporation into the highly viscous Alg/MC blend, NICC were mixed with the material, plotted into macroporous 3D scaffolds and analysed for morphology, distribution, metabolic activity, presence of insulin and survival (Figure 46). Unplotted NICC in Alg/MC, unplotted NICC in plain alginate, and NICC in suspension culture served as controls for the material and plotting process. In all conditions, NICC were homogeneously distributed inside the material and presence of insulin and metabolic activity could be detected by DTZ and MTT staining, respectively. Neither the incorporation, nor the material, nor the plotting process seemed to have an influence on general morphology of cell clusters (Figure 46 A). Distinctly visible in a qualitative analysis of live/dead stained NICC (Figure 46 B) is a relatively high number of dead cells independent of incorporation into the material and plotting process but the proportion of live to dead cells was comparable between all tested conditions.

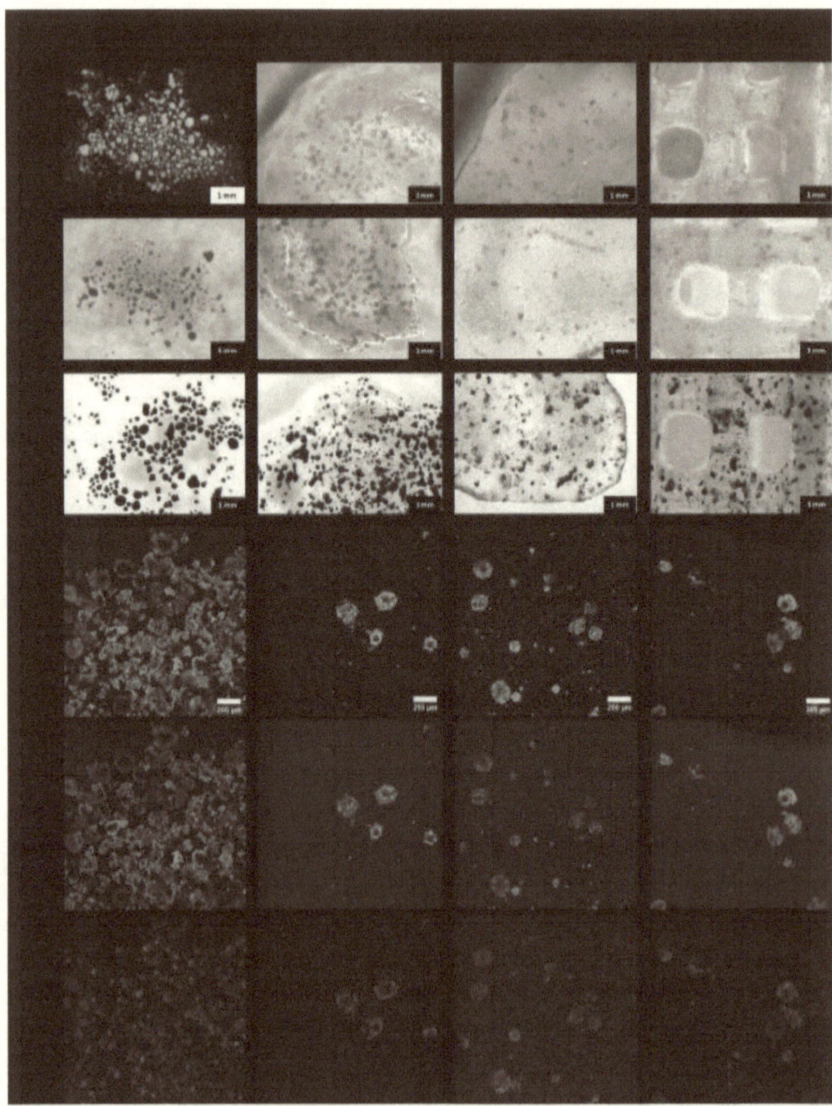

Figure 46: Metabolic activity and viability of NICC in reaction to the material and the plotting process. Plotted NICC in Alg/MC scaffolds, unplotted NICC in Alg/MC, NICC in plain alginate beads, all crosslinked with 70 mM SrCl$_2$, and free control NICC in suspension culture. All samples were incubated in RPMI$^+$ under cell culture conditions for 3 days. A) Representative images of the general distribution (top), presence of insulin (DTZ), and metabolic activity (MTT). Scale bars = 1 mm. B) Representative images of islets stained for live (green) and dead (red) cells. Scale bars = 200 μm.

Following investigation of the general compatibility of NICC and the Alg/MC blend, presence of insulin and metabolic activity in plotted and free control NICC were observed over the course of one week in culture (Figure 47). Throughout the entire time of incubation both, plotted and control NICC showed presence of insulin and metabolic activity. NICC were evenly distributed throughout the scaffolds.

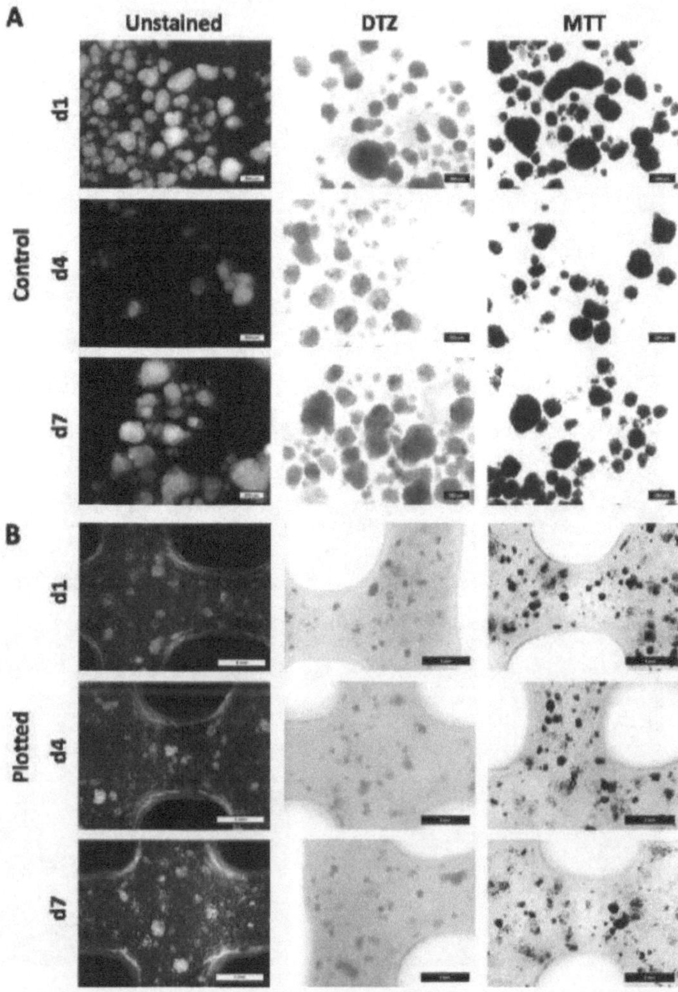

Figure 47: Metabolic activity and insulin content of NICC. Plotted NICC in clinical-grade Alg/MC scaffolds crosslinked with 70 mM SrCl$_2$ and control islets in suspension culture incubated in RPMI$^+$ under cell culture conditions for up to 7 days. Representative images of unstained NICC and NICC stained for presence of insulin (DTZ) and metabolic activity (MTT). A) Free control islets. Scale bars = 200 µm. B) Islets in plotted Alg/MC scaffolds. Scale bars = 1 mm.

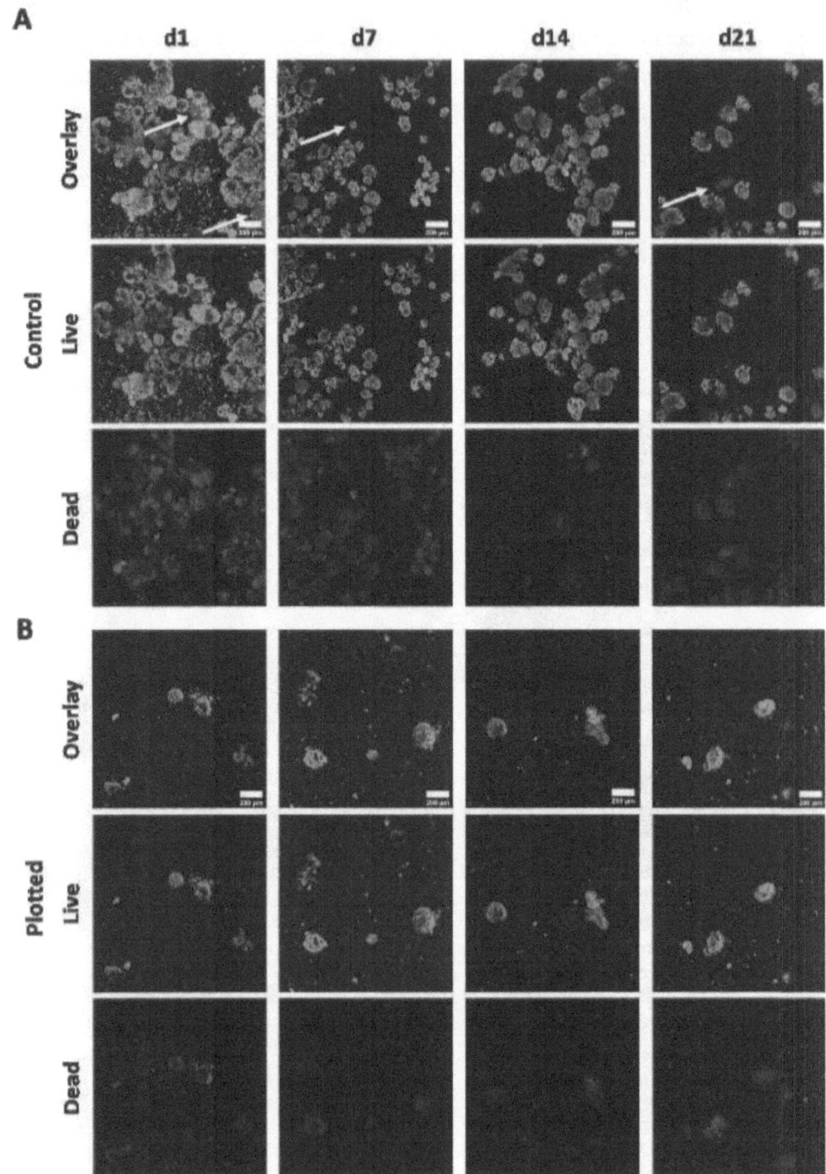

Figure 48: Qualitative viability of NICC. Plotted NICC in clinical-grade Alg/MC scaffolds crosslinked with 70 mM SrCl₂ and control islets in suspension culture incubated in RPMI⁺ under cell culture conditions for up to 21 days. Representative images of islets stained for live (green) and dead (red) cells. A) Free control islets, the white arrows indicate single islets with a majority of dead cells. B) Islets in plotted Alg/MC scaffolds. Scale bars = 200 µm for all.

In-depth examination of survival of plotted islets was done through the qualitative and quantitative analysis of staining for live vs dead cells (Figure 48 & Figure 49). While the main focus lay on survival for up to seven days analogous to murine islets, with respect to the maturation time necessary for neonatal islets, NICC were additionally observed until day 21 after plotting for selected isolations.

As previously observed in the experiments with murine islets, in most cases live/dead staining (Figure 48) revealed that the complete surface area visible in the images of the islets showed green staining indicating live cells at all timepoints and in both sample types (free control and plotted), and limited red signal distributed over the single islet-like clusters. In contrast to murine islets, a noticeable number of NICC consisted of a majority of dead cells (Figure 48 A, control, indicated by white arrows).

The semi-quantitative evaluation of live/dead stainings (Figure 49) demonstrated a comparable rate of survival between control and plotted NICC. For both conditions, percentage of survival remained mainly constant for up to 10 days and peaked at day 14 after plotting, before decreasing again towards day 21. This decrease was much stronger in plotted than control NICC though. Overall rate of survival lay between 60 and 86 % for control, 60 and 76 % for plotted NICC with the highest difference between the conditions after 3 weeks of incubation. Semi-quantitative assessment was performed on stainings of 1-4 different isolations pooled from three neonates each, but at least two replicate experiments for the first three timepoints.

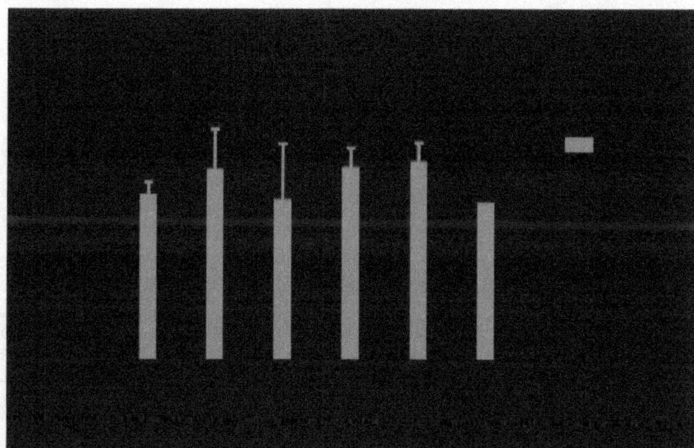

Figure 49: Quantitative viability of NICC. Plotted NICC in clinical-grade Alg/MC scaffolds crosslinked with 70 mM $SrCl_2$ and control islets in suspension culture incubated in RPMI⁺ under cell culture conditions for up to 21 days. Semi-quantitative assessment of islet viability on the basis of live/dead stainings as shown in Figure 48. Mean ± SD. Control: n = 2 isolations for day 1-7. Plotted: n = 3 isolations for day 1 & day 4, n = 2 isolations for day 7 & day 10. n = 1 for bars w.o. SD. 30-530 islets.

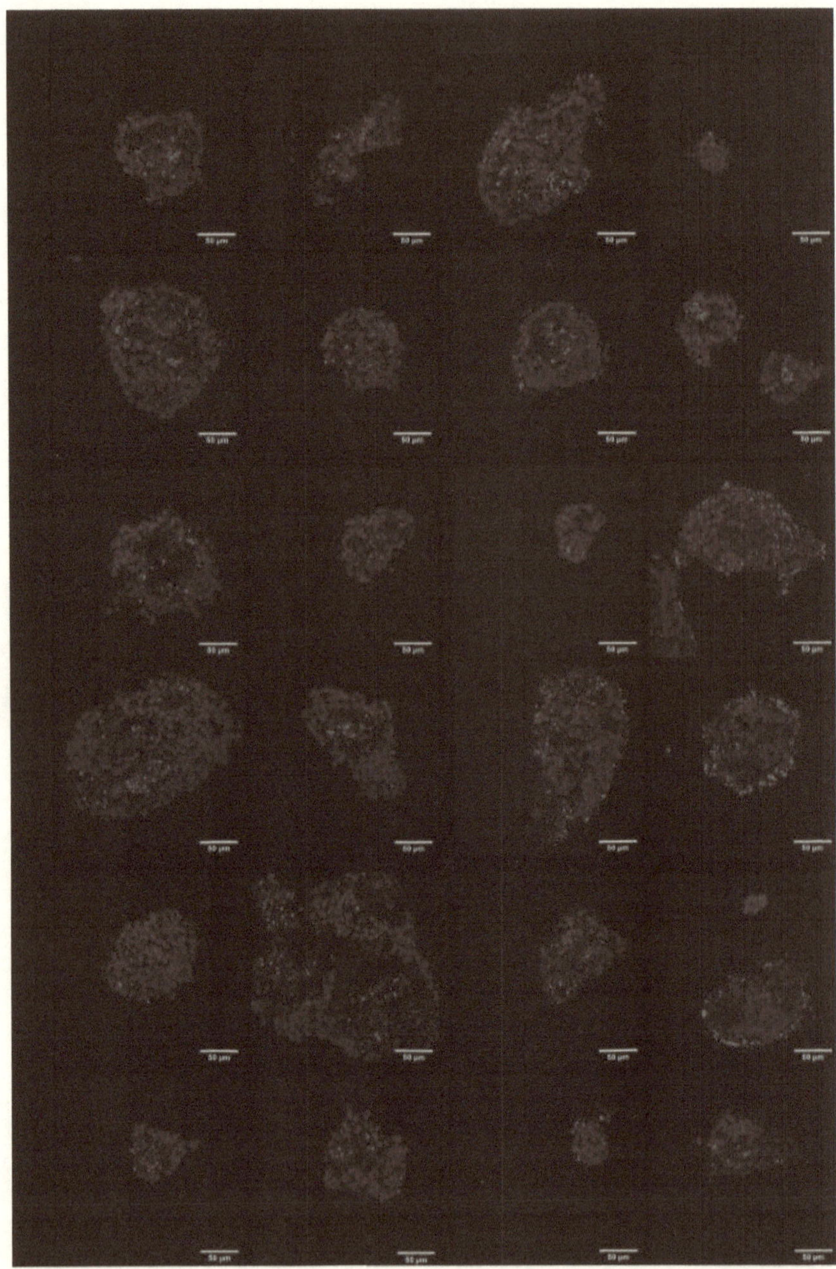

Figure 50: Qualitative depiction of intact and apoptotic nuclei in NICC. Plotted NICC in clinical-grade Alg/MC scaffolds crosslinked with 70 mM SrCl$_2$ and control islets in suspension culture incubated in RPMI$^+$ under cell culture conditions for up to 7 days. Representative images of TUNEL and DAPI stained cryosections. Scale bars = 50 µm.

TUNEL-staining for apoptotic nuclei observed for up to 7 days is qualitatively depicted in Figure 50 and quantitatively depicted in Figure 51. In qualitative analysis, it was apparent that in all conditions the vast majority of islets retained their spherical morphology and apoptotic nuclei were located throughout the whole islets with apoptotic cores present in all conditions. In plotted NICC the number of unattached single cells was visibly lower than in murine islets, but especially at later timepoints, in some islets the outer border was entirely composed of dead cells. Independent of condition and timepoint, many NICC displayed empty areas, which are within the boundaries of the islets, but contain neither DAPI nor TUNEL stained nuclei, indicating prior complete cell death. Quantitative analysis of islet size and percentage of apoptotic nuclei are determined from cryosections stained with DAPI for nuclei and TUNEL for apoptotic nuclei. Overall, size distribution is comparable between control and plotted NICC, with an approximately even number of smaller and larger islets. While size of control islets remained mostly constant over time in culture though, for plotted islets there was a significant decrease in size between day 4 and day 7 of cultivation, and therefore a significant difference between control and plotted NICC on day 7 (Figure 51 A). Percentage of apoptotic cells was comparable between control and plotted NICC on day 1, with an average of 30 % and 25 %, respectively, but continuously increased to 47 % for plotted islets and continuously decreased to 20 % in the free control on day 7 after plotting (Figure 51 B). On day 7 after plotting, plotted islets contained significantly more apoptotic nuclei than control NICC.

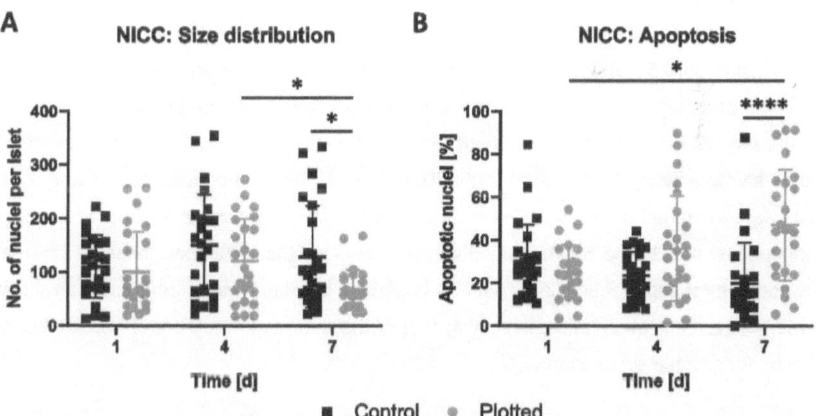

Figure 51: Size distribution and quantitative depiction of intact and apoptotic nuclei in NICC. Plotted NICC in clinical-grade Alg/MC scaffolds crosslinked with 70 mM $SrCl_2$ and control islets in suspension culture incubated in $RPMI^+$ under cell culture conditions for up to 7 days. A) Size of NICC determined by means of counting nuclei in DAPI stained 2D cross-sections. Mean ± SD, n=1 isolation, 25 islets. B) Percent apoptotic nuclei per islet calculated from TUNEL and DAPI stained cryosections. Mean ± SD, n=1 isolation, 25 islets. Significances in all graphs indicate *$p<0.05$, ****$p<0.0001$.

4.4.2 Functionality of bioplotted NICC

Despite their comparatively low number of β-cells and the need for maturation before NICC are able to normalise blood glucose levels *in vivo* (MacKenzie et al., 2003; Emamaullee et al., 2006; Elliott et al., 2007; Köllmer et al., 2016), they do contain insulin and can show a functional response *in vitro* early on (Britt et al., 1981; Korbutt et al., 1996). For this book, the functionality of NICC was assessed by analysing the production and localisation of insulin inside the islet, and the release of insulin in response to glucose stimulation.

Figure 52 depicts exemplary cryosections of free control and plotted islets fixed on day 1, day 4, and day 7 after plotting, which were immunohistochemically stained for insulin (green), glucagon (red), and somatostatin (grey), as well as for nuclei by DAPI (blue). All three hormones could be detected in all analysed NICC of both, control and plotted samples throughout the whole time of observation. In contrast to murine islets from adult rats, in neonatal porcine islet-like clusters the hormones were only prevalent in small amounts and select cells within the islets. This was for the most part independent of islet size or shape, and cells positive for insulin, glucagon, and somatostatin were distributed randomly throughout the NICC.

The detection of insulin-positive cells in the majority of NICC analysed was followed up by investigation of a functional reaction to glucose stimulation of free control and plotted NICC in clinical-grade Alg/MC scaffolds.

First considerations included a comparison between NICC incorporated into plain alginate and Alg/MC with control islets (Figure 53 A) as well as an investigation of incubation times for stimulation (Figure 53 B). While SI of NICC was very low overall, even more so after incorporation into plain alginate beads, no difference between control and islet clusters incorporated into the Alg/MC-blend could be observed (Figure 53 A). In general, NICC release less insulin and do so more slowly than mature islets (Korbutt et al., 1996), therefore, control and plotted NICC were screened for insulin release during stimulation with glucose for 3 h (analogous to murine islets), 4.5 h and 6 h (Figure 53 B). For none of the incubation times, a difference between control and plotted islets could be observed, but there was a trend towards a lower SI with longer incubation times, indicating that of the analysed conditions 3 h is the optimal duration for glucose stimulation.

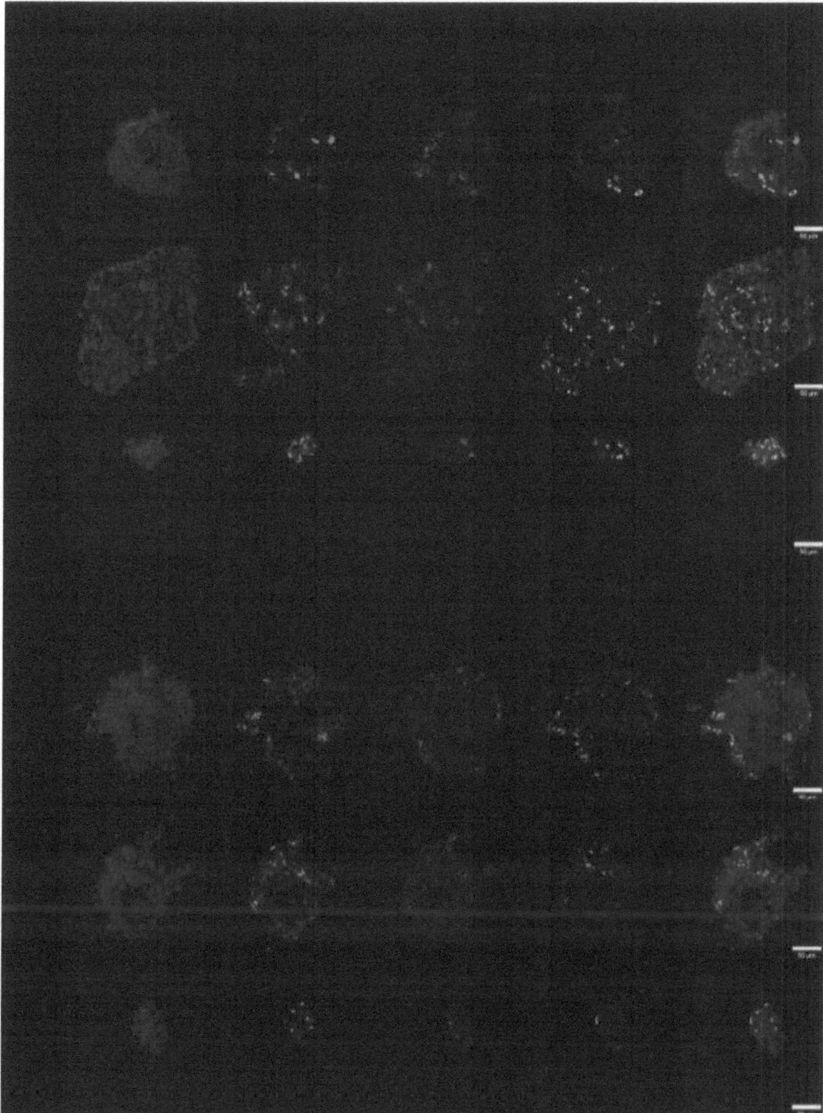

Figure 52: Presence of pancreatic hormones in NICC. Plotted NICC in clinical-grade Alg/MC scaffolds crosslinked with 70 mM SrCl$_2$ and control islets in suspension culture incubated in RPMI$^+$ under cell culture conditions for up to 7 days. Representative images of islets immunofluorescently stained for insulin (green), glucagon (red), and somatostatin (grey). Nuclei (blue) were stained with DAPI. A) Free control islets. B) Islets in plotted Alg/MC scaffolds. Scale bars = 50 µm for all.

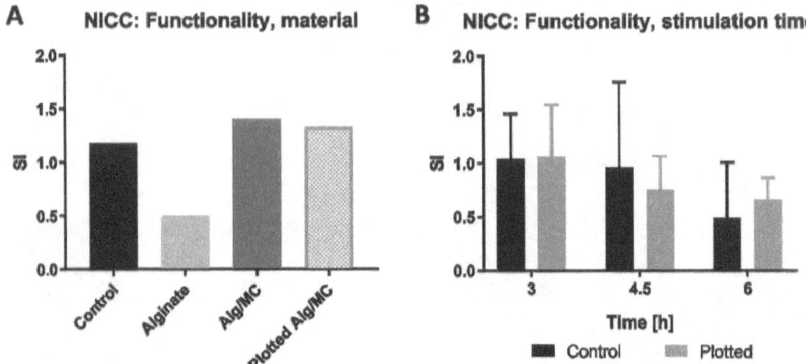

Figure 53: GSIR of NICC for parameter optimisation. Plotted NICC in clinical-grade Alg/MC scaffolds crosslinked with 70 mM SrCl$_2$ and control islets in suspension culture incubated in RPMI$^+$ under cell culture conditions for 3 days. A) SI of control and plotted samples in dependence of material. n = 1. B) SI of control and plotted samples in dependence of incubation time. Mean ± SD, n = 1 isolation, 8 samples for control; n = 1 isolation, 3 samples for plotted samples.

Having observed no influence of incorporation into the Alg/MC-blend on the resulting SI, free control and plotted NICC were exposed to glucose stimulation on day 1, 4, and 7 after plotting. Figure 54 A & Figure 55 A depict insulin released in response to low and high glucose stimulation and the SI calculated from these values, respectively. The most striking difference in comparison to adult murine islets is the overall amount of insulin released, which was below 0.1 ng / 100 ng DNA in all cases, and below 0.05 ng in case of plotted scaffolds. As observed in previous experiments with NICC, the ratio of insulin released during high to low glucose stimulation was below 2 at all observed timepoints and while a trend towards a slightly higher SI in control than in plotted samples was visible on day 1 and day 7, there was no significant difference between any of the conditions.

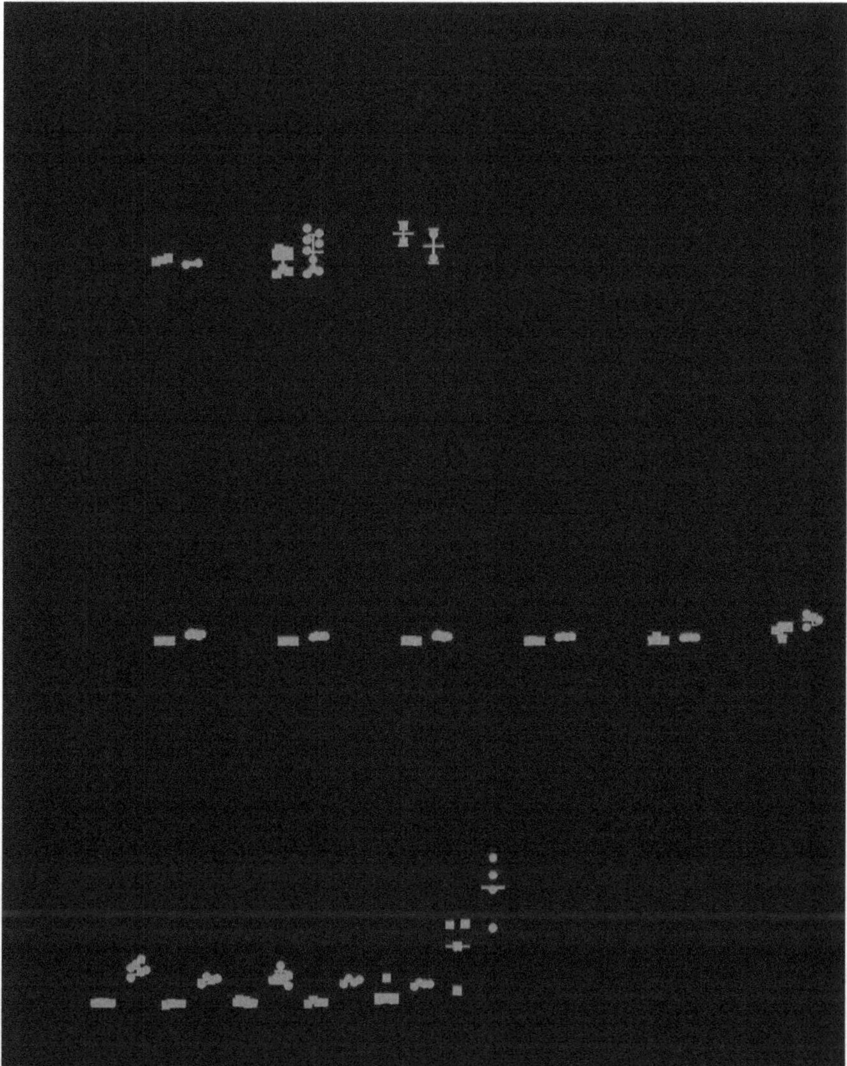

Figure 54: Insulin release of NICC. Plotted islets in clinical grade Alg/MC scaffolds crosslinked with 70 mM $SrCl_2$ and control islets in suspension culture incubated in RPMI⁺ under cell culture conditions for up to 21 days. Single values of ng insulin released in response to either low (3.3 mM) or high (16.4 mM) glucose stimulation normalised to 100 ng DNA. A) GSIR performed with low or high glucose. B) GSIR performed with low or high glucose and liraglutide, control and plotted samples. C) GSIR performed with low or high glucose and liraglutide, only plotted samples from B for better visibility. Data points for each isolation depict replicate samples. For an overview over the calculated values refer to Table 11 & Table 12, addendum.

As mentioned, as a general rule, neonatal islets need to mature before they become functional, but it is possible to induce insulin release by exposure to glucagon-like peptide-1 (Mourad et al., 2017). Liraglutide, a long-lasting GLP-1 analogue, was added to NICC for further long-term stimulation experiments (Figure 54 B&C, Figure 55 B). Generally, the amount of insulin released in response to high-glucose stimulation was a magnitude higher, the vast majority of samples still released less than 1 ng insulin per 100 ng DNA though. Analogous to murine islets, control NICC released a higher amount of insulin than plotted NICC in most cases. Over time, insulin released from control islets increased until day 14, followed by a decrease until day 21, whereas insulin released from plotted samples remained constant until day 14 and increased until day 21.

The SI from samples exposed to liraglutide on the other hand was highest on day 1 after plotting and continually decreased over time of observation. Until day 10 of culture, the SI was > 5 in all cases with no difference between control and plotted islets. After 14 and 21 days of incubation, the SI of plotted NICC fell below 2 although SI of control NICC still lay between 2.5 and 4. With the small sample size analysed here no significant differences could be detected, neither between the conditions, nor over time.

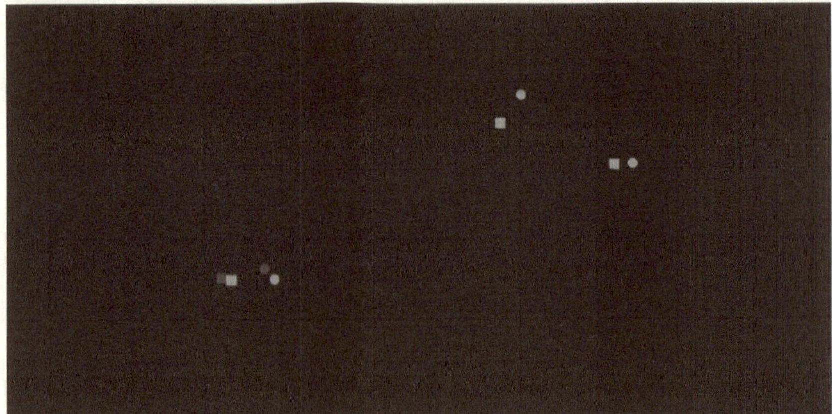

Figure 55: **GSIR of NICC.** Plotted islets in clinical-grade Alg/MC scaffolds crosslinked with 70 mM SrCl$_2$ and control islets in suspension culture incubated in RPMI$^+$ under cell culture conditions for up to 21 days. A) SI of up to three different islet isolations, GSIR performed with low or high glucose. B) SI of up to two different islet isolations, GSIR performed with low or high glucose and liraglutide. Different isolations are differentiated by colour.

5 Discussion

The main aim of this book was to develop a method for the 3D plotting of functional pancreatic islets in order to enable the fabrication of stable macroporous constructs with encapsulated islets. Encapsulation of pancreatic islets in hydrogels either in microcapsules containing single islets or in macrocapsules containing the entire transplant volume, is an established method to achieve immunoprotection (Duvivier-Kali et al., 2001; De Vos et al., 2003; Schneider et al., 2005; Veiseh et al., 2015). Microcapsules support viability and function of islets through a large surface-to-volume ratio and thereby short diffusion distances, but have the disadvantages of an overall increased transplant volume (Zhu et al., 2018), and a tendency to clump when transplanted together, which in turn increases the diffusion distance (Bochenek et al., 2019). In macrocapsules on the other hand, a large number of islets is packed comparatively densely, but the diffusion distance, especially to central areas, is much higher than in microcapsules. This means they often require external support with oxygen (Barkai et al., 2013) and react more slowly to changes in the blood glucose level. Despite dense packaging upscaling of macrocapsules to curative doses of islets remains challenging though (Hwa & Weir, 2018). With the use of 3D plotting, it could be possible to combine the advantages of both approaches and generate macroporous macrocapsules with a high packing density and short diffusion distances.

The hydrogel chosen for this application was a highly viscous Alg/MC blend, developed previously in this lab (Schütz et al., 2017). This blend is a promising material combination since it combines plottability with biological inertness in the human body. The two components are alginate and MC. Alginate, the matrix-forming component, is biocompatible, provides a hydrated environment to cells through its high capacity for binding water and cannot be degraded in human body, but also lacks cell attachment sequences (chapter 2.2.3, page 17 ff.). MC, the thickening component, is non-bioactive, only allows for limited protein and cell adhesion (Stabenfeldt et al., 2006), and can get released from the scaffolds (Schütz et al., 2017; Hodder et al., 2019) as it remains non-crosslinked by divalent cations.

Among the steps taken towards the 3D plotting of functional islets, the hydrogel composition first had to be adapted for clinical application. The materials used are in principle approved for clinical use, however they were previously neither used in clinical-grade quality and sterility nor with endocrine cells, and a change in material composition and cell type necessitates further characterisation of material and scaffold properties. Additionally, the workflow had to be optimised for the incorporation of pancreatic islets which are sensitive macroscopic cell clusters. Subsequently, the hydrogel blend was used in proof-of-concept experiments with adult murine islets which are known to show a good functional response *in vitro*. Since murine islets are unsuitable for clinical use though, this book will conclude with a first foray into the plotting of the potentially clinically translatable neonatal porcine islet-like clusters.

5.1 <u>Cell-free Alg/MC</u>

In terms of 3D cell culture in hydrogels, a number of factors are highly relevant for the survival of embedded cells. Among these are the hydrogel itself, with its chemical composition, water-content and mechanical properties; the mode of crosslinking which for alginate is physical crosslinking via divalent cations; the scaffold composition over time, concerning the stability but also the possible release of non-crosslinked components or degradation products; and the permeability of the gel for nutrients, oxygen and cellular waste products. Especially relevant for the functionality of plotted islets is hereby the permeability of the hydrogel for glucose and insulin molecules which had proven to be an obstacle in previous approaches to islet plotting (Marchioli et al., 2015; Liu et al., 2019). For the Alg/MC blend some of these factors, such as the influence of the hydrogel itself and the scaffold composition over time were known for the plotting of single cells (Schütz et al., 2017), or were investigated with collaboration of the author of this book (Hodder et al., 2019). Nevertheless, with regard to clinical applicability the mate-rials used need to be sufficiently purified to prevent an immune response in reaction to the material itself (chapter 2.2.3.1, page 17 ff.) and should be manufactured under GMP guide-lines. Alginate is commercially available in clinical-grade purity and manufactured under GMP guidelines (Dupont, 2018a). MC on the other hand is listed by the U.S. Food and Drug Ad-ministration (FDA) as an inactive ingredient if ingested orally (U.S. Food and Drug Adminis-tration, 2020) but, to the best of the author's knowledge, not yet approved for transplantation. In light of this, the MC used for the present book was of research-grade quality but sterilised via autoclaving which is a clinically approved sterilisation method.

Taking into account that the adaptation of the blend, from preparation with research-grade alginate to preparation with clinical-grade alginate, could influence material properties, the adapted blend was further characterised in terms of viscosity, crosslinking density of the algi-nate, scaffold composition over time, and permeability for glucose and insulin.

5.1.1 Gel viscosity and crosslinking of alginate

The high viscosity and shear-thinning behaviour of the Alg/MC blend prepared with research-grade alginate which enables plotting with high shape fidelity, have previously been shown to be compatible with the survival of single mammalian cells (Schütz et al., 2017). Overall, the viscosity of the blend results almost exclusively from the presence and Mw of MC: Different studies showed that the polymer content of alginate contributes only marginally to the viscosity of the material (Ahlfeld et al., 2017; Li et al., 2017; Schütz et al., 2017) whereas a strongly reduced chain length of MC molecules led to a drastic reduction of viscosity and thereby plottability of the blend (Hodder et al., 2019). Accordingly, the change from research-grade to clinical-grade alginate in this book did not significantly change the viscosity of the blend and plotting of the blend prepared with either type of alginate was possible with pressures below

80 kPa, i.e. with pressure ranges which have been reported to result in high cell survival after plotting (Schütz et al., 2017; Hodder et al., 2019).

After plotting, hydrogel scaffolds need to be crosslinked to gelate which is necessary to achieve long-term stability. Crosslinking of alginate can be accomplished with a number of divalent cations, among them Ca^{2+}, Sr^{2+}, and Ba^{2+}. The most widely used ion for crosslinking of alginate remains Ca^{2+}, which has been used successfully for the encapsulation of islets (chapter 2.2.3, page 17 ff.). In a concentration of 100 mM, $CaCl_2$ was reported to neither influence insulin secretion from freshly isolated murine islets after encapsulation in 1.2 % alginate, nor when free islets were resuspended in the solution (Fritschy et al., 1991). Contrary to this report, other groups showed that while the presence of extracellular Ca^{2+} is required for sustained insulin release, the optimal concentration for non-encapsulated murine (Hellman, 1975) and human islets (Squires et al., 2000) is between 1 and 5 mM and higher concentrations led to a reduced insulin secretion (also reviewed by Wollheim *et al.* previously (Wollheim & Sharp, 1981)). Generally, the use of Ca^{2+} for crosslinking of alginate does not impair function of microencapsulated islets (Langlois et al., 2009; Basta et al., 2011; Qi et al., 2012), likely because most of the ions are bound by the alginate matrix and cannot be internalised by the islet cells. However, Ca^{2+} has previously been shown to have a pro-inflammatory function (Chan & Mooney, 2013) so it would be preferably to avoid the use of high concentrations of Ca^{2+} in materials for transplantation. Furthermore, in previous works showing stability of Ca^{2+}-crosslinked Alg/MC scaffolds over time, the mammalian cells had been cultured in DMEM+ (Schütz et al., 2017; Hodder et al., 2019), whereas murine islets require culture in RPMI+ medium. For culture in RPMI+, crosslinking with Ca^{2+} was not considered adequate for Alg/MC scaffolds in this book because of insufficient scaffold stability during incubation (Figure 11 A, page 38), which indi-cated the necessity for a stronger crosslinking ion.

Strength of crosslinking ions, which can be used for cell encapsulation because they are not inherently cytotoxic (Smidsrød & Skjåk-Braek, 1990), increases from Ca^{2+} via Sr^{2+} to Ba^{2+}. As explained in a previous chapter (chapter 2.2.3.1, page 17 ff.), the ionic crosslinking of alginates occurs by divalent cations binding to different sections of the alginate chains, preferably blocks of α-L-guluronate (GG-blocks). This results in a characteristic structure of the crosslinked gel chains, termed "egg-box" model by Grant *et al.* in 1973 (Grant et al., 1973). The general mechanism of crosslinking is the ionic interaction between the divalent cations and two carboxy as well as two hydroxy groups of the alginate (Schweiger, 1962). Especially the carboxy groups are in closer vicinity in the "buckle-shaped" GG- than in MM-blocks which results in a higher density of charges and therefore a stronger interaction with the crosslinking ions (DeRamos et al., 1997). Furthermore, in MM-blocks one of the oxygens involved in the binding of crosslinking ions is a ring oxygen instead of a hydroxy group, which results in a weaker interaction (DeRamos et al., 1997). Nevertheless different crosslinking ions can bind to different sections of the alginate whereby Sr^{2+} exclusively binds to GG-block, whereas Ca^{2+} additionally binds to MG-blocks and Ba^{2+} additionally to MM-blocks (Figure 56). Affinity of Ca^{2+} for MG-blocks is very weak though and can usually be neglected. Overall, the affinity of crosslinking ions to the alginate increases with increasing ionic radius (DeRamos et al., 1997), in terms of visualisation this has also been described as the ionic radius fitting more closely into the space of the "egg-box" structure (Al-Musa et al., 1999).

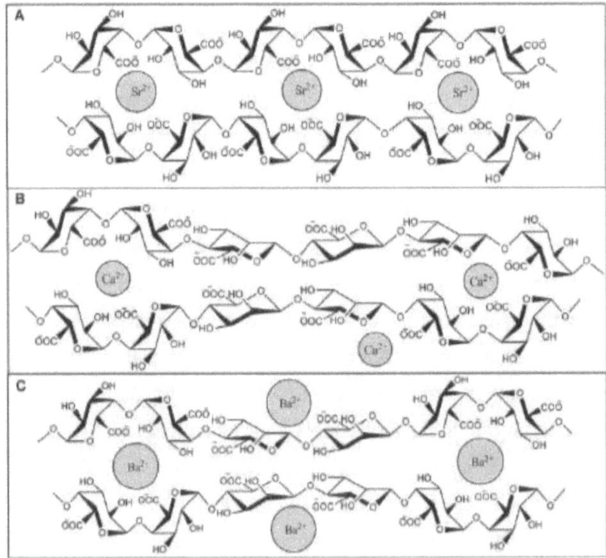

Figure 56: Binding of different crosslinking ions to alginate. Crosslinking of alginate occurs in specific conformations. From A-C: Sr^{2+} ions bind to GG-blocks, Ca^{2+} ions bind to GG- and MG-blocks, Ba^{2+} ions bind to GG- and MM-blocks. (Paredes Juárez et al., 2014)

Crosslinking can occur between, but also within alginate chains, whereby the inter-chain binding between GG-blocks of different alginate chains is responsible for the actual gel formation. This formation of junctions increases with increasing affinity between ion and alginate (Smidsrød, 1974), likely because the length of blocks required for sufficient binding of ions decreases with increasing affinity (Stokke et al., 1991) and the number of junctions that can be expected to form between alginate chains increases accordingly (Mørch et al., 2006). Another reason for increased gel stability when crosslinking is achieved with Sr^{2+} or Ba^{2+} instead of Ca^{2+} is that Ca^{2+} has a stronger affinity to chelating agents such as phosphate than to alginate (Santos et al., 2010). Furthermore, mainly due to its low affinity, there is a constant exchange between Ca^{2+} and monovalent non-gelling ions such as Na^+ in saline solutions (Martinsen et al., 1989) which results in osmotic swelling. The osmotic swelling can be greatly reduced by use of Ba^{2+} (Darrabie et al., 2006), but also by addition of other polymers to the alginate such as the MC used in this book, which results in a blend with minimal swelling of scaffold strands over time (Figure 73, addendum). Alginate capsules crosslinked with 10 mM Ba^{2+} have been successfully employed for the immunoisolation of allogeneically transplanted murine pancreatic islets (Duvivier-Kali et al., 2001). Ba^{2+} is the strongest crosslinking ion which is not cytotoxic at low concentrations, but has been reported to lead to the inhibition of K^+-channels as was reviewed by Santos *et al.* (Santos et al., 2010). While release from alginate capsules crosslinked with 50 mM $BaCl_2$ remained below this threshold and did not induce a response in mice (Montanucci et al., 2015), it has also been reported that Ba^{2+} ions leaking from alginate capsules crosslinked with only 20 mM $BaCl_2$ have been found to accumulate in the femur and blood of mice after transplantation (Mørch et al., 2006). Furthermore, due to the speed of crosslinking with Ba^{2+} it is challenging to prepare homogeneous samples. For microbeads this can be achieved with the injection of crystalline $BaCl_2$ (Zimmermann et al., 2003), but the use of crystals could lead to additional shear stress during plotting.

Sr^{2+} ions crosslink alginate in a strength in between Ca^{2+} and Ba^{2+} (Smidsrød & Skjåk-Braek, 1990) and a concentration of 70 mM has been successfully used for the encapsulation of murine islets in alginate (Ludwig et al., 2012). In general, not much information about the effect of Sr^{2+} on islets can be found: Sr^{2+} ions can be a substitute for Ca^{2+} ions in glucose-stimulated insulin release (Henquin, 1980; Hellman et al., 1997) although with a slightly lower affinity (Ribalet & Beigelman, 1981), but other effects on islets, if they were investigated, have not been published. While little is known for the direct effect of Sr^{2+} on pancreatic islets, there is plenty of research on its overall biological effect, which has been reviewed by S. Nielsen in 2004. In general, it can replace Ca^{2+} in many biological processes even though the result tends to be slightly weaker (Nielsen, 2004). Furthermore, it stimulates angiogenesis *in vivo* (Zhao et al., 2018) and has immune-modulatory effects through downregulating the expression of pro-inflammatory cytokines (Wei et al., 2018) as well as modulating macrophage phenotypes towards the anti-inflammatory M2 type (Wei et al., 2018; Zhao et al., 2018). There is evidence of cytotoxicity of Sr^{2+} at concentrations above 5 mM for continuous exposure in direct cell culture (Schumacher, 2014), which implies the concentration of 70 mM $SrCl_2$, used for the crosslinking of scaffolds here, could have a strong negative impact on cell survival. On the other hand, when used for the crosslinking of alginate, 70 mM $SrCl_2$ had no impact on the survival of pancreatic islets (Ludwig et al., 2012; Barkai et al., 2013) nor adrenocortical cells (Balyura et al., 2015). Indeed, the use of 100 mM $SrCl_2$ even supported long-term survival and proliferation of chondrocytes encapsulated in alginate (Abbah et al., 2008). This discrepancy can likely be attributed to the vast majority of the Sr^{2+} ions being bound by the alginate matrix and therefore likely not accessible to the embedded cells. Furthermore, high concentrations of ions are only present in the supernatant during the actual crosslinking, which is usually limited to 10-15 min. When exposure to 70 mM $SrCl_2$ for 10 min was used for crosslinking of Alg/MC in the present book, embedded hTERT-MSC displayed a viability rate of 60 % and 90 % on day 1 and day 21 of culture respectively (data not shown), which exceeded the viability for human MSC in Alg/MC scaffolds crosslinked with $CaCl_2$ reported by Schütz *et al.* (Schütz et al., 2017). More-over, even repeated exposure to 70 mM $SrCl_2$ for 10 min every other day did not impact viability of hTERT-MSC compared to a control which was crosslinked only once (data not shown). When applied to the culture of murine islets, viability of islets embedded in Sr^{2+}-crosslinked Alg/MC scaffolds with repeated crosslinking every 4 days, was comparable to the viability of free control islets not exposed to Sr^{2+} at all (Figure 74, addendum).

Overall, the pancreas is a rather soft organ, expressed in a Young's modulus of 3-5 kPa, therefore a soft hydrogel like alginate is an optimal choice for pancreatic tissue engineering approaches (Liu et al., 2015). Yet, for alginate-based hydrogels, a reduction of mechanical stability over time due to the affinity of crosslinking ions to chelating agents and an exchange with monovalent ions can be observed (Kuo & Ma, 2008). On the other hand, *in vivo* studies showed long-term stability of islet-containing alginate-based capsules after transplantation, whereby Ca^{2+}-crosslinked alginate-polylysine-alginate capsules remained stable for 2 years in rats (De Vos et al., 2003) and for 3 years in human patients (Basta et al., 2011), and Ba^{2+}-crosslinked alginate capsules were followed up for 10 months in mice (Schneider et al., 2005). A reduction in stability has also been shown for the Alg/MC blend (Schütz et al., 2017; Hodder et al., 2019), but a quicker degradation than that observed for plain alginate samples seems unlikely, since the stability of Alg/MC is almost exclusively based on the alginate component with the MC only contributing marginally if at all. Nevertheless, it was reasonable to investigate the crosslinking density of Alg/MC scaffolds and the release of crosslinking ions over time *in vitro*. Rheology of crosslinked scaffolds one day after plotting indicated complete crosslinking for both research-grade and clinical-grade alginate whereby storage modulus of clinical-grade scaffolds was slightly lower indicating a slightly lesser crosslinking density. The difference in crosslinking density is likely a result of a differing ratio of M to G residues of the alginate molecules: For the medium viscosity clinical-grade alginate this is defined by the manufacturer as at least 50 % M (Dupont, 2018b). For the high viscosity research-grade alginate with which the blend was originally developed and characterized, this ratio is not defined by the manufacturer, but previous results from our lab with an older batch showed a content of 30 % M residues (unpublished data, personal notice from Michael Gelinsky, TU Dresden).

In contrast to scaffolds crosslinked with 100 mM $CaCl_2$, all scaffolds crosslinked with 70 mM $SrCl_2$ remained stable even during handling over 21 days in RPMI[+], despite measurable loss of crosslinking ions. Overall, the release kinetics of ions are comparable between the different alginates (research-grade and clinical-grade) and the different ions used for crosslinking (Sr^{2+} and Ca^{2+}). The burst release within the first day after crosslinking observed in all conditions, albeit in different strengths, can in all likelihood be traced back to the presence of excess crosslinking solution on the surface of the scaffolds which had not been aspirated completely during transfer to medium. When scaffolds crosslinked with either Sr^{2+} or Ca^{2+} were incubated in $DMEM^+$, a distinct difference in the release of the ions could be observed, with a lesser and more sustained release of the stronger crosslinker Sr^{2+}. In $RPMI^+$, due to aforementioned lack of stability of Ca^{2+}-crosslinked scaffolds, only the release of Sr^{2+} could be analysed.

As mentioned, a decrease in stability of crosslinked alginates can usually be traced back to the presence of chelating agents and exchange with monovalent ions, it therefore seems reasonable to assume that the media used contain components which can either substitute for or react with the crosslinking ions and that this concentration is higher in $RPMI^+$. Hypothetically, release of Sr^{2+} should therefore be higher during incubation in $RPMI^+$ than in $DMEM^+$, yet the actual release measured was faster but lower (Figure 12, page 39). The hypothesis of a reaction between chelating agents and crosslinking ions with a higher likelihood for the reaction with Ca^{2+} is supported by the observation of a precipitate that forms immediately after the transfer of Ca^{2+}-crosslinked scaffolds into $RPMI^+$ and which could be replicated by the addition of either 100 mM $CaCl_2$ or 70mM $SrCl_2$ solution to the different media in equal volumes. The quantity of precipitate decreased in the following order: Ca^{2+}-$RPMI^+$ > Sr^{2+}-$RPMI^+$ > Ca^{2+}-$DMEM^+$ > Sr^{2+}-$DMEM^+$ (Figure 62, addendum). Since Ca^{2+} is a weaker crosslinker of alginate, it can get substituted from the scaffolds more quickly than Sr^{2+}. At the same time, Ca^{2+} has a slightly stronger electronegativity than Sr^{2+}, which would facilitate a quicker and stronger reaction with bases in the media. Both media contain a number of bases but the one strong base in which they differ in concentration with a higher amount in the $RPMI^+$ is phosphate (800 mg/l in $RPMI^+$ vs 140 mg/l in $DMEM^+$). Both media contain one other strong base, carbonate. Carbonate is present in a higher concentration in $DMEM^+$ though (3.7 g/L vs 2 g/L in $RPMI^+$), where a lesser precipitation was observed. Considering the release of ions from plotted scaffolds in light of these facts, there is a high probability for the formation of calcium or strontium phosphate depending on the ion used for crosslinking. The precipitation of calcium phosphate when alginate was crosslinked with Ca^{2+} ions and phosphate was present in the surrounding medium has been reported before (Gombotz & Wee, 1998). Especially strontium phosphate has a very low solubility in water (0.6 mg/L), so it seems likely that there is precipitation of strontium phosphate after incubation of Sr^{2+}-crosslinked scaffolds in $RPMI^+$ which is not visible to the bare eye. The precipitate cannot be detected in the assay used (Fluitest CA CPC), which was developed for the detection of Ca^{2+} but can also be used for other divalent cations. Preliminary spectroscopic data indeed indicate the presence of phosphate in the precipitate, this should be verified in future analyses though.

Taken together, the data for crosslinking density and release of ions indicate that the use of 70 mM $SrCl_2$ for crosslinking enables the fabrication of stable Alg/MC scaffolds without impacting viability of single cells or murine islets.

5.1.2 Release of MC

As mentioned above, orally ingested MC is considered non-toxic for human beings (U.S. Food and Drug Administration, 2020) but has not yet been approved for transplantation, though it has been reported to be biocompatible and biodegradable also in terms of TE (Sannino et al., 2009). However, the biodegradation of MC has so far not been fully elucidated and the human body does not produce the cellulases necessary for the degradation of MC into glucose monomers. Hence, if MC chains are released from implanted scaffolds and are not physically degraded and metabolised, they would need to be extracted via renal clearance. That MC is indeed partially released from plotted Alg/MC scaffolds over time has been strongly indicated by previous results from our lab (Schütz et al., 2017; Hodder et al., 2019), whereby it could be shown that quantity of release is dependent of the Mw of MC. MC which had been exposed to γ-irradiation had an Mw of 20 kDa and a numerical molecular weight (Mn) of 6 kDa, i.e. while long MC chains were present, the weight of the majority of chains was around 500 Da. Autoclaved MC on the other hand, had an Mw of 94 kDa and an Mn of 14 kDa. Of the differently sterilised MCs the shorter γ-treated was released almost completely, the longer autoclaved only to 35 %. (Hodder et al., 2019) For the present book, autoclaved MC similar to the one Hodder *et al.* reported on was used. This MC contains a broad distribution of chain lengths whereby a majo-rity lay around 10-15 kDa, but a sizeable fraction also exceeded a size of 90 kDa. For renal excretion, the released molecules would need to be below the molecular weight cut-off (MWCO) of the glomerular filter in the kidney, which is 50 kDa (Al-Shamkhani & Duncan, 1995; Lang & Lang, 2007). Although seems likely that that longer MC chains remain in the scaffold, with these parameters they could possibly be retained in the body if they are released from implanted scaffolds after all. It would therefore be preferable to determine the amount of MC present in and released from plotted scaffolds *in vitro* with the eventual possibility of tailoring the parameters to a maximal release before implantation.

The fundamentals of MC are well-known and have been summarised in a number of reviews over the years (Sannino et al., 2009; Nasatto et al., 2015; Ahlfeld et al., 2020b). In general terms, MC is a water-soluble molecule, prepared from cellulose through the substitution of hydroxy groups with methyl groups, which allows for the incorporation of water molecules otherwise hindered by the crystalline structure of cellulose. The extent by which hydroxy groups are substituted is thereby described by the degree of substitution (DS), which is defined as the average number of substituted groups per glucose monomer. The DS directly influences water solubility because the addition of methyl groups disturbs the formation of hydrogen bonds in the cellulose, thereby allowing the incorporation of water molecules, yet the methyl groups are non-polar and a higher amount of non-polar groups reduces the hydrophilicity. The highest water solubility of MC can be achieved with a DS of 1.5-1.9, which is the DS of the MC used for this book according to the manufacturer.

Apart from solubility, release of MC could be influenced by its gelation properties. MC is an inversely thermo-gelling polymer with high solubility at low and gelation at high temperatures. Hereby the gelation temperature is lowered by an increase in the Mw, concentration, and DS of MC, whereas the presence of salts can lower or increase it (Heymann, 1935). According to T. Wüstenberg, the gelation mechanism has not been fully elucidated thus far, but one of the most prominent hypotheses is based on hydrophobic hydration of methyl groups (Figure 57): In general, hydrophobic side chains have an ordering effect on water (Burchard, 1983), and if MC is in solution water molecules are ordered around the methyl side chains in a structure that has been described as "cage-like" (Wüstenberg, 2015). With an increase in temperature and thereby an increase in the entropy, the hydrogen bonds between these structures can break and the hydrophobic side chains can associate which has previously been described as "dehydration" (Heymann, 1935). Within the MC chains, the substituted groups are distributed heterogeneously (Arisz et al., 1995), resulting in regions with different solubilities, whereby gelation is enhanced in highly substituted regions through a higher likelihood of hydrophobic interactions (Desbrières et al., 1998). In addition to DS, a higher Mw and higher concentration of MC also increase this likelihood and thereby lower the gelation temperature.

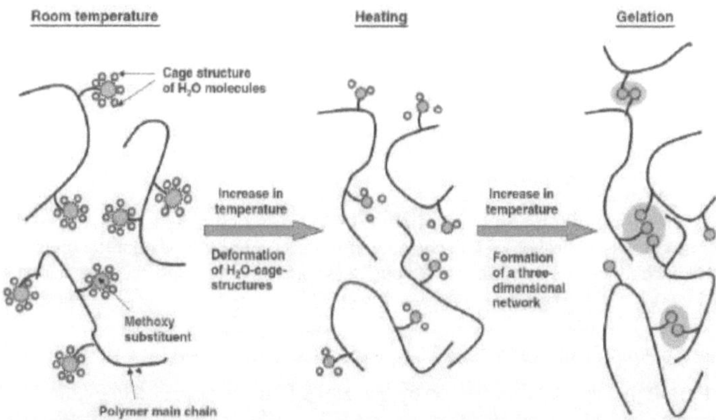

Figure 57: Proposed mechanism for the thermal gelation of MC. In solution the hydrophobic methyl substituents are surrounded by a cage-like structure of water molecules. With increasing temperature, these structures break apart and a network of MC chains forms through association of the methyl groups. (Illustration from T. Wüstenberg (Wüstenberg, 2015) adapted from M. Knarr (Knarr, 2003).)

Furthermore, gelation properties strongly depend on the presence of salts in the supernatant as first observed by E. Heyman who correlated the effect different salts had on an increase or decrease of the gelation temperature of MC with the lyotropic, or Hofmeister series of salts (Heymann, 1935). The Hofmeister series dates back to the end of the 19th century and describes the effect of different ions on the precipitation of proteins from solutions, which has also been termed "salting-out" (Hofmeister, 1888). The effect has often been attributed to a competition of ions and MC for water molecules, whereby some ions have a greater affinity for water. This reduces the hydration of MC (Sarkar, 1979) and thereby increases the likelihood of hydrophobic interactions, which in turn decreases the gelation temperature (illustrated by Liang *et al.* as depicted in Figure 58 (Liang et al., 2004)).

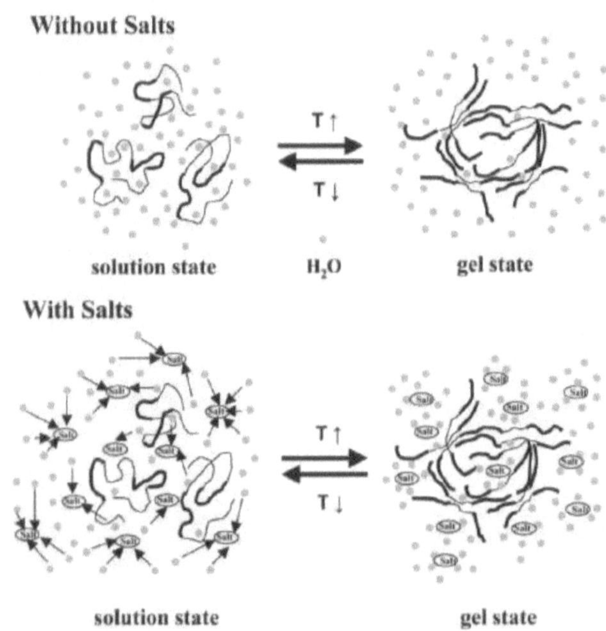

Figure 58: The effect of ions on the hydration of MC. Through a higher affinity to water select ions in solution reduce the hydration of MC chains and thereby lower the gelation temperature through an increased likelihood for hydrophobic interactions between the methyl substituents. (Liang et al., 2004)

Over time the Hofmeister series has been expanded and refined by a number of researchers, a recent thorough compilation of which by Mazzini & Craig is depicted in Figure 59. As reported by E. Heyman (Heymann, 1935), and later reproduced by other groups, for example Hirrien *et al.* (Hirrien et al., 1996) in general, the effect of salts on the gelation temperature of MC follows the Hofmeister series. However, if salt mixtures are investigated instead of single salts, a synergistic instead of an additive effect on gelation temperature has been observed (Bain et al., 2012), indicating that the effect of more complex salt mixtures, such as are present in cell culture media, are challenging to estimate. Nevertheless, an attempt shall be made for the present book. As E. Heyman (Heymann, 1935) observed that the influence of salts on gelation temperature of MC is mainly dependent on the presence of anions with marginal influence of cations which could later be reproduced by other groups (Xu et al., 2004), only anions will be discussed here.

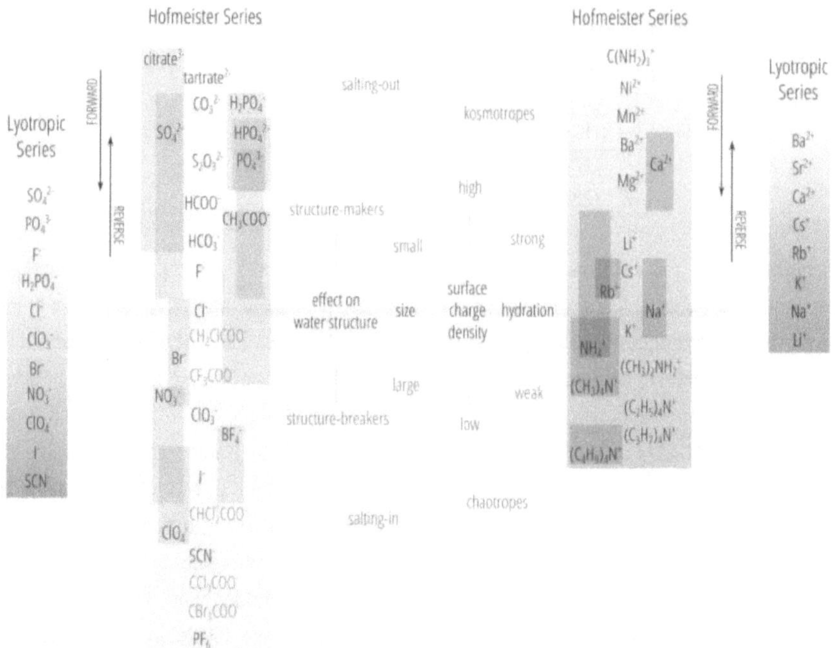

Figure 59: A recent summary of the lyotropic / Hofmeister series. The terms lyotropic series and Hofmeister series are oftentimes used interchangeably, but have been denoted as different series by Mazzini & Craig who compiled a summary of different reports about the Hofmeister series. As the order or ions can vary depending on the experimental conditions the ions are positioned in the order most reported in the literature and the variations in position are denoted by darker bars. Halo-acetates are depicted in grey. The grey horizontal bar denotes the approximate point at which the effect of the ions reverts from salting-out proteins, i.e. decreasing the solubility, to salting-in, i.e. increasing the solubility. (Mazzini & Craig, 2017)

Cell culture media are complex mixtures of amino acids, vitamins and salts and contain a num-ber of anions, which are listed for the media relevant for this book in Table 2. Anions reported
to have a salting-out effect on proteins which should lower the gelation temperature are listed above, anions with the opposite effect below the grey row, which contains Cl^-. According to
Mazzini & Craig this anion is precisely at the turning point of the effects. In reports in the litera-
ture the effect of different salt mixtures, though less complex ones than found in cell culture media, on the gelation temperature was investigated: Bain *et al.* described a temperature of 36°C for 1 % MC in the presence of 200 mM citrate and tartrate, whereas 100 mM of each ion separately led to a gelation temperature of 44°C and 47°C respectively (Bain et al., 2012).
Chen *et al.* used 8 % MC dissolved in PBS containing 10 mM HPO_4 and approximately

Table 2: Anions present in the cell culture media RPMI⁺ and DMEM⁺ in mM. Anions reported to have a salting-out effect above, those reported to have a salting-in effect below Cl⁻.

Anion	RPMI⁺	DMEM⁺
$(H_2PO_4)^-$		0.9
$(HPO_4)^{2-}$	5.6	
$(SO_4)^{2-}$	0.4	0.8
$(HCO_3)^-$	24	44
$(Cl)^-$	109	119
$(NO_3)^-$	0.8	7.5

In both studies, the MC used was of undisclosed Mw but with a comparable viscosity to the one used here, which in the present book corresponds to an Mw of 90 kDa. The anions repor-ted in these studies have stronger salting-out effects than any of those present in the culture media investigated here and/or are present in far higher concentrations. Thirumala *et al.* on the other hand, reported a gelation temperature of approximately 37°C for 8 % MC with an Mw of 15 kDa dissolved in PBS (Thirumala et al., 2013). Keeping further in mind that the different anions present could have a synergistic effect, and an MC with a medium Mw was used at a concentration of 9 % for the present book, there is a possibility for limited gelation of MC at 37°C incubation temperature. This is corroborated by the presence of fibre deposits within hydrogel strands over time (Figure 75, addendum), the partial release observed for MC with a comparable Mw to the one used here (90 kDa) by Hodder *et al.* (Hodder et al., 2019), and an increased release of MC if scaffolds are stored at 4°C (Figure 76, addendum). For MC with an Mw of 20 kDa, i.e. in range of the one used by Thirumala *et al.* (15 kDa), Hodder *et al.* observed complete release, which indicates non-gelled MC, however, Hodder *et al.* also worked in DMEM⁺ with a lower concentration of phosphate than PBS.

The methods used previously for retention and release of MC in our lab, one of which was established with collaboration of the author of this book, were the qualitative staining of MC molecules with the iodine from a chlorine–zinc–iodine (CZI) solution and the quantitative mea-surement with Mykoval™. The Mykoval™ assay, marketed as fluorophore for the detection of cellulose and chitin in fungal cell walls (Koch & Pimsler, 1987; Rasconi et al., 2009), was shown to lead to a concentration-dependent fluorescent signal in samples of dissolved MC and therefore adapted for quantitative measurements (Hodder et al., 2019). In earlier studies, the results generated with both of these methods correlated nicely. Schütz *et al.* reported a com-plete release of gamma-sterilised MC detected via CZI-staining (Schütz et al., 2017), which Hodder *et al.* observed with both methods as well. Hodder *et al.* also reported that other ste-rilisation methods led to up to 50 % release of MC detected with Mykoval™ and dark staining of these scaffolds with CZI, indicating that the qualitative analysis via iodine is prone to 103 oversaturation (Hodder et al., 2019). The quick oversaturation and somewhat erratic nature of the CZI staining restricts its use though, for the present book focus was therefore on quanti-tative determination with Mykoval™.

Released MC was quantified from the supernatant of scaffolds prepared with research-grade and clinical-grade alginate, crosslinked with $SrCl_2$ or $CaCl_2$, and incubated in DMEM[+], RPMI[+] or 10 mM $SrCl_2$ over 3 weeks, in two repeat experiments. This choice of parameters could elucidate differences in MC release for alginates with differing M:G ratios and scaffolds with different crosslinking densities caused by a change in and loss of crosslinking ions. In the present book, release of MC could be shown for all analysed conditions, which correlates with the previous study by Hodder *et al.* who could show partial release independent of sterilisation method and Mw. However, with the results presented here, it was apparent that the rate of release varied strongly between but also within repeat experiments, and had high standard deviations. The release values observed in the present book were 60-80 % and 5-20 % in two repeat experiments performed in cell culture media (Figure 13, page 41) which is approximate-ly twice and half of the release observed by Hodder *et al.* (Hodder et al., 2019). Within the 2nd experiment with a release of 5-20 % in medium, incubation in 10 mM $SrCl_2$ resulted in a release of 20-30 %, which is consistent with the theoretical considerations concerning gelation tempe-rature delineated above: the kosmotropic anions present in the media likely lower the gelation temperature compared to the ambivalent Cl^- in the crosslinking solution. Storage in 10 mM $SrCl_2$, where crosslinking ions but no chelating agents are present, should result in a stronger crosslinking of alginate than storage in RPMI[+] with its high concentration of phosphate. The results are therefore an indicator for a stronger influence of MC gelation on release of MC, than of alginate crosslinking, or indeed M:G content of the alginate. In general, the partial release of MC observed in the present book and by Hodder *et al.*, despite the MC remaining non-crosslinked in the ionically crosslinked Alg/MC scaffolds could, in all likelihood, be due to gelation of MC as discussed above. It could also be caused by a possible interaction between the alginate and MC molecules, or simple mechanical retention. An interaction between alginate and MC is unlikely, as Schütz *et al.* and Hodder *et al.* observed complete release of MC with a lower Mw (Schütz et al., 2017; Hodder et al., 2019), and osmometry measurements even indicate repelling forces between alginate and MC molecules (personal notice from Julia Emmermacher, TU Dresden). It is therefore likely that the partial retention of MC can be attri-buted to a combination of gelation and steric retention.

An explanation for the large differences in released MC between different experiments could be the use of different batches of MC which might change the Mw and distribution of substituted methyl groups thereby changing the gelation temperature slightly, or slight atmospheric dif-ferences during paste preparation such as a change in room temperature. Information gained from these analyses might be more reliable if the experiments were conducted repeatedly with the same batch of MC or a more stringent control of parameters such as temperature during paste preparation, however, the variations and especially the high standard deviation observed in some cases beg the question as to whether the release of MC is highly variable or whether the analysis method(s) are not completely reliable. It was therefore attempted to establish an alternative method for the detection of MC, such as digestion with cellulases.

Cellulases are a group of enzymes produced by bacteria and fungi which cleave cellulose macromolecules down to glucose monomers. The different sub-species exoglucanase, endo-glucanase and β-glucosidase recognise different chain lengths but all sub-species hydrolyse the β-glycosidic linkage between connected glucose monomers (Cao & Tan, 2002), which is schematically depicted in Figure 77, addendum. Cellulases have the ability to digest cellulose in its crystalline form (Byrt et al., 2013) and have also been reported to digest the water-soluble carboxymethyl-cellulose (Cao & Tan, 2002) and MC (Melander et al., 2006) which differ from cellulose only in a number of side chains. Indeed, for the determination of endoglucanase activity carboxymethyl-cellulose is often used as a standard (Juturu & Wu, 2014). Within this book, cellulases from three different sources, *Aspergillus niger*, *Trichoderma species*, and *Trichoderma reesei*, were investigated for their capacity to digest MC. For the detection of digestion products the DNS-assay was chosen, which detects reducing ends. (For a more detailed description of the cellulases and detection method please refer to chapter "Mechanism of digestion with cellulase", page 189, addendum.) After exposure of a dilution series of MC to the cellulases, a strong reduction in viscosity of the solution could be observed, indicating an at least partially successful cleavage. For two of the cellulases tested a concentration dependent signal could be detected in the DNS (Figure 78, addendum), but the overall rate of digestion was vanishingly low with a digestion product of 0.5 % of the calculated maximum. This rate could not be improved by an increase in cellulase concentration, or digestion time, a change of solvent, nor a more sensitive glucose oxidase based assay. A complete degradation of MC, despite successful reports from the literature, is unlikely, since the methyl side chains can interfere with the binding of cellulase, and a higher DS has been shown to decrease degradability by cellulases (Melander et al., 2006). On the other hand, even for an MC with a DS higher than the one chosen for this book (2.1 vs 1.5-1.9), at least a partial degradation down to glucose monomers has been described (Saake et al., 2004). For MC with a DS of 1.8, Melander *et al.* described a digestion efficiency to cellobiose and cellotriose of 2 % (Melander et al., 2006) a rate which could not be replicated here. With respect to detection of MC by digestion with cellulases, it might be possible to measure degradation products with mass spectrometry (MS) as described in the literature however, this would require careful establishment of a protocol and is generally performed for MC dissolved in water (Melander et al., 2006; Schagerlöf et al., 2007). Furthermore, the application of this method for heteroge-neous samples such as the presence of carbohydrates in a multitude of different chain lengths and the presence of ions can be challenging, as summarised in a number of reviews (Kailemia et al., 2014; Urban, 2016). To reduce the degree of complexity, the different degradation products within samples of MC digested with cellulases could be sorted by chromatographic methods such as high-pressure liquid chromatography (HPLC). Unfortunately, in a preliminary trial 1 % of undigested MC led to a clogging of the HPLC column though, and with the uncertainty in the rate of digestion presented here there is a high danger of recurrent clogging.

Promising avenues to be explored in future work are the complexation of MC with Zn^{2+} and fluorescent labelling of the MC. In case of complexation with Zn^{2+}, MC and either zinc chloride or zinc acetate are exposed to hydrothermal treatment possibly with additives such as NaOH (Richards & Williams, 1970; Xu & Chen, 1994; Musuc et al., 2015). According to results from the literature, MC-Zn complexes should precipitate and it might be possible to correlate concentration of MC with a reduction of Zn^{2+} in the supernatant through measurement of Zn^{2+} via inductively coupled plasma optical emission spectrometry. In preliminary experiments, the formation of a precipitate but only a slight concentration-dependent reduction of Zn^{2+} could be observed, the protocol for the precipitation should therefore be refined further.

With respect to future work, it might also be a possibility to detect MC via labelling of the molecules prior to paste preparation and measurement of fluorescent signal in the supernatant. An approach for the labelling of MC could be the covalent binding of fluorescently labelled hydrazine to the reducing ends (Hummert et al., 2013). However, this labelling would need to be conducted in an aqueous environment and MC is used in a dry state for paste preparation, requiring further optimisation of the paste preparation or the MC would need to be dried again without damage to the fluorescent label. Furthermore, since the labelling would need to be conducted in the beginning of the experiment rather than retrospectively, it would be necessary to characterise the stability of the label under cell culture conditions for at least one week. Preliminary results for this approach indicate successful labelling of the MC and a stable signal after lyophilisation but an inhomogeneous viscosity after dissolution of the labelled MC in alginate solutions. This approach will also be followed up on further.

5.1.3 Permeability for glucose & insulin

Permeability of a hydrogel is an important parameter for any sort of cell encapsulation, but especially so for islets, which are not only highly dependent on sufficient oxygenation, their entire function is based on recognizing elevated glucose levels in their surroundings and releasing insulin in reaction to that. A key feature of any hydrogel for islet encapsulation is the permeability for glucose and insulin, but at the same time the impermeability for components of the immune system. Plain alginate gels have been shown to be promising candidates, which barely impact the diffusion of glucose and insulin, yet protect encapsulated cells. For example the diffusivity for glucose through 3 % alginate gels has been reported as 87 % of the diffusivity through water (Axelsson & Persson, 1988), and there is a multitude of research on encapsulated pancreatic islets which retained their functionality and were protected from the immune system for extended time periods (Lanza et al., 1995; Rayat et al., 2000; Omer et al., 2003; de Vos et al., 2006; Bochenek et al., 2019). Even in plain alginate the diffusion has been shown to be directly influenced by the polymer density though, with a reduced diffusivity for glucose from 1.5 % to 2. 5 % alginate (Najdahmadi et al., 2018) and 0.5 % to 6.5 % alginate (Grassi et al., 2009). Furthermore, previous publications on the plotting of islets indicated that a high polymer content and reduced diffusivity result in a lack of functionality of plotted islets (Marchioli et al., 2015; Liu et al., 2019). Marchioli *et al.* used a gel consisting of 4 % alginate with 5 % gelatin, and Liu *et al.* a mix of 2 % alginate with 7.5 % methacrylated gelatine. The Alg/MC blend with its 3 % alginate / 9 % MC has an even higher polymer content that those blends, which could indeed hinder diffusion. On the other hand, scaffolds prepared with this blend show a high microporosity (Schütz et al., 2017; Hodder et al., 2019) which could hypothetically promote diffusion. Because of their composition, the permeability of Alg/MC gels for glucose and insulin is an unknown parameter which should be characterised for an assessment of applicability of this blend for islet plotting.

In general, the parameters used for characterisation in terms of permeability are the MWCO or the diffusion coefficient. The MWCO describes the maximum Mw of molecules which can still traverse the membrane and is a helpful tool to estimate the possibility of immune components accessing the encapsulated cells. For plain alginate gels with a low polymer content, the MWCO is summarised in the literature as 40-100 kDa for alginate beads crosslinked with Ca^{2+} (Holte et al., 2006), but has also been reported to be as large as 600 kDa for alginate beads crosslinked with Ba^{2+} (Omer et al., 2005). Glucose and insulin, with molecular weights of 180 Da and 5.7 kDa respectively, should therefore be able to pass through the gel, while most of the components of the immune system such as cells (usually > 10 µm in diameter) and components of the complement system (most of which are > 170 kDa as summarised by Rokstad *et al.* (Rokstad et al., 2014)) should be restricted from passage. However, while IgG, the smallest antibody has a size of 150 kDa and should therefore be restricted from entering alginate beads, different reports in the literature (Lanza et al., 1995; Mørch et al., 2006) as well as the author of the present book (data not shown) have observed permeability of up to 3 % alginate gels for labelled IgG. The main reason for this discrepancy is that the MWCO is most often measured by utilizing polysaccharides of different Mw, such as dextrans. However, the Mw alone is not sufficient to universally estimate permissiveness for molecules as denoted in several reviews over the years (Nafea et al., 2011; Rokstad et al., 2014; Hwa & Weir, 2018): Polysaccharides are generally neutral and in linear conformation, whereas proteins are often charged molecules and have a much smaller actual size compared to their Mw due to their folded conformation. Therefore, permeability for proteins is often underestimated when only the MWCO is considered. It is theoretically possible to use the MWCO gleaned from polysaccharides to calculate permissiveness for proteins if the hydrodynamic radius of the proteins is known (Briššová et al., 1996). If the hydrodynamic radius is considered, 3 % alginate gels with a mesh size reported as 5 nm (Grassi et al., 2009) to 17 nm (Klein et al., 1983), but also with a distribution of mesh sizes ranging from 5-150 nm (Andresen et al., 1977), should be permissive for insulin and possibly also for IgG. Insulin has a hydrodynamic radius of approximately 1 nm (Robitaille et al., 2000; Yousefi et al., 2016), whereas IgG is described to have the typical dimensions of approximately 14.5 × 8.5 × 4.0 nm according to Tan *et al.* (Tan et al., 2008). Mesh size is hereby defined as the size of the aqueous phase between the crosslinked alginate molecules, not to be confused with the microporosity of Alg/MC scaffolds mentioned above.

Overall permeability can also be analysed through the speed of diffusion of defined molecules. Concerning the diffusion, it is important to keep in mind that while crosslinked hydrogels appear to be a solid substance macroscopically, the water content of the gels is up to 90 %. The most prevalent hypothesis concerning the mechanism of diffusion is that the solute permeates by traversing through the water phase, i.e. through the pores in between the meshwork of polymer chains and the gels are therefore regarded as a fluid in this case. (Andersson et al., 1997; Gehrke et al., 1997; Remuñán-López & Bodmeier, 1997)

It is important to keep in mind that hydrogels do have a polymer content though, which influences permeability. The main driving force for diffusion of a molecule is the concentration gradient. In addition, diffusion through hydrogels is influenced by a number of factors such as movement of the polymer chains, polymer distribution, membrane heterogeneity, solute size, pore size, and path length the solute needs to traverse, as well as residual charges, ions, and polar and hydrophobic interactions between solute and polymer. These factors all affect diffusion in hydrogels to varying degrees, but are difficult to analyse separately, especially macroscopically. This makes it difficult to calculate diffusivity from mathematical models as in many cases the results gleaned from diffusion experiments differed from expectations based on models. It is therefore recommended to analyse the specific solute-hydrogel combination in permeability testings for each application. (Gehrke et al., 1997; de Vos et al., 2009; Hwa & Weir, 2018)

If the hydrogel is considered a fluid, the diffusion coefficient D can be derived from Fick's 1st law, whereby the solute flux, i.e. the amount of molecules traversing the gel in a given time, the concentrations, and the diffusion distance are used for the calculation (Aslani & Kennedy, 1996; Andersson et al., 1997). As mentioned though, it is important to keep the polymer content of hydrogels in mind. For more precise calculations of diffusion in hydrogels, many researchers derived models from Fick's 1st law, such as the pseudo-steady state model or the lag-time model (Hannoun & Stephanopoulos, 1986; Gehrke et al., 1997). The pseudo-steady state model has been reported as easier to experimentally maintain than the lag-time model (Gehrke et al., 1997), it is highly dependent on the precise diffusion area though. Hannoun & Stephanopoulos reported deviations between the model and the experimental results simply from the presence of a protective wire around the gel disc (Hannoun & Stephanopoulos, 1986). For the present book, this model was disregarded as a precise determination of area had not been possible due to gel curvature (for a more thorough explanation of gel curvature refer to page 195, addendum). The lag-time model presented by Hannoun & Stephanopoulos is based on the assumption of constant concentrations on either side of the gel disc, with a complete exchange of chamber filling instead of sampling. The authors considered this factor negligible for large chamber systems though, and reported it to be more precise than the pseudo-steady state model. This model has also been used to calculate diffusion coefficients for gels for the plotting of islets previously (Marchioli et al., 2015). On the other hand, the lag-time model has also been reported to have a very high error probability (Gehrke et al., 1997).

In light of these difficulties, it was decided to forego calculating D as a universal parameter for the present book, and permeability is solely compared between gels measured with the sys-tem presented here. Permeability is hereby determined from the amount of solute in the accep-tor chamber, i.e. the amount of solute diffused through the hydrogel disc over time. This ap-proach has previously been used by Remuñán-López & Bodmeier (Remuñán-López & Bod-meier, 1997). In the present book, the model used by Remuñán-López & Bodmeier was ap-plied to data from two different approaches to assess permeability of the gels. Those approach-es were static uptake and release, and dynamic diffusion chamber measurements. Of those, uptake and release assays are quick and easy to perform, and allow for conditions mimicking islet plotting experiments as closely as possible, i.e. the analysis of plotted scaffolds incubated under static conditions in the relatively small volume of 1 ml supernatant. Furthermore, this system is likely a good approximation for extravascular macroencapsulation devices which are supplied by diffusion under mostly static conditions *in vivo* (Hwa & Weir, 2018). For a direct comparison between Alg/MC and plain alginate gels with this system model gel discs with retrospectively added macropores were used, as 3 % alginate is not viscous enough for plotting into macroporous scaffolds. Disadvantages of the system, are that the retrospective addition of macropores might influence permeability by artificially inducing breaks in the crosslinked alginate chains, and that release experiments require prior saturation.

For a more general characterisation of Alg/MC gels concerning their diffusion characteristics, measurements in a diffusion chamber were performed additionally. The use of this system eliminates the formation of a concentration gradient at the surface of the gel, which is an in-fluencing factor in diffusion, demonstrates definitive transition of the molecules through the complete gel layer, and allows for a more precise characterisation of differently aged gels since

109

no prior saturation is required. The main disadvantage of this system is that the gel discs are necessarily thin to achieve a high surface-to-volume ratio, which makes them fragile and assembly of the chamber system challenging and prone to systematic errors. The general para-meters chosen for the diffusion chamber system established within this book are the use of bulk gels and constant stirring during the chamber runs, so that the driving force for diffusion is the concentration gradient between the chamber halves, not within one half.

Glucose

For the permeability for glucose the influence of a variety of different parameters was investigated, whereby focus lay on the parameters presence of MC, type of alginate, gel age, and type of incubation, all of which were investigated with both approaches introduced above. Presence of MC was hereby analysed through a comparison between plain alginate and Alg/MC gels, type of alginate through a comparison between gels prepared with research-grade and clinical grade alginate, gel age through a comparison between gels incubated for 1-7 days after preparation, and type of incubation medium through a comparison between gels stored in RPMI 1640, HBSS, 10 mM $SrCl_2$, and KRB. Further parameters, those analysed solely in the chamber system, were the influence of diffusion distance, different crosslinking ions (Ca^{2+} and Sr^{2+}) and the concentration of alginate (1 % and 2 %).

For the general kinetics of glucose diffusion in the chamber system, it could be shown that overall diffusion, independent of gel type, followed the normal course of diffusion through hydrogels observed by other groups previously: A lag-phase during which the glucose permeates the hydrogel without arriving in the acceptor compartment was followed by a linear increase in concentration in said compartment before entering a saturation phase close to equilibrium where this increase slows down again (Hannoun & Stephanopoulos, 1986; Aslani & Kennedy, 1996; Gehrke et al., 1997; Remuñán-López & Bodmeier, 1997; Malusis et al., 2001). In the present book, observations were that, after a short lag-time of 30-60 min, an overview over the linear phase can be achieved with observation over 4 h, and that near-equilibrium between the chamber halves can be reached after approximately 30 h.

Unsurprisingly a comparison of different gel heights, i.e. different diffusion distances, observed for plain alginate gels showed a strong difference. During the establishment of the workflow, the preparation of the gel discs was optimised as to the creation of sufficiently homogeneous discs. It was not possible to achieve complete homogeneity between gels, especially between plain alginate and Alg/MC gels though. According to Fick's law the speed of diffusion is inversely proportional to the diffusion distance (Helmich, 2018). The comparison between gel heights presented here approximately confirmed this relationship between concentration in the acceptor compartment and gel height, therefore proportionality was assumed within the premises of this book. To factor in the inversely proportional dependence of gel height and thereby eliminate this factor for the comparison between gel types, the height of all discs was measured precisely (chapter 3.2.7.2, page 31). This value was then multiplied with the concentration in the acceptor compartment.

Influence of the presence of MC: In uptake and release experiments (Figure 14, page 43), a comparison of alginate and Alg/MC discs with the same surface area did not show a difference in the release of glucose. In experiments with the chamber system (Figure 23, page 53), no significant difference could be detected either, although research-grade gels on day 1 after preparation showed a trend for quicker diffusion. This trend was present but far less pronounced after longer incubation times, and not visible for clinical-grade gels. An obvious explanation for slightly better permeability of plain alginate compared to Alg/MC gels would be the higher polymer content, which, as explained above, can influence diffusivity of hydrogels. The influence of polymer content on permeability of the gels analysed here, was subsequently tested with 1 % and 2 % plain alginate, and 2 % Alg/MC gels (Figure 80, addendum). At these concentrations, Grassi *et al.* observed a distinct reduction in diffusivity of alginate for glucose (Grassi et al., 2009). In general, a higher permeability for glucose in gels with a lower polymer content could not be shown as the concentration of glucose in the acceptor compartment was lower than in the previous experiments with 3 % alginate. On the other hand, no significant difference but a trend for lower permeability in Alg/MC gels was also observed when 2 % plain alginate gels were compared with 2 % Alg/MC gels. To further investigate the possibility of not a higher polymer content in general, but specifically the presence of MC being the cause of this trend for reduced permeability, 3 % Alg/MC gels were incubated at 4°C or at 37°C. As explained in detail in chapter 5.1.2 (page 99 ff.), this should result in a lower MC content in the gels stored at 4°C (for a reduced MC content in Alg/MC gels after storage at 4°C also refer to Figure 76, addendum). Concerning permeability, no significant difference, nor indeed a trend could be observed between gels stored at the different temperatures. It might be possible to further investigate the influence of different concentrations of MC by adding different amounts of MC during gel preparation instead of trying to increase MC release. However, interpretation of the data would not be trivial, as the amount of MC might change crosslinking density and microporosity simply by steric hindrance, and it is impossible to analyse the factors independently. For influence of the presence of MC on the permeability for glucose, the results of uptake and release, and diffusion chamber measurements are largely in accordance and a significant influence can be excluded.

Influence of the incubation time: In uptake and release experiments (Figure 15, page 44), uptake of glucose increased when plotted Alg/MC scaffolds were incubated longer between gel preparation and observation of release, whereby the increase rose steadily between day 1 and day 7. If release was observed instead of uptake, gels of different ages did not differ. For experiments in the chamber system (Figure 65, addendum), no significant differences were detected between differently aged gels either, and the only slight trend detected was a slightly lower permeability of Alg/MC gels incubated for 1 day compared to those incubated for 4 or 7 days. As scaffolds analysed on later timepoints were saturated over a longer timeframe for uptake experiments, the increased uptake over time could indicate incomplete saturation after 24 h. However, 2.5 % alginate gels have previously been shown to be saturated with 150 kDa dextrans in less than 1 h (Najdahmadi et al., 2018), incomplete saturation with a molecule of 180 Da is therefore unlikely. It could also indicate an increase in storage capacity of the scaffolds for glucose over time, possibly correlated to a release of crosslinking ions (chapter 5.1.1, page 93 ff.) or a release of MC (chapter 5.1.2, page 99 ff.) and an associated increase in mesh size. Release of MC can in all likelihood be excluded as a possible cause though: As explained in the previous section, presence of MC does not have an influence on the permeability for glucose. To further investigate the possibility of a difference in crosslinking density causing the higher capacity for uptake, diffusion was observed through gels crosslinked with Ca^{2+} or Sr^{2+}, ions of different affinities for alginate (chapter 5.1.1, page 93 ff.). That crosslinking density can influence diffusion through alginate gels for smaller proteins (in the range of 15-70 kDa) with reduced influence for the diffusion of larger proteins (150 kDa) has been shown by Shoichet et al. (Shoichet et al., 1996). In the present book choice of crosslinking ion did not influence permeability for glucose. It is therefore unlikely that the increased capacity for uptake is caused by a reduced crosslinking density over time.

Except for the increased capacity for uptake, the results from both approaches applied for permeability analyses are in agreement, which allows for the conclusion that a significant influence of incubation time on permeability for glucose is improbable.

Influence of the type of alginate: In uptake and release experiments (Figure 15, page 44), the capacity for uptake was comparable between the alginates, but a significantly greater release could be detected from clinical-grade Alg/MC scaffolds. For experiments in the diffusion chamber on the other hand (Figure 24, page 54), no significant differences but a strong trend for quicker diffusion through research-grade plain alginate than through clinical-grade plain alginate gels was apparent. This trend was also present, though reduced by far, in Alg/MC gels. A higher permeability of research-grade alginate is a logical effect when seen in light of the stability data: As mentioned, the research-grade alginate scaffolds have a higher crosslinking density and presumably a higher G-content (chapter 5.1.1, page 93). Yet, while it might seem counterintuitive, more stable alginate gels with a high G-content also have a higher porosity. G-blocks are rather stiff segments of the alginate chains and, through their inability to bend, lead to the formation of larger pores as shown by Martinsen et al. and later reviewed by Ertesvåg & Valla, and Rokstad et al. among others (Martinsen et al., 1989; Ertesvåg & Valla, 1998; Rokstad et al., 2014). A visualisation of the concept is depicted in Figure 60. That the addition of MC negates this effect could be due to the simple presence of MC fibres within the alginate mesh, in visualisation Alg/MC gels are likely comparable with alginates with a high M-content. The flexibility of gels with a high M-content might result in higher movement of chains, and thereby constantly changing pore sizes. While this could promote diffusion through the generation of larger pores it is more likely that the increased mobility increases the length of the path the molecule needs to traverse and thereby slows diffusion as reviewed by Gehrke *et al.* (Gehrke et al., 1997).

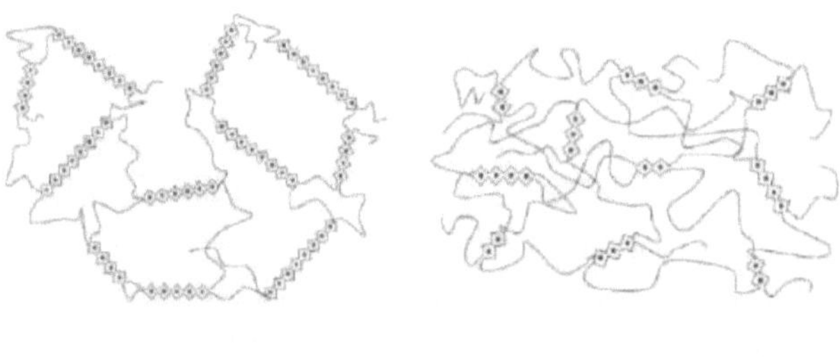

Figure 60 Schematic depiction of the microporosity in alginate gels with a high G-content and a high M-content. Crosslinked alginate gels with a high G-content have a larger mesh size than those with a high M-content as crosslinked G-blocks are stiff segments, whereas especially non-crosslinked M-blocks are flexible and add elasticity. (Santos et al., 2010)

For influence of the type of alginate, the approaches tested led to contrasting results, with a significantly higher release from clinical-grade Alg/MC scaffolds and a significantly higher diffusion through research-grade plain alginate discs but no difference in the diffusion through Alg/MC discs. It has to be kept in mind though, that the experimental conditions for the approaches and thereby probably the crosslinking density and MC content of the scaffolds for release and the discs in the chamber system were different. From solely this data no definitive conclusion as to the influence of type of alginate can be drawn.

Influence of incubation medium: In uptake and release experiments (Figure 14, page 43 & Figure 15, page 44), release was tested for alginate and Alg/MC discs in HBSS, and for plotted Alg/MC scaffolds in RPMI 1640, whereby an overall higher capacity for uptake normalised to weight was detected in HBSS. For experiments in the diffusion chamber (Figure 25, page 55), where 10 mM $SrCl_2$ were compared with KRB, no significant differences, nor indeed a trend were visible, rather the concentrations in the acceptor compartment were almost identical for both incubation media. Differences caused by the medium can logically only be explained by a reduced crosslinking density due to chelating agents in the medium. The concentration of chelating agents is higher in RPMI than in HBSS though and incubation in 10 mM $SrCl_2$ should result in an increased crosslinking density compared to KRB. Furthermore, as detailed above, crosslinking density does not appear to influence permeability for glucose.

Although a comparison between the approaches does not lead to conclusive evidence for a possible influence of incubation medium, in light of the other results presented here, it can be assumed that incubation medium does not influence permeability for glucose.

Overall, the approaches applied for analysing permeability for glucose are largely in accordance and there was no strong evidence for influence of either of the factors tested. In cases where the results generated with both methods are in disagreement, there are logical hypotheses to explain the results from the diffusion chamber, but not for the results from uptake and release experiments. Although the results should be examined for reproducibility in future, for the case presented here the diffusion chamber system appears to be more reliable for the testing of permeability for glucose. All in all, permeability for glucose does not seem impaired in the Alg/MC gels.

Insulin

For the permeability for insulin, the parameters presence of MC, type of alginate, and gel age were analysed analogous to permeability for glucose. While permeability for insulin is an important parameter for the suitability of a hydrogel for islet encapsulation, the analysis of this is complicated by the fact that insulin is a peptide. For preliminary insulin diffusion experiments, 10 mM $SrCl_2$ were used as a chamber filling and, to create a large concentration gradient, 25 µg/ml of human insulin was added to the donor compartment. With these parameters, a linear increase of insulin in the acceptor compartment could only be detected after 7 h, and the values measured in the acceptor compartment at similar timepoints varied up to 10-fold between the experiments but also between the different chambers in one experiment. Furthermore, presence of insulin was randomly detected in the acceptor compartment at timepoints that are within the lag-phase. To exclude that this could be caused by tears in the gel matrix, the chambers were thoroughly checked for tightness with phenol red, a small molecule of 350 Da, more in the range of glucose than insulin.

The most reasonable assumption for the early detection of insulin in the acceptor compartment is adsorption and desorption to the chamber walls, which is corroborated by the observation that the use of 25 ng/ml instead of 25 µg/ml insulin led to a complete loss of signal in both chamber compartments and the gel disc. Interestingly, the timeframe for this loss ranged from t = 0 h to t = 24 h. It is known that the amphiphatic insulin can adhere to the hydrophilic and, in aqueous solutions negatively charged, borosilicate glass surface (Jeworrek et al., 2009; Goebel-Stengel et al., 2011), though less strongly than to hydrophobic plastic surfaces (Sefton & Antonacci, 1984; Goebel-Stengel et al., 2011), and that this binding is reversible (Hill, 1959; Mansur et al., 2000). On the other hand, the chamber were thoroughly cleaned between runs, which has been shown to remove bound insulin even from plastic surfaces (Twardowski et al.,

1983). Furthermore, this possible adsorption and desorption seems highly irregular, since immediate detection of insulin in the acceptor compartment was only present in approximately 50 % of the chamber runs and could not logically be correlated to the amount of possible residue, nor could it be replicated in different borosilicate glass containers.

Adsorption of proteins can generally be prevented or at least reduced by prior coating of the surfaces, silicate glass in this case, with a blocking protein, the most used of which is BSA. For adsorption to glass, BSA has sometimes been reported as adhering only weakly (Sagvolden et al., 1998). This effect might be charge-dependent, since the isoelectric point of BSA is at a pH of 5.6, at neutral pH it is therefore negatively charged. Silicate glass contains a high number of silanol groups (Si-OH) on its surface which can dissociate to Si-O$^-$ in aqueous solutions, and dissociation increases with an increase in pH (Horn & Onoda, 1978). Weak adhesion of BSA could therefore be caused by electrostatic repulsion between the silicate glass and the protein. On the other hand, BSA is a so-called "soft protein" with low structural stability and can therefore adhere to most surfaces, even under unfavourable electrostatic conditions (Höger, 2014; Benavidez et al., 2015) and has been used for successful coating at the neutral pH relevant for the present case (Hyman & Mitchison, 1993; Jeyachandran et al., 2010). Furthermore, BSA coating has been shown to have a protective effect against insulin adsorption even at con-centrations of 1 %. Coating with 2.5 % BSA in KRB in the present book did also show a protective effect against adsorption of 25 ng/ml insulin, this effect was only present for a limited time though, the concentration still dropped slightly after 6 h and strongly after 24 h. It is theo-retically possible that BSA also desorbs from the surface and some insulin can then bind to the uncoated area. To reduce the relative loss of insulin, its concentration was adjusted to 250 ng/ml. With this concentration and BSA coating, it was possible to avoid major loss of insulin and reach the linear phase of diffusion in a reasonable timeframe, yet a flattening of the curves was still detected in some chamber runs. Exchanging BSA as a coating protein for a protein with an isoelectric point in the basic range, which would be positively charged at neutral pH and has been shown to adhere strongly to borosilicate glass, could potentially improve blocking efficiency (Gutenwik et al., 2004; Höger, 2014).

Studies concerning the permeability for insulin were mainly conducted with KRB as storage medium and chamber filling. KRB had been tested against 10 mM SrCl$_2$ in terms of glucose diffusion and stability of research-grade Alg/MC gels and no differences had been detected. However, while Alg/MC gels as well as research-grade plain alginate gels remain stable in KRB, this was not true for clinical-grade plain alginate gels. Due to their generally softer nature, only Alg/MC gels had been chosen for stability testing in KRB, however, stability of Alg/MC gels over time actually seems to be enhanced compared to plain alginate gels, which could hypothetically be attributed to simple mechanical retention of the alginate molecules by coiled structures of longer MC chains. That research-grade plain alginate gels but not clinical-grade plain alginate gels remain stable is likely caused by the higher G-content of the research-grade alginate as discussed above (chapter 5.1.1, page 93 ff.). Interestingly, this stability effect is already apparent at day 1 after preparation, indicating that the loss of crosslinking ions and MC within the first 24 h has a far stronger effect on gel stability than the sustained release over time. Due to the unpredictable nature of adsorption/desorption and the lack of stability of clinical-grade plain alginate gels the results described for diffusion of insulin within the chamber system presented here are only preliminary and need to be verified in further experiments.

Influence of the presence of MC: In uptake experiments (Figure 16, page 45), insulin was quantified within the samples after 30 min and 2 h in RPMI[+]. No significant difference between any of the samples could be observed after 30 min of incubation. After 2 h however, there was a distinct difference between plain alginate samples and samples containing MC, whereby the Alg/MC samples took up more insulin irrespective of geometry and time in culture. These results indicate that the speed of insulin uptake is comparable between hydrogels with and without MC, but that the Alg/MC blend has a higher capacity for overall uptake of insulin. This higher capacity is likely due to the microporosity that can be seen in Alg/MC but not in plain alginate samples (Schütz et al., 2017) but could possibly also be related to electrostatic interactions between the insulin and the gel. At neutral pH both, the alginate (You et al., 2001) and the insulin (as mentioned by Jeworrek *et al.* (Jeworrek et al., 2009)) molecules are negatively charged and therefore likely repulse each other. Addition of the neutral polysaccharide MC into the pores could hypothetically shield the negative molecules from each other and thereby reduce this repulsion, which in turn could increase the capacity for insulin uptake. Measurement of permeability for insulin within the diffusion chamber system (Figure 26, page 56 & Figure 27, page 57) eliminates the factor of uptake capacity. For two out of three timepoints tested, permeability for insulin was significantly reduced through Alg/MC gels compared to plain alginate gels. It is highly probable that this difference between the gel compositions is due to the increased polymer content through addition of MC. This difference had not been observed for the permeability for glucose, but glucose is a much smaller uncharged molecule. From the comparison of both approaches applied it can be concluded that the addition of MC significantly increases the overall capacity for uptake of insulin (possibly through a reduction in electrostatic interactions), at the same time this significantly reduces the permeability of the gel for insulin though.

Influence of the incubation time: In uptake experiments (Figure 16, page 45), insulin was quantified within gels aged 1 day and 7 days and no significant differences were detected between those storage times. For experiments in the diffusion chamber on the other hand (Figure 26, page 56), there was a strong difference in the permeability for insulin when gels were analysed at day 1 after preparation vs day 4 or 7 after preparation. Permeability of research-grade plain alginate as well as Alg/MC gels on day 1 was exceedingly low though, even compared to clinical-grade Alg/MC gels on day 1. The lag-time is comparable for all gels aged 1 day, however while the slope of the linear phase of clinical-grade Alg/MC gels was comparable to the slopes at other timepoints, that of research-grade alginate and Alg/MC gels was 5-6 times lower. Furthermore, diffusion through research-grade plain alginate gels entered a plateau. A difference between differently aged gels could be attributed to changing gel properties, i.e. the release of crosslinking ions and a lower polymer content through release of MC molecules over time. Then again, this change over time was neither visible for permeability for insulin when clinical-grade Alg/MC discs were tested in the chamber system, nor in uptake and release studies. Taken together with all other results presented here this strongly indicates insufficient coating resulting in adsorption. Nevertheless as the plateau was only visible for research-grade gels on day 1, there is a possibility that diffusion through these gels is indeed impaired in fresh gels, which should be verified in future experiments.

From the preliminary data presented here it can be assumed that gel age does not influence permeability of the gels for insulin, the results need to be verified with optimised coating though to allow for a more robust conclusion.

Influence of the type of alginate: In uptake experiments (Figure 16, page 45), capacity for uptake was overall comparable between the alginates, independent of gel age and incubation time for uptake. For experiments in the diffusion chamber (Figure 27, page 57), the permeability of research-grade and clinical-grade Alg/MC gels was comparable for gels aged 4 days and 7 days, though significantly higher for clinical-grade gels on day 1 after preparation. As explained above, the permeability of research-grade gels aged one day was improbably low and should be verified in future experiments before any definitive conclusions can be drawn. For permeability for the small molecule glucose a trend between the alginate types had been observed, which had been attributed to a difference in pore size. Hypothetically, this effect should be more pronounced for the permeability for the larger molecule insulin, however, it has so far not been possible to analyse the difference between plain alginate gels stored in KRB due to a lack of stability.

Similar to the influence of incubation time, the preliminary data presented here indicates no influence of alginate type on the permeability for insulin, these results urgently need to be verified in future experiments though.

In summary, for all gels tested permeability for glucose and insulin could be shown, the Alg/MC blend therefore meets the requirements for encapsulation of pancreatic islets in general. The permeability for glucose is comparable between plain alginate and Alg/MC gels. Permeability for insulin on the other hand, was found to be reduced in Alg/MC gels compared to plain alginate but this should be verified in further experiments with optimised conditions for coating of the chamber surface, under storage conditions which better support gel stability, and with a higher number of repetitions to eliminate lingering adsorption effects. Despite the probability for slightly reduced permeability for insulin the results presented here suggest adequate diffusion characteristics of the Alg/MC blend for the crucial molecules for function of pancreatic islets. If reports on islet plotting in the literature describe impaired functionality, analyses in those reports showed reduced permeability for the small molecule glucose (Marchioli et al., 2015; Liu et al., 2019), whereas in the present book reduced permeability was only indicated for the larger molecule insulin. In light of this, in a next step the Alg/MC blend was used for encapsulation and 3D plotting of cells and pancreatic islets.

5.2 Cell incorporation into Alg/MC

5.2.1 Incorporation of β-cells

The Alg/MC blend has previously been shown to be suitable for the plotting of single mesenchymal cells (Ahlfeld et al., 2017; Schütz et al., 2017; Ahlfeld et al., 2020a), chondrocytes (Hodder et al., 2019), and fibroblasts (Li et al., 2017) but has to the best of the author's knowledge not been investigated for pancreatic cells. All studies with mesenchymal cells used autoclaving for the sterilisation of alginate solution or dry powder and especially autoclaving of alginate solutions is also an established method for the preparation of sterile alginate gels for encapsulation of chondrogenic cells (Jeong et al., 2012; Kundu et al., 2015; Park et al., 2017). For MC on the other hand, Hodder *et al.* could show a strong influence of the sterilisation method on viability of chondrogenic cells and their capacity for the production of ECM components (Hodder et al., 2019). To establish a baseline of cytocompatibility of the material for endocrine cells, the insulin producing INS-1 were used as a model cell line in preparation for islet plotting experiments. For the sterilisation of MC, the three methods which had produced plottable gels in the study by Hodder *et al.*, i.e. autoclaving, scCO$_2$ treatment, and UV-irradiation, were compared to their effect on viability and behaviour of INS-1. For this, metabolic activity, as well as percent viability, cell count, and overgrown area of INS-1 in plotted scaffolds were observed over 21 days and analysed qualitatively (Figure 28, page 59) as well as quantitatively (Figure 29, page 61). Overall, INS-1 seem to be more sensitive to the process of embedding and plotting as indicated by staining for metabolic activity which is barely present on day 1 after plotting, while other cell types such as hTERT-MSC often present a high metabolic activity at that timepoint (Figure 81, addendum). INS-1 cells recover their metabolic activity until day 7 after plotting though. It has furthermore been observed previously that mammalian cells in Alg/MC scaffolds remain single cells and while the viability stays constant over time, the overall cell count decreases (Ahlfeld et al., 2017) generally accredited to the lack of cellular attachment sites in the alginate gel (Andersen et al., 2015). For INS-1, a contrasting behaviour could be observed in the Alg/MC: These cells were able to proliferate and form large metabolically active clusters over the course of 21 days. Cluster formation is a behaviour which can also be observed in 2D cell culture of INS-1, which were isolated from an insulinoma, a rare pancreatic tumour, which is naturally prone to cluster growth (Asfari et al., 1992). For culture in alginate-based gels, this natural tendency likely supports cell proliferation as, in contrast to other adherent cell types, these cells seem to be able to adhere to each other comparably to cellular attachment sites. Cluster formation of INS-1 in alginate gels has been observed previously *in vitro* (Dang et al., 2009) and *in vivo* (Bloch et al., 2011). Concerning the comparison between the tested sterilisation methods INS-1 in gels prepared with autoclaved and UV-irradiated MC behaved similarly with formation of cell clusters and an increase in DNA and overgrown area over time, with the small difference that cell count peaked at day 14 and at day 21 in gels prepared with UV-irradiated and autoclaved MC respectively. In contrast to that, in gels prepared with $scCO_2$-sterilised MC no cluster formation could be observed and DNA content decreased gradually. These results are in accordance with the results presented by Hodder *et al.* where survival of chondrocytes and especially production of sulphated glycosaminoglycans was significantly reduced in gels prepared with $scCO_2$-sterilised MC (Hodder et al., 2019). As reported by Hodder *et al.* the negative influence of $scCO_2$-sterilisation can likely be attributed to traces of hydrogen peroxide, an additive necessary for the sterilisation process, remaining in the dry MC powder. This could likely be alleviated by letting the MC air out for a longer timespan before use. Considering that autoclaving is a simpler and quicker method for sterilisation than $scCO_2$-irradiation, and, other than UV-irradiation, is clinically approved for the sterilisation of materials, all further experiments conducted for this book used autoclaved MC.

5.2.2 Incorporation of pancreatic islets

As discussed in the beginning of this chapter, the gel characteristics are comparable between the alginates and the pressures used are in ranges which do not negatively impact single cells via shear stress (Emmermacher et al., 2020). However, islets are larger cell clusters and one concern in islet printing is damage through shear stress (Kim et al., 2019) because even the purification process after isolation leads to some fragmentation (Shintaku et al., 2008). For pancreatic islets, shear damage has been reported to decrease the functionality (Silva et al., 2013), which has resulted in strong recommendations to use a catheter of 700 µm inner dia-meter for intraportal transplantations (Daly et al., 2004). In contrast to that, some research groups fragment pancreatic islets on purpose since islets tend to autonomously re-aggregate into functional clusters (Halban et al., 1987; Jun et al., 2019). The resulting clusters are usually of a smaller and more uniform size which is considered beneficial because small islets experi-ence less hypoxia and release more insulin in relation to their size than large ones (MacGregor et al., 2006; Lehmann et al., 2007; Komatsu et al., 2017). As concisely described in a review by Kelly *et al.*, normal patterns of insulin release at least partially depend on the architecture of the islets, mainly through intracellular communication. If islets are dispersed into single cells *in vitro*, they lose their ability to react to glucose stimulation, stimulation is possible in re-aggregated pseudoislets though. Furthermore, islet cell types seem to have an inherent ability to form anatomically correct pseudoislets, which is beneficial for appropriate insulin secretion. (Kelly et al., 2011) Adams *et al.* could later show that a change in islet morphology in mice affects insulin release patterns, chiefly through a disruption of synchronized oscillations of Ca^{2+} (Adams et al., 2020). However, despite this natural tendency of islet cells to form islets, re-aggregation within a hydrogels with high polymer content such as the Alg/MC blend can likely not be guaranteed. Since different groups also showed that maintaining islet morphology is beneficial in transplantation in rodents (Morini et al., 2006; Rackham et al., 2013), for this book it was considered desirable to maintain islet morphology to the greatest extent possible during incorporation into the Alg/MC blend and plotting. As mentioned, a great deal of research con-cerns the encapsulation of islets in alginate, which has a viscosity approximately ten times low-er than that of the Alg/MC blend (Schütz et al., 2017), at least at the concentrations used for encapsulation. In light of the high viscosity of this paste, it was crucial to optimise the incorpo-ration and the plotting process for islets.

The method habitually used for the incorporation of single cells led to a large percentage of islets with damaged morphology and was not suitable to achieve a homogeneous distribution, therefore a more gentle method had to be established. Of the incorporation methods investigated closely, two were based on manual incorporation with a spatula, one of which was the method used for incorporation of single cells as a control (stirring), and one was a gentle folding in. Two further methods chosen were based on mixing of gel and cell suspension via movement within a syringe-based system with respect to the harsh edge of the spatula used for stirring/folding and the aim of creating a homogeneous mixture with as little movement as possible, as well as possibly avoiding the step of manual transfer from falcon to cartridge with respect to sterility and shear stress. In a comparison between the methods, gentle folding in was superior to the habitual stirring and to syringe-based mixing (Figure 30, page 63) which was chosen as a standard method for islet incorporation. Compared to free control islets a certain amount of damage could not be avoided even with the gentlest method, but the extent decreased with practice of handling and, as discussed later, did not impact survival or function. Other parameters that could result in mechanical damage to islets are the plotting process itself and the needle diameter. To analyse influence of the plotting process, islets folded in were compared to islets folded in followed by plotting and it was found that the extrusion process did not influence islet morphology further. This is in accordance with the results reported by Emmermacher *et al.* who proposed a greater influence of the incorporation process than of the short exposure to shear stress during the plotting for mesenchymal single cells (Emmermacher et al., 2020). Concerning the needle diameter, hypothetically a size of 400 µm should be sufficient since islet size, independent of species, usually lies between 100-200 µm with a maximum of 400 µm (Jo et al., 2007). With this rationale, previous publications on islet plotting reported the use of plotting needles with an inner diameter of 410 µm (Marchioli et al., 2015) and 450 µm (Liu et al., 2019) without major damage to plotted islets. In the present book on the other hand, a diameter of 610 µm impacted maintenance of morphology qualitatively as well as quantitatively compared to a diameter of 840 µm. This might be due to a larger number of islets being exposed to the edges of the needle where the shear stress is greatest as re-ported by Emmermacher *et al.* (Emmermacher et al., 2020). With smaller needle diameter, the centre of the strands where islets are protected from most of the shear stress becomes smaller and holds fewer islets. The discrepancy between needle diameters in this book could be an indicator that plotting of the highly viscous blend does lead to some shear damage after all, however due to the process of optimization it is impossible to completely separate effects of incorporation method from effects of needle diameter and possibly effects of alginate type. Yet, with respect to choosing the gentlest method possible, it was decided to use 840 µm for islet plotting for this book despite the somewhat smaller surface-to-volume ratio of larger strand diameters.

5.3 Plotting of adult murine pancreatic islets

Following material adaptation and method optimisation, the suitability of the material for the survival and function of primary islets was investigated. The gold-standard for islet transplantation studies remains the use of human islets which are difficult and expensive to obtain though. Due to the existence of an established protocol for the isolation of murine islets and the preferable size of rats compared to mice, primary murine islets from rat were chosen as a model for proof-of-concept plotting experiments.

Islets cultured *in vitro* deteriorate rapidly after isolation, e.g. reported as a decreased number and decreased insulin release from mouse islets over 7 days of culture (Andersson, 1978), or a significantly decreased IEQ of isolated human islets after 20 h of culture (Kin et al., 2008), which was also reviewed by Noguchi *et al.* (Noguchi et al., 2015). With respect to this, the main focus for analyses in the present book was on survival and functionality for up to 7 days, a timepoint up to which functionality of rodent islets has been reported (Andersson, 1978). How-ever, in light of the fact that islet-containing scaffolds need to preserve survival and function of islets over a long period of time for medical applicability, preliminary data for both was also collected until day 14 of culture, as a first indicator for long-term behaviour of plotted islets.

5.3.1 Distribution, morphology and viability of bioplotted murine islets

Distribution of islets across plotted scaffolds and within the individual hydrogel strands was sufficiently homogeneous. Embedding in the hydrogel prevented the aggregation of islets spo-radically observed over all timepoints in control islets (Figure 40, page 73). This protective function of embedding in a hydrogel has previously been suggested by other authors (Marchioli et al., 2015) and is thought to decrease the probability of islet aggregation leading to hypoxic regions, which in turn results in necrosis. This phenomenon has been reported for the intra-peritoneal transplantation of non-encapsulated rat islets into mice, but not for encapsulated islets in the same study (Lacy et al., 1991). Furthermore, while a considerable number of islets was located near the outer rim of the hydrogel strands in this book, none were observed to protrude from the gel macroscopically, which indicates protection from the environment.

The survival as measured by live/dead staining was comparable between free control and plotted islets for up to 7 days (Figure 35, page 69). When plotted islets were observed over a timeframe of 14 days (Figure 37, page 71), survival was highest by trend on day 7, but no significant difference in viability could be observed between the analysed timepoints (day 1, 7, and 14). In the vast majority of islets, the bulk of islet area was viable, but a limited number of dead cells could be detected, resulting in a generally high rate of survival with 75-90 % live cells. Live/dead stainings were assessed by semi-quantitative analysis of the images through visual sorting into viability categories (Karaoz et al., 2010) which is a relatively quick and easy way to assess overall viability but limited in sensitivity. Since quantitative analysis of green and red area in ImageJ did not result in a different outcome though, the method was considered reliable. By trend, the viability in the control was slightly higher than in the plotted scaffolds at all timepoints and an increase of percent viability over time could be observed in both groups. As mentioned for the analysis of single cells (chapter 5.2.1, page 118 f.), this increase is a re-curring theme in (plotted) alginate-based scaffolds in our lab (Ahlfeld et al., 2017). Interestingly, in islet experiments there is a shift of when the main increase happens, between day 1 and day 4 in the control vs between day 4 and day 7 in the plotted scaffolds. This could possibly be ascribed to the physical barrier of the hydrogel: when islets are freely floating in media, dead cells from the outer area can detach and get removed with the media changes, which is not possible in plotted scaffolds, where dead cells remain until endocytosis by neighbouring cells. Quantitative analysis of survival, by counting of apoptotic nuclei stained for TUNEL (Figure 39, page 73), shows the same general trend as live/dead staining, albeit more pronounced: Islets in plotted scaffolds contained slightly more apoptotic cells, but a constant presence of dead or dying cells could be observed in almost all samples. Taken together with the fact that β-cells (in contrast to β-cell lines such as INS-1 as also observed in the present book) have low turnover even *in vivo* (Skelin et al., 2010) and very limited ability to proliferate in culture (Rush et al., 2004), this corresponds to the reduction of DNA observed over time in plotted scaffolds (Table 1, page 69). This reduction was not apparent in all analysed isolations, however, since the DNA at different timepoints was necessarily extracted from different scaf-folds, this is likely an indicator that distribution of islets between scaffolds was sufficiently, but not completely, homogeneous.

Especially in larger free islets, apoptotic nuclei were often observed in the central area, something that could not be observed in plotted ones (Figure 38, page 72). This indicates a higher amount of central necrosis in larger control islets which has been observed especially for larger islets in suspension culture, for example isolated islets from rat cultured at 21 % O_2 (MacGregor et al., 2006), or human islets which had been exposed to hypoxia for 24 h (Giuliani et al., 2005). The concept of central hypoxia in larger islets has also been modelled by Buchwald *et al.* who calculated a reduced oxygenation for islets of 200 µm and larger diameters and Komatsu *et al.* who detected reduced oxygenation even for islets of 150 µm in diameter (Buchwald, 2009; Komatsu et al., 2017). Central hypoxia is generally observed when isolated islets are supplied via diffusion, but does not occur *in vivo* where pancreatic islets are supplied by an extensive network of capillaries and a high blood flow as reviewed by Jansson *et al.* (Jansson et al., 2016). In smaller islets, here more prevalent in the plotted scaffolds but also visible in the free control, the apoptotic cells could rather be found in the periphery, not the centre. While this could be attributed to shear stress during incorporation and plotting, reports in the literature indicate it might be a common factor in smaller islets (MacGregor et al., 2006), but do not hypothesize on the cause. Another important phenomenon observed in islet culture is the reduction of islet size over time, for which apoptosis of individual cells from islets is the likeliest explanation. In general, plotted islets were slightly smaller than control ones, a difference which was significant on day 1 and 4 after plotting, but not as pronounced after 7 days of culture. While the difference in size between free control and plotted islets at early timepoints could mean that larger islets are indeed damaged by the embedding/plotting process, no effect on metabolic activity (MTT-staining) and presence of insulin (DTZ-staining) could be observed. Furthermore, the trend for a decrease in number of islets with more than 200 nuclei between day 1 & 4 and day 7 of culture which was observed in control islets, indicates a loss of larger islets in suspension culture over time. Large control islets with apoptotic cores but without the support of the surrounding hydrogel could lose structural integrity and break apart, resulting in smaller slightly non-round but complete islets in microscopy images. Loss of islet volume *in vitro* is partially promoted by a higher percentage of large islets, and has been attributed to islet fragmentation as a result of central necrosis previously (Kin et al., 2008). Furthermore, for pancreatic islets from rat, a loss of cells from the islet periphery has also been described in the literature (Morini et al., 2006), which would also result in smaller islets at later timepoints and concur with the apoptotic cells in the outer areas observed in this book.

Overall, no significant difference in survival of islets between free control and plotted scaffolds could be observed. The main differences were the localisation of apoptotic nuclei and the islet size, which could even have a positive effect, since small islets have been reported to contribute more to glucose responsiveness than large ones over the years (MacGregor et al., 2006; Lehmann et al., 2007; Fujita et al., 2011).

5.3.2 Functionality of bioplotted murine islets

In native rodent islets, α-cells, which produce glucagon in response to low blood-glucose, surround a core of β-cells, which produce insulin in response to high blood-glucose (Cabrera et al., 2006; MacGregor et al., 2006; Carter et al., 2009; Rorsman & Braun, 2013). Morphological assessment of plotted islets indicated that both cell types remain appropriately located (Figure 41, page 75) which, as mentioned, some sources report to have a beneficial effect on function (Morini et al., 2006; Rackham et al., 2013). Furthermore, both hormones are continuously produced and still present in the cytoplasm in sufficient amounts, even after 7 days in culture, at least as far as can be inferred from qualitative imaging. Apart from size and amount of detached cells around the edges, the main morphological difference visible between control and plotted islets in the fixed cryosections is that control islets do not seem to be as dense as plotted ones. This is especially visible in the insulin/glucagon stainings. Part of this can probably be attributed to the necrotic core in larger islets, but the empty spaces visible are not only in the central area. On the other hand, empty spaces within islets, often where they used to be connected to blood vessels, have been observed before (Tal et al., 1992; Cabrera et al., 2006; Bosco et al., 2010) and could plausibly also be artefacts created during cryosectioning. That this is not visible in the plotted scaffolds could probably be traced back to the limited space or the higher stability inside the hydrogel scaffold.

Healthy β-cells in pancreatic islets react to the presence of increased blood-glucose with the release of corresponding amounts of insulin from secondary granules (Fu et al., 2012). To investigate whether plotted islets still carry out this function, GSIR assays were performed, where the insulin release in hypoglycaemic conditions (3.3 mM, "low glucose") is compared to that in hyperglycaemic conditions (16.4 mM, "high glucose") (Steffens, 1970; Andersson, 1978). The absolute amount of insulin released into the supernatant was normalised to the DNA content of each sample to eliminate the factor of differences in cell number. While islets for free control samples were always manually counted, IEQ still differed between the samples Furthermore, for plotted scaffolds, it was not possible to guarantee the same number of islets per scaffold as discussed previously (5.3.1, page 121 ff.). Furthermore, plotted scaffolds contained a higher number of islets than control samples. Normalisation was therefore imperative for a reliable comparison between the variants. The proportion of the insulin released in response to low and high glucose stimulation is called stimulation index, SI. For healthy pancreatic islets from rat, the SI should be between 2 and 20 (Carter et al., 2009) but has, for the concentrations used in this study, also been published as slightly below 2 (Zekorn et al., 1992). Any value greater than 1 for the SI denotes a higher release of insulin when islets were exposed to high glucose, which is in agreement with their biological function.

Within the scope of this book, functionality tests for control and plotted islets were performed on day 1, 4, 7, 11, and 14 after plotting over a total of seven isolations (Figure 43, page 77 &

Figure 44, page 78; see also page 182 ff., addendum), whereby not all timepoints could be analysed for each isolation due to shortage of samples. As analyses to the distribution of plotted islets between scaffolds had demonstrated a minimal requirement of 3000 IEQ per gram material for sufficiently homogeneous distribution, the number of scaffolds from each batch was limited to a maximum of 15. For these basic parameters, islets of 10 rats were pooled for each isolation. Each isolation is depicted as amount of insulin normalized to the DNA, and as the SI calculated from that. Overall, the most striking contrast between control and plotted islets is the total amount of insulin released, which is considerably higher in the control, indicating that either reaction of plotted islets or diffusion of insulin is impaired. The occurrence of outliers could also be attributed to dying islets within the sample which is more noticeable in control samples than in plotted ones which contained a higher number of islets. For the plotting of islets in hydrogels that are likely to offer immunoprotection, it was not possible to show functionality so far, which has been ascribed to impaired diffusion of even glucose and thereby likely insulin to a greater extent, through the dense hydrogel consisting of 4 % alginate with 5 % gelatin, or 2 % alginate with 7.5 % methacrylated gelatine (Marchioli et al., 2015; Liu et al., 2019). As mentioned previously in this book, it was possible to demonstrate that the addi-tion of MC does not influence the permeability of the gel for glucose (chapter 5.1.3, page 106 ff.). For insulin on the other hand, the Alg/MC blend had a higher capacity for uptake in static assays, possibly due to the presence of micropores or lesser repulsive forces between the alginate and the insulin as discussed in chapter 5.1.2 (page 99 ff.). Then again, diffusion of insulin through Alg/MC discs in a chamber system was decelerated compared to plain alginate discs (Figure 27, page 57). The overall lower release of insulin from plotted scaffolds than from the free control islets can likely be ascribed to this impaired diffusion. Many groups over the years observed that microencapsulation with alginate does not impair function as exemplarily reviewed by De Vos *et al.* (de Vos et al., 2006). On the other hand, Trivedi *et al.* did indeed observe a marked difference between macro-encapsulated islets and islets in suspension cul-ture, with overall performance after encapsulation reduced to approximately 6 ng/ml insulin compared to 25 ng/ml released from control islets. However, they could show that even with the distinctly longer diffusion distances due to the macrocapsule, transplanted islets were still capable of restoring normoglycaemia in diabetic rodents (Trivedi et al., 2001).

In a comparison of the SI instead of the quantity of insulin (Figure 44, page 78), functionality of control islets continually decreases between day 1 and day 7 of culture. Plotted islets on the other hand had an SI below that considered healthy for rats on day 1 in most isolations, but the average SI increased until day 4 before again decreasing slightly until day 7. On day 4, the average SI is similar in control and plotted samples (4.8 vs 4.5), on day 7 it is even slightly higher for islets in Alg/MC scaffolds (2.4 vs 1.8). Between day 4 and 11, in most isolations free and plotted samples reacted similarly, i.e. functionality was observed in both or none. Overall, both, control and plotted samples, have to be considered non-functional at later timepoints. This is not surprising since primary islets are known to lose their ability to respond to glucose stimulation over time *in vitro*, which manifests in a strong decrease in SI. This has for example been reported as a reduction of 62 % when human islets were incubated for 14 days (Schmied et al., 2000), and a reduction of approximately 40 % when rat islets were incubated for 7 days (Chen et al., 2007). The low SI for plotted islets on day 1 is likely not due to material properties as MC is not cytotoxic nor can this be ascribed to impaired diffusion since incubation time of clinical-grade plotted scaffolds and gel discs in permeability studies did not influence said permeability. Therefore, if this was due to impaired diffusion, no change in functionality should be observed over time in culture. It is rather more likely that this low SI could be due to the stress of incorporation into the material in addition to the stress of isolation which all islets undergo. Furthermore, plotted islets stimulated on day 1 and day 4 release very similar amounts of insulin in response to high glucose, but not low glucose where values on day 4 are only one third of those on day 1 on average. The trend that the low SI on day 1 is not due to islets releasing too little insulin in high glucose, but rather reacting too strongly to low glucose has also been noted previously by Marchioli *et al.* (Marchioli et al., 2015). In general, our approach to islet plotting is very similar, however, direct comparisons remain difficult since different timepoints and islets from different species were investigated. In the present study, islets from rat were utilized whereas the previous report concentrated on human islets. Species differences might have an impact on function of embedded islets, however it is likely that choice of timepoint for analysis also plays a role in the observation of functionality: The highest SI in plotted islets was observed on day 4 after plotting in this work, whereas Marchioli *et al.* analysed functionality on day 1 and day 7. Furthermore, it is interesting to note that Marchioli *et al.* mainly worked with research-grade alginate, but also could not show functionality in clinical-grade alginate. When research-grade alginate was used for the preparation of Alg/ MC for plotting of rat islets in this book, no appropriate reaction to glucose stimulation could be observed in this book either, despite live/dead imaging showing no difference between islets in the different alginates, nor permeability of Alg/MC gels being affected by the alginate type. To further investigate whether plotted islets not only react to glucose stimulation, but also follow an approximation of the normal course of glucose stimulation in the body, where blood glucose increases after a meal but then decreases again islets were also exposed to low-high low stimulation on days 1 and 4. Day 7 after plotting was excluded since previous experiments had shown a strongly reduced reaction after one week in culture. With this low-high-low stimulation protocol for the same sample, it was possible to show that plotted islets truly sense changes in external glucose levels and react accordingly. From the results presented here for the plot-ting of adult murine islets as proof-of-concept it can be concluded that viability and functionality of islets can be retained during incorporation into the Alg/MC blend and 3D plotting and that plotted macroporous scaffolds are a promising system for the preparation of islet-containing scaffolds with a high surface-to-volume ratio.

5.4 <u>Plotting of neonatal porcine islet-like cell clusters (NICC)</u>

The advantages of using porcine islets and especially neonatal porcine islet-like clusters for xenotransplantation have been illustrated in detail in previous chapters (chapter 2.2.2, page 15 ff.). To the best of the author's knowledge, no studies on plotting of porcine islets, be they adult or neonatal, have been published as of now. There are a number of promising studies on the encapsulation of adult (Duvivier-Kali et al., 2004; Vériter et al., 2014) and neonatal (Elliott et al., 2000; Omer et al., 2003; Matsumoto et al., 2016) porcine islets, all of whom could show an improvement in blood-glucose control for a limited amount of time after transplantation. For the present discussion, the focus will be on NICC though. For all analyses performed with NICC, the timepoints stated are the days elapsed since the day of plotting. NICC were generally plotted after 8 days of culture following isolation to allow for the formation of distinct islets. In the neonatal pancreas, insulin- and glucagon-positive cells are scattered throughout the pancreas rather than located in distinct islet clusters. This has been illustrated via immunostainings by Hassouna *et al.* (Hassouna et al., 2018), although it was already mentioned by Yoon *et al.* in 1999, that "porcine neonatal pancreas cell clusters (NPCCs) [...] form when pancreatic digests are kept in culture" (Yoon et al., 1999).

5.4.1 Distribution, morphology and viability of bioplotted NICC

Analogous to adult murine islets, NICC were homogeneously distributed throughout the material, remained metabolically active, and stained positive for presence of insulin over a cultivation period of 7 days (chapter 4.4.1, page 80 ff.). This was independent of material composition and shear stress, as the results were comparable between free control NICC, NICC incorporated in plain alginate, NICC incorporated in Alg/MC, and NICC in plotted Alg/MC scaffolds.

Size of NICC as derived from counted DAPI-stained nuclei (Figure 51, page 86) in general was broadly distributed with number of nuclei ranging from 15-300 within each group with no clear trend, and no difference between control and plotted islets nor between the different timepoints. The only significant difference detected in islet size was a drop in the size of plotted NICC between day 4 and day 7 after plotting, leading to a significant size difference between control and plotted NICC on day 7. In general, NICC measured from a similar sample size as islets from rat (Figure 33, page 67), were smaller than murine islets with a maximum of 350 compared to a maximum of 500 nuclei (with an outlier of 700 nuclei within the murine samples). The observed reduction in size over time could be due to a loss of larger NICC in the plotted scaffolds likely due to a beginning maturation. Yoon *et al.* previously observed a reduced DNA mainly attributed to the loss of exocrine cells (Yoon et al., 1999), and Luca *et al.* reported a slight reduction in size of NICC between day 9 and day 21 of culture (Luca et al., 2005), corres-ponding to day 1 and day 12 after plotting in the present book. It is not probable that a com-plete loss of larger NICC from plotted scaffolds such that they were not visible in the qualitative imaging is the sole cause of the size difference between control and plotted NICC. In all likeli-hood this effect is enhanced by the fusion of smaller control NICC into fewer but bigger clusters which has been observed in light microscopic quality checks during cell culture for this book and also been reported previously for NICC in suspension culture (Tatarkiewicz et al., 2001). General survival of NICC in alginate-based capsules *in vitro* has been reported for at least 5 weeks as measured by oxygen consumption (Kitzmann et al., 2012). In the present book, viability was observed by live/dead staining during the entire time of observation of 21 days after plotting (29 days after isolation). Semi-quantitative analysis (Figure 49, page 84) showed a relatively high amount of cell death compared to murine islets, with an overall viability of 60 % for the first week after plotting and a slight increase towards day 14. Overall viability determined from live/dead stainings did not differ between control and plotted NICC neither in amount nor distribution, with most islets showing a majority of live but also a fair amount of dead cells. Interestingly, the control samples contained a low number of completely dead NICC, which was not detected for plotted NICC though. In the quantitative analysis of TUNEL/ DAPI stainings, on the other hand, viability on day 1 after plotting was also comparable be-tween control and plotted NICC with 25 % and 30 % apoptotic nuclei, respectively, but overall higher than in live/dead analyses. However, while viability remained constant over one week of culture in analysis of live/dead stainings, TUNEL staining (Figure 51, page 86) revealed a decrease in apoptotic nuclei over time in the control from 25 % to 20 %, whereas percentage increased from 30 % to 47 % in the plotted samples, This resulted in a highly significant dif-ference between control and plotted samples on day 7 after plotting. Overall viability observed is comparable to values reported in the literature, although a bit lower in the plotted samples on day 7: Reports of the viability of NICC in culture vary between 80-90 % after 8 days in culture (Yoon et al., 1999; Luca et al., 2005; Park et al., 2012), 75 % after 7 days (Harb & Korbutt, 2006), and 50 % after 20 days (Hassouna et al., 2018). As mentioned above, these timepoints are approximately comparable to the day of plotting and day 12 after plotting. The slightly higher rate of apoptosis compared to murine islets can likely be attributed to the pro-cess of maturation with a high loss of exocrine cells as discussed above. In qualitative analysis of TUNEL/DAPI stained cryosections (Figure 50, page 85), it was ap-parent that almost all NICC contained some apoptotic nuclei distributed throughout the islets. Some plotted NICC on the other hand had an outer ring of apoptotic nuclei surrounding a core of healthy cells which was not visible on control NICC. While this might be attributed to shear stress, it first became apparent on day 4 after plotting. Furthermore, among the plotted NICC the vast majority retained their spherical morphology. In comparison to plotted murine islets, a far lower number of samples showed unattached single cells around the islets as far as can be inferred from qualitative images (Figure 38, page 72 vs Figure 51, page 86). It could therefore be hypothesized that the shear stress applied during the incorporation and plotting has even less effect on NICC than on adult murine islets. It could also be that the proficiency of the researcher in performing the incorporation has a greater influence than anticipated and NICC were exposed to reduced shear stress during handling compared to murine islets. As the distribution of apoptotic nuclei is otherwise comparable between control and plotted NICC, it is likely that free NICC also contain apoptotic cells at the borders but that those can detach in free floating culture. Additionally, both, control and plotted NICC contained large apoptotic areas, apoptotic cores and empty areas. This is in accordance with the eventual disintegration of dying cells and has been observed by other groups in the past, especially for central necrotic areas after 7 days of culture (Nielsen et al., 2003; Hassouna et al., 2018).

A reduction of viability of NICC was also visible in measurements of DNA content (Table 13, addendum) between the day of plotting and day 1, 4, and 7 after plotting, although in contrast to staining for apoptosis where control samples showed a significantly higher viability, the reduction of DNA was far stronger in the free control. Hereby only 30 % of the original DNA content of NICC in suspension culture could be recovered after 1 week, whereas plotted samples still contained 70 % DNA compared to the day of plotting. Such a strong reduction was not visible in the viability stainings and can only be interpreted as complete disintegration of some NICC in the control, which did not happen in plotted samples. A strong loss of DNA is a characteristic feature of NICC in suspension culture, which can lose between 50 and 90 % of their original DNA content within 10 days (Korbutt et al., 1996; Otonkoski et al., 1999; Tatarkiewicz et al., 2001), yet sometimes have also been reported to still contain 80 % of their original DNA content after 7 days (Harb & Korbutt, 2006). Interestingly, earlier reports also could not detect a difference between free-floating control and NICC encapsulated in alginate gels (Tatarkiewicz et al., 2001). It has to be noted though, that in general loss of DNA is strongest in the first few days after isolation, i.e. timepoints prior to the delivery of NICC to Dresden.

As mentioned, compared to reports in the literature, NICC used for experiments within this book showed a slightly higher rate of cell death, even in the control but more pronounced in the plotted samples. This cannot be attributed to the Alg/MC material itself, which has been shown to be non-toxic, or the shear stress they were exposed to as discussed above. In the static culture performed, cell death could also be caused by hypoxia but NICC are known to be relatively resistant against exposure to hypoxia (Emamaullee et al., 2006) because they do not contain the enzyme inducible nitric oxide synthase, which is responsible for the production of nitric oxide and has been suggested as a mechanism for β-cell destruction in diabetes (Feng et al., 2000; Harb et al., 2007). This also indicates that the transport of NICC from Munich to Dresden should not affect viability (also confirmed by personal notice from Elisabeth Kempter,

Gene Center Munich). On the other hand, as mentioned the NICC were slightly larger than the murine islets and qualitatively showed more central necrosis (Figure 38, page 72 vs Figure 51, page 86). The presence of larger islets is known to result in central necrosis (Tatarkiewicz et al., 2001; Nielsen et al., 2003) and the fusion of smaller islets into larger clusters has been reported for adult rat (De Haan et al., 2003) and foetal porcine islets (Otonkoski et al., 1999), factors which could result in increased cell death as observed in this book. Furthermore, a higher cellular density can easily result in hypoxic regions – employing simulations, the maximal density of islets per cm^2 that can be used without leading to hypoxia, has been determined as 500-760 IEQ (Johnson et al., 2009; Colton, 2014). Depending on the experiment, density of NICC used for the present book was usually in this range or slightly higher. With respect to clinical application, a high islet density is required though: the curative dose of human islets is between 5000 and 10.000 IEQ/kg body weight (McCall & Shapiro, 2012; Ludwig et al., 2013), for a patient of 70 kg this equals up to 700.000 IEQ, the equivalent of 15-25 islet isolations from neonatal pigs. The number of islets used for this book were usually three isolations per experiment divided between suspension culture and plotted samples. To reach curative doses, a higher density and a scaling up of scaffold size is therefore required. Plotted scaffolds have the advantage of macroporosity which increases the surface-to-volume ratio and thereby al-lows for a higher cell density, this needs to be verified for NICC in future experiments though.

Taken together, the viability data suggest that the Alg/MC blend largely maintains viability and morphology of NICC equivalent to suspension culture but that the material should be refined further to support not only survival of NICC but also their inherent capacity for expansion of neonatal β-cells which has been described by many researchers (Yoon et al., 1999; Hassouna et al., 2018). This could possibly be achieved with the incorporation of human plasma (Ahlfeld et al., 2020a) or components of the ECM, which have been reported as improving survival and function of (encapsulated) islets (Daoud et al., 2010; Jun et al., 2013; Llacua et al., 2018; Child et al., 2020).

5.4.2 Functionality of bioplotted NICC

When NICC were analysed for functionality in the present book, a low number of insulin-, glucagon-, and somatostatin-positive cells were detected in all NICC over the whole time of observation and in both conditions (Figure 52, page 88). That NICC only contain a very limited amount of hormone-positive cells is a well-established fact. NICC have been reported to con-tain only 3-10 % insulin-positive but 90 % non-endocrine cells (MacKenzie et al., 2003; Nielsen et al., 2003). Of the insulin-positive cells, many additionally stain for other markers such as cytokeratin 7, a marker of ductal cells, indicating their immature state (MacKenzie et al., 2003). Over time, neonatal porcine islet-like cluster mature from loose clusters with a majority of exocrine cells into defined islet-like structures with a majority of endocrine cells *in vitro* as well as *in vivo*. This drastic change in composition occurs through the death of exocrine cells but also the formation of new β-cells. For the culture time relevant for this book, i.e. between 7 and 20 days after isolation, NICC have been reported to contain 17-24 % β-cells (Korbutt et al., 1996; Yoon et al., 1999; Nielsen et al., 2003; Harb & Korbutt, 2006). Furthermore, the localisation of endocrine cells within NICC changes: Over a cultivation time of 20 days, glucagon- and somatostatin-positive cells have been reported to become preferentially localised in the periphery (Nielsen et al., 2003). This was not observed in the present book, where all cells stained positive for either of the three hormones were randomly scattered throughout the islets over the whole time of observation. In future experiments, number and localisation of hormone-containing cells therefore need to be analysed quantitatively over a longer timeframe.

In light of the low number of β-cells and in accordance with the literature (Korbutt et al., 1996), 50-100 free NICC per replicate, and a density of 10,000-40,000 IEQ per gram material were used for stimulation experiments in the present book. Even with this high number of NICC the SI indicated non-functionality (Figure 55, page 91), although insulin is indeed present in NICC as shown in this book via immunohistochemical stainings (Figure 52, page 88), and reported in the literature as insulin recovered per pancreas or normalised to the DNA-content (Korbutt et al., 1996). Non-functionality of glucose-stimulated NICC has been observed previously (Niel-sen et al., 2003), although Korbutt *et al.* reported an SI of 5 for stimulation of NICC on day 9 of culture, equivalent to day 1 after plotting (Korbutt et al., 1996). The purpose of pancreatic β-cells is the release of insulin in response to elevated glucose levels, a functional response which only develops after birth though, foetal islets do not react to stimulation. An impaired reaction to increased extracellular glucose levels by NICC (Rorsman & Braun, 2013) and islets of non-insulin dependent diabetic rats (Portha et al., 1988) has been attributed to a reduced oxidation of glucose at the mitochondrial level. Through this impaired metabolism the rise in the ATP/ADP ratio necessary for the closure of ATP-sensitive K^+-channels, and the following depolarization which initiates the process of insulin release is hampered (chapter 2.1.2, page 7 ff.). In neonates, the functional response develops over a period of several weeks, which is reflected in transplantation studies where NICC have been shown to regulate blood-glucose levels only after several weeks *in vivo* (Korbutt et al., 1996; Yoon et al., 1999; Trivedi et al., 2001; Harb & Korbutt, 2006; Hassouna et al., 2018). Encapsulation in alginate-based matrices does not hamper this maturation *in vivo* (Omer et al., 2003) nor *in vitro* (Mourad & Gianello, 2019). If NICC are implanted early, the maturation period without regulation of blood-glucose levels involves exposure to elevated glucose levels for several weeks. However, while long-term hyperglycaemia is toxic to adult islets *in vivo* (Kaneto et al., 1999; Harb & Korbutt, 2006; Narang & Mahato, 2006) and *in vitro* (Federici et al., 2001), NICC actually increase their β-cell mass via differentiation of progenitor cells (Harb & Korbutt, 2006) and mature quicker (Kin & Korbutt, 2007) when exposed to continuous levels of high glucose.

Even in the immature state, NICC can be driven to insulin secretion in response to high glucose in combination with agents increasing levels of cyclic adenosine-monophosphate such as theophylline (Korbutt et al., 1996; Cooper et al., 2016; Mourad et al., 2017) or GLP-1 analogues (Mourad et al., 2017). As mentioned before (chapter 2.1.2, page 7 ff.), the regular pathway for insulin secretion is the oxidation of glucose to ATP, a raise in the ATP/ADP ratio which leads to the closure of ATP-dependent K^+-channels, followed by depolarization of the cell which leads to the opening of voltage-gated Ca^{2+}-channels, which in turn triggers the exocytosis of insulin-containing granules. As reviewed by Rorsman & Braun and Tengholm & Gylfe (Rorsman & Braun, 2013; Tengholm & Gylfe, 2017), the main pathway through which agents such as GLP-1 potentiate insulin secretion is an elevation of intracellular cAMP, which activates the protein kinase A signalling pathway. The resulting phosphorylation of ATP-dependent K^+-channels mediates their function as shown by Lin *et al.* for HEK293 cells (Lin et al., 2000). To promote insulin secretion in response to glucose stimulation, liraglutide, a long-lasting GLP-1 analogue (Wang et al., 2013) was employed in this book. With the addition of liraglutide, the amount of insulin released increased by a magnitude from 0.05 to 0.5 ng per 100 ng DNA (Figure 55, page 91) although this is still not comparable to insulin levels released by adult murine islets. Amount of released insulin from control NICC increased until day 14 of culture followed by a strong drop, whereas the amount released by plotted NICC only increased between 14 and 21 days of culture. This could possibly be correlated to a beginning maturation. This hypothesis would be corroborated by an increase in the number of β-cells; in future experiments the relative number of β-cells per islet cluster should therefore be quantified. With the addition of liraglutide, the SI of NICC was between 9 and 10 for both, control and plotted samples on day 1 after plotting. The SI was generally comparable between the conditions, but decreased continually over time in culture. Despite their natural tendency to mature, a loss of insulin response of NICC over 2 weeks in culture has been reported previously (Tatarkiewicz et al., 2001). Overall, the SI observed here with the addition of liraglutide was still comparatively low, for example Korbutt *et al.* reported an SI of 40 after the addition of theophylline (Korbutt et al., 1996), but does indicate functionality for at least 3 weeks in culture.

The preliminary experiments for the plotting of NICC show the general feasibility of the concept although the experiments should be repeated in a higher number and the material composition leaves room for improvement concerning survival and maturation and thereby functionality. Possible avenues to promote maturation *in vitro* are optimization of the material itself, for exam-ple with ECM-components such as collagen which has been shown to preserve functionality of NICC (Mourad & Gianello, 2019). Further approaches could be exposure to high glucose during culture (Harb & Korbutt, 2006), pre-treatment with GLP-1 receptor agonists (Wang et al., 2013), or the stepwise exposure to specialised maturation media with an assortment of growth factors and supplements (Hassouna et al., 2018). Maturation of NICC *in vitro* is not imperative for the eventual regulation of blood-glucose levels *in vivo*, but it could still have a beneficial effect to increase the number of β-cells, reduce apoptosis and necrosis to prevent the release of pro-inflammatory molecules (Rock & Kono, 2011), and reduce the expression of α-Gal (chapter 2.2.2, page 15 ff.) which is expressed in much higher levels on NICC than adult porcine islets (Rayat et al., 2003).

Reduction of immunogenicity is a key factor of xenotransplantation even for encapsulated islets. On the one hand, alginate-based encapsulation has been shown to protect xenogeneic islets because while the membrane is permeable for IgG (Lanza et al., 1995; Mørch et al., 2006), it is impermeable for IgM, the main xeno-reactive antibody type as well as larger components of the complement system (Rayat et al., 2000), which prevents hyperacute rejection. On the other hand, as summarised in different reviews, despite sufficient immunoprotection hydrogel capsules usually cannot completely prevent an immune response due to the leakage of antigens, protruding cells, micropores, and even the surgery itself (Rokstad et al., 2014; Korsgren, 2017). Especially the release of antigens is a crucial factor in xenotransplantation, because the dominant mechanism for porcine xenograft rejection is antigen presentation by CD4[+] T-cells (Olack et al., 2002) which results in activation of macrophages and production of inflammatory cytokines. The difficulties in preventing the diffusion of cytokines into the hydrogel capsule while retaining permeability for insulin have been summarised by O. Korsgren with the bleak statement that "from a theoretical point of view, it is almost impossible to avoid the problem with indirect antigen presentation most likely limiting the application of encapsulation for islet xenotransplantation" (Korsgren, 2017). On the other hand, as mentioned in a previous chapter (chapter 2.2.2, page 15 ff.), genetic modifications to reduce immunogenicity of porcine islets have led to promising results but were so far not sufficient to completely preserve function and prevent rejection. Yet, there have been encouraging studies on the simultaneous support for viability and functionality of islets and the immune-modulating capacity of pre-culture (Rackham et al., 2014), co-encapsulation (Vériter et al., 2014), and co-transplantation (Hayward et al., 2017) of MSC. Furthermore, immature porcine islet cluster naturally have a high resistance against human cytokines (Bai et al., 2002; Harb et al., 2007). In the opinion of this author, none of the strategies discussed here are likely to succeed separately. Yet, a combination of approaches, such as could be achieved with the co-encapsulation of MSC and NICC in plotted scaffolds, perhaps even the encapsulation of genetically modified NICC could eventually result in the long-term immune-compatibility of xenogeneically transplanted pancreatic islets.

Summary

Background/Aim

To prevent long-term complications in T1D, donor islets can be transplanted; this requires life-long strict immunosuppressive regimens though. Encapsulation of islets can circumvent immunosuppression but upscaling is difficult.

The aim of this book was to develop a strategy for the plotting of scalable semi-permeable macroporous scaffolds with a large surface-to-volume ratio, containing viable and functional pancreatic islets.

Methods

The hydrogel used for bioprinting in this book was a blend of 3 % alginate (Alg) with 9 % methylcellulose (MC) as a thickener to create a plottable paste. The existing blend had to be adapted for the use of highly purified, i.e. non-immunogenic ("clinical-grade") alginate instead of the cell-compatible but less stringently purified ("research-grade") alginate used previously. Comparisons for the characterisation of the cell-free blend were always drawn between pastes prepared with the two different alginates. Stability was tested with rheological measurements, and release of ions and MC. Permeability for glucose and insulin was analysed with uptake and release assays as well as in a diffusion chamber system developed for this book. As alginate gels have been shown to be sufficiently permeable and encapsulated islets retain their functionality, comparisons for the permeability were drawn between plain alginate and Alg/MC gels.

Alg/MC has previously been shown to be compatible with the plotting of single cells of mesenchymal origin. To test compatibility with endocrine cells the β-cell-line INS-1 was incorporated into the blend prepared with differently sterilised MC. For pancreatic islets, which as cell clusters are more sensitive to shear stress than single cells, a workflow for the incorporation into the highly viscous blend was successfully developed. Hereby the islets were carefully folded into the material with a spatula and a needle with an inner diameter of 840 µm was used for plotting.

Plotting of islets was performed with adult murine islets as well as neonatal porcine islet-like clusters (NICC) which were tested for distribution, viability, apoptosis, and presence of hormones with stainings. Functional response was analysed via glucose-stimulated insulin release assays (GSIR) with detection of insulin in the supernatant released in response to hypoglycaemic (3.3 mM glucose) or hyperglycaemic (16.4 mM glucose) conditions.

Results

Pastes prepared with the different alginates showed a comparable viscosity suitable for the plotting of stable structures. Clinical-grade scaffolds had a slightly reduced crosslinking density which was attributed to differences in the M:G-ratio. Scaffolds crosslinked with 70 mM $SrCl_2$ remained stable over 21 days in $RPMI^+$. Over time in culture release of crosslinking ions is sustained and independent of alginate-type, but dependent on the type of medium used. Within the ionically crosslinked scaffolds the inversely thermo-gelling MC is likely partially gelled at 37°C. Release of non-gelled MC could be shown to be temperature-dependent and was observed from all tested scaffold variations in varying quantities.

In permeability analyses overall kinetics of diffusion observed in the chamber system followed the normal course of diffusion through hydrogels. The permeability for glucose was comparable between the materials, i.e. no influence of the alginate-type and crosslinking density, nor the presence and release of MC over time could be detected. The permeability for insulin needs to be verified in further experiments due to binding to the diffusion chamber and a lack of stability of gel discs. A preliminary conclusion from the results presented here is a slight reduction in permeability in Alg/MC gels compared to plain alginate gels.

INS-1 were successfully incorporated and plotted. Viability directly after plotting was comparatively low considering viability rates of immortalised mesenchymal stem cells, they recovered within a week and proliferated into large metabolically active cell clusters within the scaffolds though. This recovery was dependent on the sterilisation method used for MC: Autoclaving and UV-irradiation resulted in pastes supporting the viability, whereas MC sterilised with supercritical CO_2 did not result in the development of cell clusters.

Metabolically active murine islets containing insulin were distributed homogeneously throughout the scaffolds. Viability was 70-80 %, comparable to control islets in suspension culture, over a total of 14 days. DNA-content in plotted scaffolds was strongly reduced over a total of 21 days. In all islets observed over 7 days a limited amount of apoptotic nuclei was present, which were preferentially located centrally in control islets, and preferentially located in the periphery in plotted islets. Number of apoptotic nuclei was not significantly different between control and plotted islets. Overall, during incorporation into the blend and plotting the morphology and viability of islets were retained.

The pancreatic hormones insulin and glucagon were detected in the appropriate ratio and locations within control and plotted islets. Stimulation of murine islets was verified over a total of 7 isolations and showed a lower total amount of insulin released from plotted than from control islets but a comparable stimulation index (SI) calculated from GSIR on day 4 and 7 of culture. Furthermore it could be shown that when islets are exposed to successive low-high-low glucose stimulation, release of insulin corresponded to glucose concentration, showing that plotted islets truly sense external glucose concentrations and react accordingly. In summary, while total release of insulin was lower from plotted than from control islets, functionality was retained in plotted scaffolds.

For validation of the results from adult murine islets the potentially clinically translatable but more sensitive NICC were used in a preliminary study. Metabolically active NICC containing insulin were distributed homogeneously throughout the scaffolds. Viability of NICC was comparatively low with approximately 60 % without any significant changes over 21 days of incubation, but equal to control NICC. All plotted NICC retained some viability, but in a limited amount of control NICC almost no signal was detected in the live staining. Number of apoptotic nuclei increased significantly over the course of 7 days for plotted but not control NICC.

The pancreatic hormones insulin, glucagon and somatostatin were detected in a low number of cells scattered randomly throughout the cell clusters over 7 days. Functional response was not impacted by the incorporation into the material nor the plotting. With amplification with a GLP-1 analogue, NICC showed a functional response which was comparable between plotted and control samples. The SI decreased over the time of observation and resulted in an SI < 2 after 14 and 21 days of culture in plotted and control samples respectively.

Conclusions

The adapted Alg/MC blend showed sufficient stability and permeability for the plotting of islets. The feasibility of 3D plotting of viable and functional pancreatic islets with the proposed hydrogel blend was demonstrated in a proof-of-concept study with adult murine islets.

Preliminary results, performed with a low number of repetitions and samples, indicate that the adapted blend is also an appropriate basis for the plotting of NICC.

Further characterisation and especially further material adaptation to support viability and maturation of NICC *in vitro* will be analysed in a subsequent study.

Zusammenfassung

Hintergrund/Ziel

Um Langzeitkomplikationen bei T1D zu verhindern, können Spenderinseln transplantiert werden, was allerdings lebenslange rigorose Immunsuppression erfordert. Durch Verkapselung der Inselzellen kann die Immunsuppression umgangen werden, aber Upscaling ist schwierig. Ziel dieser Arbeit war es, eine Strategie für das Plotting skalierbarer, semipermeabler, makroporöser Scaffolds mit einem großen Oberfläche-zu-Volumen-Verhältnis zu entwickeln, um lebensfähige und funktionsfähige Pankreasinseln zu Plotten.

Methoden

Die für diese Arbeit verwendete Hydrogelmischung bestand aus 3 % Alginat mit 9 % Methylcellulose (MC) als Verdickungsmittel, um eine plottbare Paste herzustellen. Die existierende Mischung musste für die Verwendung von hochaufgereinigtem, d. h. nicht immunogenem ("clinical-grade") Alginat anstelle des zuvor verwendeten zellverträglichen, aber weniger streng aufgereinigten ("research-grade") Alginates adaptiert werden. Für die Charakterisierung der zellfreien Mischung wurden immer Vergleiche zwischen Pasten gezogen, die mit den beiden verschiedenen Alginaten hergestellt wurden. Die Stabilität wurde über rheologische Messungen und die Freisetzung von Ionen und MC bestimmt. Die Permeabilität für Glukose und Insulin wurde mittels Aufnahme- und Freisetzungs-Assays sowie in einem für diese Arbeit entwickelten Diffusionskammersystem analysiert. Da sich Alginatgele als ausreichend permeabel erwiesen haben und eingekapselte Inseln ihre Funktionalität behalten, wurde die Permeabilität von Alginat- und Alg/MC-Gelen verglichen.

In früheren Veröffentlichung wurde Alg/MC bereits als kompatibel mit dem Plotting von Einzelzellen beschrieben. Um die Kompatibilität mit endokrinen Zellen zu testen, wurde die β-Zelllinie INS-1 verwendet und in Alg/MC Pasten, die mit unterschiedlich sterilisierter MC hergestellt worden waren, getestet. Für pankreatische Inseln, die als Zellcluster empfindlicher auf Scherstress reagieren als Einzelzellen, wurde erfolgreich ein Workflow für das Einbringen in die hochviskose Mischung entwickelt. Dabei wurden die Inseln mit einem Spatel vorsichtig in das Material gefaltet und mit einer Nadel mit einem Innendurchmesser von 840 µm geplottet.

Das Plotten pankreatischer Inseln wurde sowohl mit adulten Inseln aus der Ratte als auch mit neonatalen insel-ähnlichen Clustern aus dem Schwein (NICC) durchgeführt und auf Verteilung, Überleben, Apoptose und das Vorhandensein von Hormonen mit Färbungen getestet. Die Funktionalität wurde über Glukose-stimulierter Insulinsekretion (GSIR) analysiert, wobei Inseln Insulin in Reaktion auf hypoglykämische (3,3 mM Glukose) oder hyperglykämische (16,4 mM Glukose) Bedingungen freisetzen, welches im Überstand nachgewiesen wurde.

Ergebnisse

Pasten, die mit den verschiedenen Alginaten hergestellt wurden, zeigten eine vergleichbare Viskosität, die für die Herstellung stabiler Strukturen geeignet ist. Clinical-grade Scaffolds hatten eine leicht geringere Vernetzungsdichte, was auf Unterschiede im M:G-Verhältnis zurückgeführt wurde. Mit 70 mM $SrCl_2$ vernetzte Scaffolds blieben in RPMI$^+$ über 21 Tage stabil. Die anhaltende Freisetzung von Vernetzungsionen über den Kultivierungszeitraum war unabhängig vom Alginattyp, aber abhängig von der Art des verwendeten Mediums. Innerhalb der ionisch vernetzten Scaffolds liegt die umgekehrt thermisch gelierende MC bei 37°C mit hoher Wahrscheinlichkeit teilweise geliert vor. Die Freisetzung von nicht gelierter MC konnte in Abhängigkeit der Temperatur gezeigt werden und wurde in allen getesteten Scaffold-varianten in unterschiedlicher Menge beobachtet.

Bei Permeabilitätsanalysen folgte die im Kammersystem beobachtete allgemeine Kinetik der Diffusion dem normalen Verlauf der Diffusion durch Hydrogele. Die Permeabilität für Glukose war zwischen den Materialien vergleichbar, d.h. es konnte weder ein Einfluss des Alginat-Typs und der Vernetzungsdichte, noch des Vorhandenseins bzw. der Freisetzung von MC über die Zeit nachgewiesen werden. Die Permeabilität für Insulin muss aufgrund der Bindung an die Diffusionskammer und der mangelnden Stabilität der Gelscheiben in weiteren Experimenten verifiziert werden. Eine vorläufige Schlussfolgerung aus den hier vorgestellten Ergebnissen ist eine leicht verringerte Permeabilität in Alg/MC-Gelen im Vergleich zu reinen Alginatgelen.

INS-1 wurden erfolgreich in Alg/MC geplottet. Die Überlebensrate direkt nach dem Plotten war in Anbetracht der Raten immortalisierter mesenchymaler Stammzellen vergleichsweise gering, INS-1 erholten sich jedoch innerhalb einer Woche und proliferierten innerhalb der Scaffolds zu großen metabolisch aktiven Zellclustern. Dies war abhängig von der Sterilisationsmethode: Die Verwendung autoklavierter sowie UV-sterilisierter MC resultierte in Pasten die das Über-leben unterstützten. Im Gegensatz dazu führte die Verwendung von mit überkritischem CO_2 sterilisierter MC nicht zur Entwicklung von Zellclustern.

Metabolisch aktive, Insulin enthaltende Ratteninseln lagen innerhalb der Scaffolds gleich-mäßig verteilt vor. Vergleichbar mit Kontrollinseln in Suspensionskultur betrug die Viabilität geplotteter Inseln über einen Zeitraum von 14 Tagen 70-80 %. Der DNA-Gehalt der Scaffolds reduzierte sich über insgesamt 21 Tage stark. In allen über 7 Tage analysierten Inseln war eine begrenzte Menge apoptotischer Kerne vorhanden. In den Kontrollinseln waren diese be-vorzugt zentral, in den geplotteten Inseln bevorzugt peripher lokalisiert. Die Anzahl der apop-totischen Kerne unterschied sich zwischen den Kontrollinseln und den geplotteten Inseln nicht signifikant. Insgesamt blieben die Morphologie und die Viabilität der Inseln während des Einbringens in die Mischung und beim Plotten erhalten.

Die pankreatischen Hormone Insulin und Glukagon wurden in der Kontrolle und der ge-plotteten Inseln in angemessener Verteilung und Lokalisation nachgewiesen. Die Stimulation der Ratteninseln wurde über insgesamt 7 Isolationen verifiziert und zeigte eine geringere ab-solute Insulinsekretion aus den geplotteten Inseln als aus den Kontrollinseln, aber an Tag 4 und 7 der Kultur einen vergleichbaren aus dem GSIR berechneten Stimulationsindex (SI).

Darüber hinaus konnte gezeigt werden, dass die Insulinsekretion bei sukzessiv variierender Stimulation mit Glukose dem Verlauf der Glukosekonzentration folgt. Dies zeigt, dass die geplotteten Inseln die externe Glukosekonzentration nachweislich wahrnehmen und entsprechend reagieren. Zusammenfassend lässt sich festhalten, dass die absolute Insulinsekretion aus den geplotteten Inseln zwar geringer war als die der Kontrollinseln, die relative Funktionalität in den geplotteten Scaffolds jedoch erhalten blieb.

Zur Validierung der Ergebnisse von adulten Ratteninseln wurden in einer vorläufigen Studie die potentiell klinisch translatierbaren, aber empfindlicheren, NICC verwendet. Metabolisch aktive, Insulin enthaltende NICC, lagen innerhalb der Scaffolds gleichmäßig verteilt vor. Die Viabilität der NICC war mit etwa 60 % vergleichsweise gering, aber vergleichbar mit der der Kontroll-NICC und änderte sich über einen Kultivierungszeitraum von 21 Tagen nicht signifikant. In allen geplotteten NICC konnten lebendige Zellen nachgewiesen werden, während eine geringe Anzahl Kontroll-NICC in der Lebendfärbung fast kein Signal zeigten. Die Anzahl der apoptotischen Kerne nahm im Verlauf von 7 Tagen bei den geplotteten, nicht aber bei den Kontroll-NICC signifikant zu.

Die pankreatischen Hormone Insulin, Glukagon und Somatostatin wurden in einer geringen Anzahl von zufällig innerhalb der Cluster verteilten Zellen über einen Zeitraum von 7 Tagen nachgewiesen. Die Funktionalität wurde weder durch das Einbringen in das Material noch durch das Plotten beeinflusst. Unter Verwendung eines GLP-1-Analogons zur Amplifikation der Reaktion zeigten geplottete und Kontroll-NICC eine vergleichbare Funktionalität. Der SI nahm im Laufe der Kultivierungszeit jedoch ab und lag nach 14 bzw. 21 Tagen Kultur in geplotteten und Kontrollproben unter 2.

Schlussfolgerungen

Die adaptierte Alg/MC-Mischung zeigte ausreichende Stabilität und Permeabilität für das Plotten pankreatischer Inseln.

In einer Proof-of-Concept-Studie mit adulten Ratteninseln wurde gezeigt, dass die hier adaptierte Alg/MC-Mischung generell für das Plotting lebendiger und funktionaler pankreatischer Inseln geeignet ist.

Vorläufige Ergebnisse, die mit einer geringen Anzahl von Wiederholungen und Proben erstellt wurden, deuten darauf hin, dass Alg/MC auch ein grundlegend geeignetes Material für das Plotten von NICC ist.

Die weitere Charakterisierung und insbesondere die weitere Materialadaption zur Unterstützung des Überlebens und der Ausreifung von NICC *in vitro* werden in einer Folgestudie vorgenommen werden.

References

Abbah, S. A., Lu, W. W., Peng, S. L., Aladin, D. M. K., Li, Z. Y., Tam, W. K., Cheung, K. M. C., Luk, K. D. K., & Zhou, G. Q. (2008). Extracellular matrix stability of primary mammalian chondrocytes and intervertebral disc cells cultured in alginate-based microbead hydrogels. *Cell Transplantation*, *17*(10–11), 1181–1192. https://doi.org/10.3727/096368908787236648

Adams, M. T., Reissaus, C. A., Szulczewski, J. M., Dwulet, J. M., Lyman, M. R., Sdao, S. M., Nimkulrat, S. D., Ponik, S. M., Merrins, M. J., Benninger, R. K. P., Mirmira, R. G., Linnemann, A. K., & Blum, B. (2020). Islet architecture controls synchronous β cell response to glucose in the intact mouse pancreas in vivo. *SSRN Electronic Journal*, *1*(1), 1–13. https://doi.org/10.2139/ssrn.3513566

Ahlfeld, T., Cidonio, G., Kilian, D., Duin, S., Akkineni, A. R., Dawson, J. I., Yang, S., Lode, A., Oreffo, R. O. C., & Gelinsky, M. (2017). Development of a clay based bioink for 3D cell printing for skeletal application. *Biofabrication*, *9*(3), 34103. https://doi.org/10.1088/1758-5090/aa7e96

Ahlfeld, T., Cubo-Mateo, N., Cometta, S., Guduric, V., Vater, C., Bernhardt, A., Akkineni, A. R., Lode, A., & Gelinsky, M. (2020a). A Novel Plasma-Based Bioink Stimulates Cell Proliferation and Differentiation in Bioprinted, Mineralized Constructs. *ACS Applied Materials and Interfaces*, *12*(11), 12557–12572. https://doi.org/10.1021/acsami.0c00710

Ahlfeld, T., Guduric, V., Duin, S., Akkineni, A. R., Schütz, K., Kilian, D., Emmermacher, J., Cubo-Mateo, N., Dani, S., von Witzleben, M., Spangenberg, J., Abdelgaber, R., Richter, R. F., Lode, A., & Gelinsky, M. (2020b). Methylcellulose – a versatile printing material that enables biofabrication of tissue equivalents with high shape fidelity. *Biomaterials Science*, *8*(8), 2102–2110. https://doi.org/10.1039/D0BM00027B

Al-Musa, S., Abu Fara, D., & Badwan, A. A. (1999). Evaluation of parameters involved in preparation and release of drug loaded in crosslinked matrices of alginate. *Journal of Controlled Release*, *57*(3), 223–232. https://doi.org/10.1016/S0168-3659(98)00096-0

Al-Shamkhani, A., & Duncan, R. (1995). Radioiodination of Alginate via Covalently-Bound Tyrosinamide Allows Monitoring of its Fate In Vivo. *Journal of Bioactive and Compatible Polymers*, *10*(1), 4–13. https://doi.org/doi.org/10.1177/088391159501000102

An, D., Chiu, A., Flanders, J. A., Song, W., Shou, D., Lu, Y. C., Grunnet, L. G., Winkel, L., Ingvorsen, C., Christophersen, N. S., Fels, J. J., Sand, F. W., Ji, Y., Qi, L., Pardo, Y., Luo, D., Silberstein, M., Fan, J., & Ma, M. (2017). Designing a retrievable and scalable cell encapsulation device for potential treatment of type 1 diabetes. *Proceedings of the National Academy of Sciences of the USA*, *115*(2), E263–E272. https://doi.org/10.1073/pnas.1708806115

Andersen, T., Auk-Emblem, P., & Dornish, M. (2015). 3D Cell Culture in Alginate Hydrogels.

Microarrays, *4*(2), 133–161. https://doi.org/10.3390/microarrays4020133

Andersson, A. (1978). Isolated mouse pancreatic islets in culture: Effects of serum and different culture media on the insulin production of the islets. *Diabetologia*, *14*(6), 397–404. https://doi.org/10.1007/BF01228134

Andersson, M., Axelsson, A., & Zacchi, G. (1997). Diffusion of glucose and insulin in a swelling N-isopropylacrylamide gel. *International Journal of Pharmaceutics*, *157*(2), 199–208. https://doi.org/10.1016/S0378-5173(97)00243-3

Andresen, I.-L., Skipnes, O., Smidsrød, O., Ostgaard, K., & Hemmer, P. C. (1977). Some Biological Functions of Matrix Components in Benthic Algae in Relation to Their Chemistry and the Composition of Seawater. In J. C. Arthur (Ed.), *Cellulose Chemistry and Technology* (pp. 361–381). https://doi.org/10.1021/bk-1977-0048.ch024

Arisz, P. W., Kauw, H. J. J., & Boon, J. J. (1995). Substituent distribution along the cellulose backbone in O-methylcelluloses using GC and FAB-MS for monomer and oligomer analysis. *Carbohydrate Research*, *271*(1), 1–14. https://doi.org/10.1016/0008-6215(95)00039-V

Aronoff, S. L., Berkowitz, K., Shreiner, B., & Want, L. (2004). Glucose Metabolism and Regulation: Beyond Insulin and Glucagon. *Diabetes Spectrum*, *17*(3), 183–190. https://doi.org/10.2337/diaspect.17.3.183

Asfari, M., Janjic, D., Meda, P., Li, G., Halban, P. A., & Wollheim, C. B. (1992). Establishment of 2-Mercaptoethanol-Dependent Differentiated Insulin-Secreting Cell Lines. *Endocrinology*, *130*(1), 167–178. https://doi.org/10.1210/endo.130.1.1370150

Aslani, P., & Kennedy, R. A. (1996). Studies on diffusion in alginate gels. I. Effect of cross-linking with calcium or zinc ions on diffusion of acetaminophen. *Journal of Controlled Release*, *42*(1), 75–82. https://doi.org/10.1016/0168-3659(96)01369-7

Atkinson, M. A., & Eisenbarth, G. S. (2001). Type 1 diabetes: New perspectives on disease pathogenesis and treatment. *Lancet*, *358*(9277), 221–229. https://doi.org/10.1016/S0140-6736(01)05415-0

Atkinson, M. A., Eisenbarth, G. S., & Michels, A. W. (2014). Type 1 diabetes. *The Lancet*, *383*(9911), 69–82. https://doi.org/10.1016/S0140-6736(13)60591-7

Axelsson, A., & Persson, B. (1988). Determination of effective diffusion coefficients in calcium alginate gel plates with varying yeast cell content. *Applied Biochemistry and Biotechnology*, *18*(1), 231–250. https://doi.org/10.1007/BF02930828

Badwaik, R. (2019). 3D Printed Organs: The Future of Regenerative Medicine. *Journal of Clinical and Diagnostic Research*. https://doi.org/10.7860/jcdr/2019/42546.13256

Bai, L., Tuch, B. E., Hering, B., & Simpson, A. M. (2002). Fetal pig β cells are resistant to the toxic effects of human cytokines. *Transplantation*, *73*(5), 714–722. https://doi.org/10.1097/00007890-200203150-00010

References

Bain, M. K., Bhowmick, B., Maity, D., Mondal, D., Mollick, M. M. R., Rana, D., & Chattopadhyay, D. (2012). Synergistic effect of salt mixture on the gelation temperature and morphology of methylcellulose hydrogel. *International Journal of Biological Macromolecules*, *51*(5), 831–836. https://doi.org/10.1016/j.ijbiomac.2012.07.028

Balyura, M., Gelfgat, E., Ehrhart-Bornstein, M., Ludwig, B., Gendlerc, Z., Barkai, U., Zimerman, B., Rotem, A., Block, N. L., Schally, A. V., & Bornstein, S. R. (2015). Transplantation of bovine adrenocortical cells encapsulated in alginate. *Proceedings of the National Academy of Sciences of the USA*, *112*(8), 2527–2532. https://doi.org/10.1073/pnas.1500242112

Barkai, U., Weir, G. C., Colton, C. K., Ludwig, B., Bornstein, S. R., Brendel, M. D., Neufeld, T., Bremer, C., Leon, A., Evron, Y., Yavriyants, K., Azarov, D., Zimermann, B., Maimon, S., Shabtay, N., Balyura, M., Rozenshtein, T., Vardi, P., Bloch, K., ... Rotem, A. (2013). Enhanced oxygen supply improves islet viability in a new bioartificial pancreas. *Cell Transplantation*, *22*(8), 1463–1476. https://doi.org/10.3727/096368912X657341

Basta, G., Montanucci, P., Luca, G., Boselli, C., Noya, G., Barbaro, B., Qi, M., Kinzer, K. P., Oberholzer, J., & Calafiore, R. (2011). Long-term metabolic and immunological follow-up of nonimmunosuppressed patients with type 1 diabetes treated with microencapsulated islet allografts: Four cases. *Diabetes Care*, *34*(11), 2406–2409. https://doi.org/10.2337/dc11-0731

Bauermeister, A. J., Zuriarrain, A., & Newman, M. I. (2016). Three-dimensional printing in plastic and reconstructive surgery a systematic review. *Annals of Plastic Surgery*, *77*(5), 569–576. https://doi.org/10.1097/SAP.0000000000000671

Benavidez, T. E., Torrente, D., Marucho, M., & Garcia, C. D. (2015). Adsorption of Soft and Hard Proteins onto OTCEs under the influence of an External Electric Field. *Langmuir*, *31*(8), 2455–2462. https://doi.org/10.1021/la504890v

Bendas, A., Rothe, U., Kiess, W., Kapellen, T. M., Stange, T., Manuwald, U., Salzsieder, E., Holl, R. W., Schoffer, O., Stahl-Pehe, A., Giani, G., Ehehalt, S., Neu, A., & Rosenbauer, J. (2015). Trends in incidence rates during 1999-2008 and prevalence in 2008 of childhood type 1 diabetes mellitus in Germany - Model-based national estimates. *PLoS ONE*, *10*(7), 2004–2008. https://doi.org/10.1371/journal.pone.0132716

Beta Cell Biology Consortium. (2004). *Insulin maturation*. Website. https://de.wikipedia.org/wiki/Datei:Insulin_Maturation.jpg

Billiet, T., Vandenhaute, M., Schelfhout, J., Van Vlierberghe, S., & Dubruel, P. (2012). A review of trends and limitations in hydrogel-rapid prototyping for tissue engineering. In *Biomaterials* 33(26), 6020–6041. https://doi.org/10.1016/j.biomaterials.2012.04.050

Bloch, K., Bloch, O., Tarasenko, I., Lazard, D., Rapoport, M., & Vardi, P. (2011). A strategy for the engineering of insulin producing cells with a broad spectrum of defense properties.

Biomaterials, *32*(7), 1816–1825. https://doi.org/10.1016/j.biomaterials.2010.11.018

Bochenek, M. A., Veiseh, O., Vegas, A. J., James, J., Qi, M., Marchese, E., Omami, M., Doloff, J. C., Mendoza-elias, J., Nourmohammadzadeh, M., Khan, A., Yeh, C., Xing, Y., Isa, D., Ghani, S., Li, J., Landry, C., Bader, A. R., Olejnik, K., … Anderson, D. G. (2019). Alginate encapsulation as long-term immune protection of allogeneic pancreatic islet cells transplanted into the omental bursa of macaques. *Nat Biomed Eng.*, *2*(11), 810–821. https://doi.org/10.1038/s41551-018-0275-1.

Böker, W., Yin, Z., Drosse, I., Haasters, F., Rossmann, O., Wierer, M., Popov, C., Locher, M., Mutschler, W., Docheva, D., & Schieker, M. (2008). Introducing a single-cell-derived human mesenchymal stem cell line expressing hTERT after lentiviral gene transfer. *Journal of Cellular and Molecular Medicine*, *12*(4), 1347–1359. https://doi.org/10.1111/j.1582-4934.2008.00299.x

Bosco, D., Armanet, M., Morel, P., Niclauss, N., Sgroi, A., Muller, Y. D., Giovannoni, L., Parnaud, G., & Berney, T. (2010). Unique arrangement of α- and β-cells in human islets of Langerhans. *Diabetes*, *59*(5), 1202–1210. https://doi.org/10.2337/db09-1177

Bottino, R., Wijkstrom, M., Van Der Windt, D. J., Hara, H., Ezzelarab, M., Murase, N., Bertera, S., He, J., Phelps, C., Ayares, D., Cooper, D. K. C., & Trucco, M. (2014). Pig-to-monkey islet xenotransplantation using multi-transgenic pigs. *American Journal of Transplantation*, *14*(10), 2275–2287. https://doi.org/10.1111/ajt.12868

Briššová, M., Petro, M., Lacík, I., Powers, A. C., & Wang, T. (1996). Evaluation of microcapsule permeability via inverse size exclusion chromatography. *Analytical Biochemistry*, *242*(1), 104–111. https://doi.org/10.1006/abio.1996.0435

Britt, L. D., Stojeba, P. C., Scharp, C. R., Greider, M. H., & Scharp, D. W. (1981). Neonatal pig pseudo-islets. A product of selective aggregation. *Diabetes*, *30*(7), 580–583. https://doi.org/10.2337/diab.30.7.580

Bruni, A., McCall, M., & Shapiro, A. M. J. (2017). Islet Cell Transplantation. In D. J. Ledbetter & P. R. V. Johnson (Eds.), *Endocrine Surgery in Children* (pp. 181–196). Springer Verlag GmbH. https://doi.org/10.1007/978-3-662-54256-9

Buchwald, P. (2009). FEM-based oxygen consumption and cell viability models for avascular pancreatic islets. *Theoretical Biology and Medical Modelling*, *6*(1). https://doi.org/10.1186/1742-4682-6-5

Buchwald, P., Tamayo-Garcia, A., Manzoli, V., Tomei, A. A., & Stabler, C. L. (2018). Glucose-stimulated insulin release: Parallel perifusion studies of free and hydrogel encapsulated human pancreatic islets. *Biotechnology and Bioengineering*, *115*(1), 232–245. https://doi.org/10.1002/bit.26442

Burchard, W. (1983). Solution thermodynamics of water-soluble polymers. In C. A. Finch (Ed.), *Chemistry and Technology of Water-Soluble Polymers* (1st ed., pp. 125–142). Springer

US. https://doi.org/10.1007/978-1-4757-9661-2

Byrt, C. S., Betts, N. S., Farrokhi, N., & Burton, R. A. (2013). Deconstructing plant biomass: Cell wall structure and novel manipulation strategies. In B. P. Singh (Ed.), *Biofuel Crops: Production, Physiology and Genetics* (pp. 135–150). CABI. https://doi.org/10.1079/9781845938857.0135

Cabrera, O., Berman, D. M., Kenyon, N. S., Ricordi, C., Berggren, P. O., & Caicedo, A. (2006). The unique cytoarchitecture of human pancreatic islets has implications for islet cell function. *Proc. Natl. Acad. Sci. U.S.A.*, *103*(7), 2334–2339. https://doi.org/10.1073/pnas.0510790103

Calafiore, R., Basta, G., Luca, G., Lemmi, A., Racanicchi, L., Mancuso, F., Montanucci, M. P., & Brunetti, P. (2006). Standard Technical Procedures for Microencapsulation of Human Islets for Graft into Nonimmunosuppressed Patients With Type 1 Diabetes Mellitus. *Transplantation Proceedings*, *38*(4), 1156–1157. https://doi.org/10.1016/j.transproceed.2006.03.014

Cantarelli, E., & Piemonti, L. (2011). Alternative transplantation sites for pancreatic islet grafts. *Current Diabetes Reports*, *11*(5), 364–374. https://doi.org/10.1007/s11892-011-0216-9

Cao, Y., & Tan, H. (2002). Effects of cellulase on the modification of cellulose. *Carbohydrate Research*, *337*(14), 1291–1296. https://doi.org/10.1016/S0008-6215(02)00134-9

Cappai, A., Petruzzo, P., Ruiu, G., Congiu, T., Dessy, E., De Seta, W., Santa Cruz, G., & Brotzu, G. (1995). Evaluation of new small barium alginate microcapsules. *International Journal of Artificial Organs*, *18*(2), 96–102. https://doi.org/10.1177/039139889501800209

Cardona, K., Korbutt, G. S., Milas, Z., Lyon, J., Cano, J., Jiang, W., Bello-Laborn, H., Hacquoil, B., Strobert, E., Gangappa, S., Weber, C. J., Pearson, T. C., Rajotte, R. V., & Larsen, C. P. (2006). Long-term survival of neonatal porcine islets in nonhuman primates by targeting costimulation pathways. *Nature Medicine*, *12*(3), 304–306. https://doi.org/10.1038/nm1375

Carlsson, P. O., Espes, D., Sedigh, A., Rotem, A., Zimerman, B., Grinberg, H., Goldman, T., Barkai, U., Avni, Y., Westermark, G. T., Carlbom, L., Ahlström, H., Eriksson, O., Olerud, J., & Korsgren, O. (2018). Transplantation of macroencapsulated human islets within the bioartificial pancreas βAir to patients with type 1 diabetes mellitus. *American Journal of Transplantation*, *18*(7), 1735–1744. https://doi.org/10.1111/ajt.14642

Carter, J. D., Dula, S. B., Corbin, K. L., Wu, R., & Nunemaker, C. S. (2009). A practical guide to rodent islet isolation and assessment. *Biological Procedures Online*, *11*(1), 3–31. https://doi.org/10.1007/s12575-009-9021-0

Castiello, F. R., Heileman, K., & Tabrizian, M. (2016). Microfluidic perfusion systems for secretion fingerprint analysis of pancreatic islets: Applications, challenges and opportunities. *Lab on a Chip*, *16*(3), 409–431. https://doi.org/10.1039/c5lc01046b

CELLINK. (2020). *CELLMIXER*. Website. https://www.cellink.com/product/cellmixer/

Chan, G., & Mooney, D. J. (2013). Ca2+ released from calcium alginate gels can promote inflammatory responses in vitro and in vivo. *Acta Biomaterialia*, *9*(12), 9281–9291. https://doi.org/10.1016/j.actbio.2013.08.002

Chen, C. H., Tsai, C. C., Chen, W., Mi, F. L., Liang, H. F., Chen, S. C., & Sung, H. W. (2006). Novel living cell sheet harvest system composed of thermoreversible methylcellulose hydrogels. *Biomacromolecules*, *7*(3), 736–743. https://doi.org/10.1021/bm0506400

Chen, X. B., Li, Y. X., Jiao, Y., Dong, W. P., Li, G., Chen, J., & Tan, J. M. (2007). Influence of heme oxygenase-1 gene transfer on the viability and function of rat islets in in vitro culture. *World Journal of Gastroenterology*, *13*(7), 1053–1059. https://doi.org/10.3748/wjg.v13.i7.1053

Chicheportiche, D., & Reach, G. (1988). In vitro kinetics of insulin release by microencapsulated rat islets: effect of the size of the microcapsules. *Diabetologia*, *31*(1), 54–57. https://doi.org/10.1007/BF00279134

Child, A., Larkin, E. J., & Fontaine, M. J. (2020). Co-encapsulation of ECM proteins to enhance pancreatic islet cell function. *Transplantation, Bioengineering, and Regeneration of the Endocrine Pancreas*, *2*, 307–313. https://doi.org/10.1016/b978-0-12-814831-0.00022-1

Clayton, H. A., London, N. J. M., Brandhorst, D., Brandhorst, H., Hering, B. J., Federlin, K., Bretzel, R. G., & Lacy, P. (1996). Survival and function of islets during culture. *Cell Transplantation*, *5*(1), 1–12. https://doi.org/10.1016/0963-6897(95)02005-5

Coffey, D. G., Bell, D. A., & Henderson, A. (2006). Methylcelluloses. In A. M. Stephen, G. O. Phillips, & P. A. Williams (Eds.), *Food Polysaccharides and Their Applications* (2nd ed., pp. 159–163). CRC Press, Taylor & Francis Group. https://doi.org/10.1201/9781420015164

Colton, C. K. (2014). Oxygen supply to encapsulated therapeutic cells. *Advanced Drug Delivery Reviews*, *67*–68(April), 93–110. Elsevier B.V. https://doi.org/10.1016/j.addr.2014.02.007

Cooper, D. K. C., Ekser, B., & Tector, A. J. (2015). A brief history of clinical xenotransplantation. *International Journal of Surgery*, *23*(Pt B), 205–210. https://doi.org/10.1016/j.ijsu.2015.06.060

Cooper, D. K. C., Ezzelarab, M. B., Hara, H., Iwase, H., Lee, W., Wijkstrom, M., & Bottino, R. (2016). The pathobiology of pig-to-primate xenotransplantation: A historical review. *Xenotransplantation*, *23*(2), 83–105. https://doi.org/10.1111/xen.12219

Cooper, D. K. C., Matsumoto, S., Abalovich, A., Itoh, T., Mourad, N. I., Gianello, P. R., Wolf, E., & Cozzi, E. (2016). Progress in Clinical Encapsulated Islet Xenotransplantation. *Transplantation*, *100*(11), 2301–2308. https://doi.org/10.1097/TP.0000000000001371

Da Silva Xavier, G. (2018). The Cells of the Islets of Langerhans. *Journal of Clinical Medicine*,

7(3), 54. https://doi.org/10.3390/jcm7030054

Daly, B., O'Kelly, K., & Klassen, D. (2004). Interventional procedures in whole organ and islet cell pancreas transplantation. *Seminars in Interventional Radiology*, *21*(4), 335–343. https://doi.org/10.1055/s-2004-861568

Dang, T. T., Xu, Q., Bratlie, K. M., O'Sullivan, E. S., Chen, X. Y., Langer, R., & Anderson, D. G. (2009). Microfabrication of homogenous, asymmetric cell-laden hydrogel capsules. *Biomaterials*, *30*(36), 6896–6902. https://doi.org/10.1016/j.biomaterials.2009.09.012

Daoud, J., Petropavlovskaia, M., Rosenberg, L., & Tabrizian, M. (2010). The effect of extracellular matrix components on the preservation of human islet function in vitro. *Biomaterials*, *31*(7), 1676–1682. https://doi.org/10.1016/j.biomaterials.2009.11.057

Daoud, J. T., Petropavlovskaia, M. S., Patapas, J. M., Degrandpré, C. E., DiRaddo, R. W., Rosenberg, L., & Tabrizian, M. (2011). Long-term in vitro human pancreatic islet culture using three-dimensional microfabricated scaffolds. *Biomaterials*, *32*(6), 1536–1542. https://doi.org/10.1016/j.biomaterials.2010.10.036

Darrabie, M. D., Kendall, W. F., & Opara, E. C. (2006). Effect of alginate composition and gelling cation on micro-bead swelling. *Journal of Microencapsulation*, *23*(1), 29–37. https://doi.org/10.1080/02652040500286144

De Groot, M., Schuurs, T. A., & Van Schilfgaarde, R. (2004). Causes of limited survival of microencapsulated pancreatic islet grafts. *Journal of Surgical Research*, *121*(1), 141–150. https://doi.org/10.1016/j.jss.2004.02.018

De Haan, B. J., Faas, M. M., & De Vos, P. (2003). Factors influencing insulin secretion from encapsulated islets. *Cell Transplantation*, *12*(6), 617–625. https://doi.org/10.3727/000000003108747226

De Vos, P., De Haan, B. J., & Van Schilfgaarde, R. (1997a). Effect of the alginate composition on the biocompatibility of alginate-polylysine microcapsules. *Biomaterials*, *18*(3), 273–278. https://doi.org/10.1016/S0142-9612(96)00135-4

De Vos, P., De Haan, B. J., Wolters, G. H. J., Strubbe, J. H., & Van Schilfgaarde, R. (1997b). Improved biocompatibility but limited graft survival after purification of alginate for microencapsulation of pancreatic islets. *Diabetologia*, *40*(3), 262–270. https://doi.org/10.1007/s001250050673

de Vos, P., Bučko, M., Gemeiner, P., Navrátil, M., Švitel, J., Faas, M., Strand, B. L., Skjak-Braek, G., Morch, Y. A., Vikartovská, A., Lacík, I., Kolláriková, G., Orive, G., Poncelet, D., Pedraz, J. L., & Ansorge-Schumacher, M. B. (2009). Multiscale requirements for bioencapsulation in medicine and biotechnology. *Biomaterials*, *30*(13), 2559–2570. https://doi.org/10.1016/j.biomaterials.2009.01.014

de Vos, P., Faas, M. M., Strand, B., & Calafiore, R. (2006). Alginate-based microcapsules for immunoisolation of pancreatic islets. *Biomaterials*, *27*(32), 5603–5617.

https://doi.org/10.1016/j.biomaterials.2006.07.010

De Vos, P., & Marchetti, P. (2002). Encapsulation of pancreatic islets for transplantation in diabetes: The untouchable islets. *Trends in Molecular Medicine*, 8(8), 363–366). https://doi.org/10.1016/S1471-4914(02)02381-X

De Vos, P., Van Hoogmoed, C. G., Van Zanten, J., Netter, S., Strubbe, J. H., & Busscher, H. J. (2003). Long-term biocompatibility, chemistry, and function of microencapsulated pancreatic islets. *Biomaterials*, 24(2), 305–312. https://doi.org/10.1016/S0142-9612(02)00319-8

DeRamos, C. M., Irwin, A. E., Nauss, J. L., & Stout, B. E. (1997). 13C NMR and molecular modeling studies of alginic acid binding with alkaline earth and lanthanide metal ions. *Inorganica Chimica Acta*, 256(1), 69–75. https://doi.org/10.1016/S0020-1693(96)05418-7

Desbrières, J., Hirrien, M., & Rinaudo, M. (1998). A calorimetric study of methylcellulose gelation. *Carbohydrate Polymers*, 37(2), 145–152. https://doi.org/10.1016/S0144-8617(98)00023-X

DiMeglio, L. A., Evans-Molina, C., & Oram, R. A. (2018). Type 1 diabetes. *The Lancet*, 391(10138), 2449–2462. https://doi.org/10.1016/S0140-6736(18)31320-5

Dimitrioglou, N., Kanelli, M., Papageorgiou, E., Karatzas, T., & Hatziavramidis, D. (2019). Paving the way for successful islet encapsulation. *Drug Discovery Today*, 24(3), 737–748. https://doi.org/10.1016/j.drudis.2019.01.020

Draget, K. I., & Taylor, C. (2011). Chemical, physical and biological properties of alginates and their biomedical implications. *Food Hydrocolloids*, 25(2), 251–256. https://doi.org/10.1016/j.foodhyd.2009.10.007

Dufrane, D., Goebbels, R. M., & Gianello, P. (2010). Alginate macroencapsulation of pig islets allows correction of streptozotocin-induced diabetes in primates up to 6 months without immunosuppression. *Transplantation*, 90(10), 1054–1062. https://doi.org/10.1097/TP.0b013e3181f6e267

Dufrane, D., Goebbels, R. M., Saliez, A., Guiot, Y., & Gianello, P. (2006). Six-month survival of microencapsulated pig islets and alginate biocompatibility in primates: Proof of concept. *Transplantation*, 81(9), 1345–1353. https://doi.org/10.1097/01.tp.0000208610.75997.20

Dupont. (2018a). *Novamatrix*. Website. https://www.novamatrix.biz/#home

Dupont. (2018b). *PRONOVA UP MVM*. Website. https://www.novamatrix.biz/store/pronova-up-mvm/

Dusseault, J., Tam, S. K., Ménard, M., Polizu, S., Jourdan, G., Yahia, L., & Hallé, J. P. (2006). Evaluation of alginate purification methods: Effect on polyphenol, endotoxin, and protein contamination. *Journal of Biomedical Materials Research - Part A*, 76(2), 243–251. https://doi.org/10.1002/jbm.a.30541

Duvivier-Kali, V. F., Omer, A., Lopez-Avalos, M. D., O'Neil, J. J., & Weir, G. C. (2004). Survival of microencapsulated adult pig islets in mice in spite of an antibody response. *American Journal of Transplantation*, *4*(12), 1991–2000. https://doi.org/10.1111/j.1600-6143.2004.00628.x

Duvivier-Kali, V. F., Omer, A., Parent, R. J., O'Neil, J. J., & Weir, G. C. (2001). Complete Protection of Islets Against Allorejection and Autoimmunity by a Simple Barium-Alginate Membrane. *Diabetes*, *50*(8), 1698–1705. https://doi.org/10.2337/diabetes.50.8.1698

Elliott, R. B., Escobar, L., Calafiore, R., Basta, G., Garkavenko, O., Vasconcellos, A., & Bambra, C. (2005). Transplantation of micro- and macroencapsulated piglet islets into mice and monkeys. *Transplantation Proceedings*, *37*(1), 466–469. https://doi.org/10.1016/j.transproceed.2004.12.198

Elliott, R. B., Escobar, L., Garkavenko, O., Croxson, M. C., Schroeder, B. A., McGregor, M., Ferguson, G., Beckman, N., & Ferguson, S. (2000). No evidence of infection with porcine endogenous retrovirus in recipients of encapsulated porcine islet xenografts. *Cell Transplantation*, *9*(6), 895–901. https://doi.org/10.1177/096368970000900616

Elliott, R. B., Escobar, L., Tan, P. L. J., Muzina, M., Zwain, S., & Buchanan, C. (2007). Live encapsulated porcine islets from a type 1 diabetic patient 9.5 yr after xenotransplantation. *Xenotransplantation*, *14*(2), 157–161. https://doi.org/10.1111/j.1399-3089.2007.00384.x

Emamaullee, J. A., Shapiro, A. M. J., Rajotte, R. V., Korbutt, G., & Elliott, J. F. (2006). Neonatal porcine islets exhibit natural resistance to hypoxia-induced apoptosis. *Transplantation*, *82*(7), 945–952. https://doi.org/10.1097/01.tp.0000238677.00750.32

Emmermacher, J., Spura, D., Cziommer, J., Kilian, D., Wollborn, T., Fritsching, U., Steingroewer, J., Walther, T., Gelinsky, M., & Lode, A. (2020). Engineering considerations on extrusion-based bioprinting: interactions of material behavior, mechanical forces and cells in the printing needle. *Biofabrication*, *12*(2). https://doi.org/10.1088/1758-5090/ab7553

Encyclopædia Britannica. (2010). *Islets of Langerhans*. Website. https://www.britannica.com/science/islets-of-Langerhans

Ertesvåg, H., & Valla, S. (1998). Biosynthesis and applications of alginates. *Polymer Degradation and Stability*, *59*(1–3), 85–91. https://doi.org/10.1201/b18990-34

Espona-Noguera, A., Ciriza, J., Cañibano-Hernández, A., Villa, R., Saenz del Burgo, L., Alvarez, M., & Luis Pedraz, J. (2019). 3D printed polyamide macroencapsulation devices combined with alginate hydrogels for insulin-producing cell-based therapies. *International Journal of Pharmaceutics*, *566*(May), 604–614. https://doi.org/10.1016/j.ijpharm.2019.06.009

Farina, M., Ballerini, A., Fraga, D. W., Nicolov, E., Hogan, M., Demarchi, D., Scaglione, F.,

Sabek, O. M., Horner, P., Thekkedath, U., Gaber, O. A., & Grattoni, A. (2017). 3D Printed Vascularized Device for Subcutaneous Transplantation of Human Islets. *Biotechnology Journal, 12*(9), 1–5. https://doi.org/10.1002/biot.201700169

Farney, A. C., Sutherland, D. E. R., & Opara, E. C. (2016). Evolution of Islet Transplantation for the Last 30 Years. *Pancreas, 45*(1), 8–20. https://doi.org/10.1097/MPA.0000000000000391

Federici, M., Hribal, M., Perego, L., Ranalli, M., Caradonna, Z., Perego, C., Usellini, L., Nano, R., Bonini, P., Bertuzzi, F., Marlier, L. N. J. L., Davalli, A. M., Carandente, O., Pontiroli, A. E., Melino, G., Marchetti, P., Lauro, R., Sesti, G., & Folli, F. (2001). High Glucose Causes Apoptosis in Cultured Human Pancreatic Islets of Langerhans. *Diabetes, 50*(6), 1290–1301. https://doi.org/10.2337/diabetes.50.6.1290

Feng, X., Yi, S., Hawthorne, W. J., Patel, A. T., Walters, S. N., & O'Connell, P. J. (2000). Inducible nitric oxide synthetase is expressed in adult but not fetal pig pancreatic islets. *Xenotransplantation, 7*(3), 197–205. https://doi.org/10.1034/j.1399-3089.2000.00060.x

Foster, N. C., Beck, R. W., Miller, K. M., Clements, M. A., Rickels, M. R., Dimeglio, L. A., Maahs, D. M., Tamborlane, W. V., Bergenstal, R., Smith, E., Olson, B. A., & Garg, S. K. (2019). State of Type 1 Diabetes Management and Outcomes from the T1D Exchange in 2016-2018. *Diabetes Technology and Therapeutics, 21*(2), 66–72. https://doi.org/10.1089/dia.2018.0384

Fritschy, W. M., Wolters, G. H. J., & Van Schilfgaarde, R. (1991). Effect of alginate-polylysine-alginate microencapsulation on in vitro insulin release from rat pancreatic islets. *Diabetes, 40*(1), 37–43. https://doi.org/10.2337/diab.40.1.37

Fu, Z., R. Gilbert, E., & Liu, D. (2012). Regulation of Insulin Synthesis and Secretion and Pancreatic Beta-Cell Dysfunction in Diabetes. *Current Diabetes Reviews, 9*(1), 25–53. https://doi.org/10.2174/157339913804143225

Fujita, Y., Takita, M., Shimoda, M., Itoh, T., Sugimoto, K., Noguchi, H., Naziruddin, B., Levy, M. F., & Matsumoto, S. (2011). Large human islets secrete less insulin per islet equivalent than smaller islets in vitro. *Islets, 3*(1), 1–5. https://doi.org/10.4161/isl.3.1.14131

Gasperini, L., Mano, J. F., & Reis, R. L. (2014). Natural polymers for the microencapsulation of cells. *Journal of the Royal Society Interface, 11*(100). https://doi.org/10.1098/rsif.2014.0817

Gehrke, S. H., Fisher, J. P., Palais, M., & Lund, M. E. (1997). Factors Determining Hydrogel Permeability. *Annals of the New York Academy of Sciences, 831*(1), 179–207. https://doi.org/10.1111/j.1749-6632.1997.tb52194.x

Giuliani, M., Moritz, W., Bodmer, E., Dindo, D., Kugelmeier, P., Lehmann, R., Gassmann, M., Groscurth, P., & Weber, M. (2005). Central necrosis in isolated hypoxic human pancreatic islets: Evidence for postisolation ischemia. *Cell Transplantation, 14*(1), 67–76.

https://doi.org/10.3727/000000005783983287

Goebel-Stengel, M., Stengelc, A., Tachéc, Y., & Reeve, Joseph R., J. (2011). The importance of using the optimal plastic and glassware in studies involving peptides. *Anal Biochem*, *414*(1), 38–46. https://doi.org/10.1016/j.ab.2011.02.009

Gombotz, W. R., & Wee, S. F. (1998). Protein release from alginate matrices. *Advanced Drug Delivery Reviews*, *31*(3), 267–285. https://doi.org/10.1016/S0169-409X(97)00124-5

Gonzalez-Fernandez, T., Rathan, S., Hobbs, C., Pitacco, P., Freeman, F. E., Cunniffe, G. M., Dunne, N. J., McCarthy, H. O., Nicolosi, V., O'Brien, F. J., & Kelly, D. J. (2019). Pore-forming bioinks to enable spatio-temporally defined gene delivery in bioprinted tissues. *Journal of Controlled Release*, *301*(May), 13–27. https://doi.org/10.1016/j.jconrel.2019.03.006

Grant, G. T., Morris, E. R., Rees, D. A., Smith, P. J. C., & Thom, D. (1973). Biological interactions between polysaccharides and divalent cations: The egg-box model. *FEBS Letters*, *32*(1), 195–198. https://doi.org/10.1016/0014-5793(73)80770-7

Grassi, M., Sandolo, C., Perin, D., Coviello, T., Lapasin, R., & Grassi, G. (2009). Structural characterization of calcium alginate matrices by means of mechanical and release tests. *Molecules*, *14*(8), 3003–3017. https://doi.org/10.3390/molecules14083003

Grosse, L., & Klaus, W. (1972). Die Analytik wasserlöslicher Celluloseäther. *Z. Anal. Chem.*, *259*(3), 195–203. https://doi.org/10.1007/BF00428439

Gusakov, A. V., Kondratyeva, E. G., & Sinitsyn, A. P. (2011). Comparison of Two Methods for Assaying Reducing Sugars in the Determination of Carbohydrase Activities. *International Journal of Analytical Chemistry*, *2011*, 1–4. https://doi.org/10.1155/2011/283658

Gutenwik, J., Nilsson, B., & Axelsson, A. (2004). Determination of protein diffusion coefficients in agarose gel with a diffusion cell. *Biochemical Engineering Journal*, *19*(1), 1–7. https://doi.org/10.1016/j.bej.2003.09.004

Halban, P. A., Powers, S. L., George, K. L., & Bonner-Weir, S. (1987). Spontaneous reassociation of dispersed adult rat pancreatic islet cells into aggregates with three-dimensional architecture typical of native islets. *Diabetes*, *36*(7), 783–790. https://doi.org/10.2337/diab.36.7.783

Hannoun, B. J. M., & Stephanopoulos, G. (1986). Diffusion coefficients of glucose and ethanol in cell-free and cell-occupied calcium alginate membranes. *Biotechnology and Bioengineering*, *28*(6), 829–835. https://doi.org/10.1002/bit.260280609

Harb, G., & Korbutt, G. S. (2006). Effect of prolonged in vitro exposure to high glucose on neonatal porcine pancreatic islets. *Journal of Endocrinology*, *191*(1), 37–44. https://doi.org/10.1677/joe.1.06812

Harb, G., Toreson, J., Dufour, J., & Korbutt, G. (2007). Acute exposure to streptozotocin but not human proinflammatory cytokines impairs neonatal porcine islet insulin secretion in vitro but not in vivo. *Xenotransplantation*, *14*(6), 580–590. https://doi.org/10.1111/j.1399-3089.2007.00427.x

Harding, J. L., Pavkov, M. E., Magliano, D. J., Shaw, J. E., & Gregg, E. W. (2019). Global trends in diabetes complications: a review of current evidence. *Diabetologia*, *62*(1), 3–16. https://doi.org/10.1007/s00125-018-4711-2

Hassouna, T., Seeberger, K. L., Salama, B., & Korbutt, G. S. (2018). Functional Maturation and in Vitro Differentiation of Neonatal Porcine Islet Grafts. *Transplantation*, *102*(10), e413–e423. https://doi.org/10.1097/TP.0000000000002354

Hayward, J. A., Ellis, C. E., Seeberger, K., Lee, T., Salama, B., Mulet-Sierra, A., Kuppan, P., Adesida, A., & Korbutt, G. S. (2017). Cotransplantation of mesenchymal stem cells with neonatal porcine islets improve graft function in diabetic mice. *Diabetes*, *66*(5), 1312–1321. https://doi.org/10.2337/db16-1068

He, S., Wang, C., Du, X., Chen, Y., Zhao, J., Tian, B., Lu, H., Zhang, Y., Liu, J., Yang, G., Li, L., Li, H., Cheng, J., & Lu, Y. (2018). MSCs promote the development and improve the function of neonatal porcine islet grafts. *FASEB Journal*, *32*(6), 3242–3253. https://doi.org/10.1096/fj.201700991R

Hellman, B. (1975). The significance of calcium for glucose stimulation of insulin release. *Endocrinology*, *97*(2), 392–398. https://doi.org/10.1210/endo-97-2-392

Hellman, B., Gylfe, E., Bergsten, P., Grapengiesser, E., Berts, A., Liu, Y. J., Tengholm, A., & Westerlund, J. (1997). Oscillatory signaling and insulin release in human pancreatic β-cells exposed to strontium. *Endocrinology*, *138*(8), 3161–3165. https://doi.org/10.1210/endo.138.8.5296

Helmich, U. (2018). *Diffusionsgesetze*. Website. http://www.u-helmich.de/bio/cytologie/05/051/seite052.html

Henquin, J. C. (1980). Specificity of divalent cation requirement for insulin release - Effects of strontium. *Pflügers Archiv European Journal of Physiology*, *383*(2), 123–129. https://doi.org/10.1007/BF00581872

Henriksson, H., Ståhlberg, J., Isaksson, R., & Pettersson, G. (1996). The active sites of cellulases are involved in chiral recognition: A comparison of cellobiohydrolase 1 and endoglucanase 1. *FEBS Letters*, *390*(3), 339–344. https://doi.org/10.1016/0014-5793(96)00685-0

Hering, B. J., Wijkstrom, M., Graham, M. L., Hårdstedt, M., Aasheim, T. C., Jie, T., Ansite, J. D., Nakano, M., Cheng, J., Li, W., Moran, K., Christians, U., Finnegan, C., Mills, C. D., Sutherland, D. E., Bansal-Pakala, P., Murtaugh, M. P., Kirchhof, N., & Schuurman, H. J. (2006). Prolonged diabetes reversal after intraportal xenotransplantation of wild-type porcine islets in immunosuppressed nonhuman primates. *Nature Medicine*, *12*(3), 301–303. https://doi.org/10.1038/nm1369

Heymann, E. (1935). Studies on sol-gel transformations. I. The inverse sol-gel transformation of methylcellulose in water. *Transactions of the Faraday Society*, *31*(846), 846–864. https://doi.org/10.1039/tf9353100846

Hill, J. B. (1959). The adsorption of I131-insulin to glass. *Endocrinology*, *65*(3), 515–517. https://doi.org/10.1210/endo-65-3-515

Hirrien, M., Desbrières, J., & Rinaudo, M. (1996). Physical properties of methylcelluloses in relation with the conditions for cellulose modification. *Carbohydrate Polymers*, *31*(4), 243–252. https://doi.org/10.1016/S0144-8617(96)00118-X

Hoang, D. T., Matsunari, H., Nagaya, M., Nagashima, H., Millis, J. M., Witkowski, P., Periwal, V., Hara, M., & Jo, J. (2014). A conserved rule for pancreatic islet organization. *PLoS ONE*, *9*(10), 1–9. https://doi.org/10.1371/journal.pone.0110384

Hodder, E., Duin, S., Kilian, D., Ahlfeld, T., Seidel, J., Nachtigall, C., Bush, P., Covill, D., Gelinsky, M., & Lode, A. (2019). Investigating the effect of sterilisation methods on the physical properties and cytocompatibility of methyl cellulose used in combination with alginate for 3D-bioplotting of chondrocytes. *Journal of Materials Science: Materials in Medicine*, *30*(1). https://doi.org/10.1007/s10856-018-6211-9

Hofmeister, F. (1888). Zur Lehre von der Wirkung der Salze. *Arch. Exp. Pathol. Pharmakol.*, *25*, 1–30. https://doi.org/10.1007/BF01838161

Höger, K. (2014). *Investigations on Protein Adsorption to Coated Glass Vials* [book]. Ludwig-Maximilians-Universität München.

Holte, O., Tønnesen, H. H., & Karlsen, J. (2006). Measurement of diffusion through calcium alginate gel matrices. *Die Pharmazie*, *61*(1), 30–34. http://www.ncbi.nlm.nih.gov/pubmed/16454203

Horn, J. M., & Onoda, G. Y. (1978). Surface Charge of Vitreous Silica and Silicate Glasses in Aqueous Electrolyte Solutions. *Journal of the American Ceramic Society*, *61*(11–12), 523–527. https://doi.org/10.1111/j.1151-2916.1978.tb16132.x

Hummert, E., Henniges, U., & Potthast, A. (2013). Fluorescence labeling of gelatin and methylcellulose: Monitoring their penetration behavior into paper. *Cellulose*, *20*(2), 919–931. https://doi.org/10.1007/s10570-013-9864-z

Hunt, N. C., Shelton, R. M., & Grover, L. M. (2009). An alginate hydrogel matrix for the localised delivery of a fibroblast/keratinocyte co-culture. *Biotechnology Journal*, *4*(5), 730–737. https://doi.org/10.1002/biot.200800292

Hwa, A. J., & Weir, G. C. (2018). Transplantation of Macroencapsulated Insulin-Producing Cells. *Current Diabetes Reports*, *18*(8). https://doi.org/10.1007/s11892-018-1028-y

Hyman, A. A., & Mitchison, T. J. (1993). An Assay for the Activity of Microtubule-Based Motors on the Kinetochores of Isolated Chinese Hamster Ovary Chromosomes. In J. M. Scholey (Ed.), *Methods in Cell Biology* (Vol. 39, Issue C, pp. 267–276). Academic Press, Inc.

https://doi.org/10.1016/s0091-679x(08)60176-4

Jansson, L., Barbu, A., Bodin, B., Drott, C. J., Espes, D., Gao, X., Grapensparr, L., Källskog, Ö., Lau, J., Liljebäck, H., Palm, F., Quach, M., Sandberg, M., Strömberg, V., Ullsten, S., & Carlsson, P. O. (2016). Pancreatic islet blood flow and its measurement. *Upsala Journal of Medical Sciences*, *121*(2), 81–95. https://doi.org/10.3109/03009734.2016.1164769

Jeong, J. Y., Park, S. H., Shin, J. W., Kang, Y. G., Han, K. H., & Shin, J. W. (2012). Effects of intermittent hydrostatic pressure magnitude on the chondrogenesis of MSCs without biochemical agents under 3D co-culture. *Journal of Materials Science: Materials in Medicine*, *23*(11), 2773–2781. https://doi.org/10.1007/s10856-012-4718-z

Jeworrek, C., Hollmann, O., Steitz, R., Winter, R., & Czeslik, C. (2009). Interaction of IAPP and insulin with model interfaces studied using neutron reflectometry. *Biophysical Journal*, *96*(3), 1115–1123. https://doi.org/10.1016/j.bpj.2008.11.006

Jeyachandran, Y. L., Mielczarski, J. A., Mielczarski, E., & Rai, B. (2010). Efficiency of blocking of non-specific interaction of different proteins by BSA adsorbed on hydrophobic and hydrophilic surfaces. *Journal of Colloid and Interface Science*, *341*(1), 136–142. https://doi.org/10.1016/j.jcis.2009.09.007

Jo, J., Moo, Y. C., & Koh, D. S. (2007). Size distribution of mouse Langerhans islets. *Biophysical Journal*, *93*(8), 2655–2666. https://doi.org/10.1529/biophysj.107.104125

Johnson, A. S., Fisher, R. J., Weir, G. C., & Colton, C. K. (2009). Oxygen consumption and diffusion in assemblages of respiring spheres: Performance enhancement of a bioartificial pancreas. *Chemical Engineering Science*, *64*(22), 4470–4487. https://doi.org/10.1016/j.ces.2009.06.028

Jun, Y., Kim, M. J., Hwang, Y. H., Jeon, E. A., Kang, A. R., Lee, S. H., & Lee, D. Y. (2013). Microfluidics-generated pancreatic islet microfibers for enhanced immunoprotection. *Biomaterials*, *34*(33), 8122–8130. https://doi.org/10.1016/j.biomaterials.2013.07.079

Jun, Y., Lee, J. S., Choi, S., Yang, J. H., Sander, M., Chung, S., & Lee, S. H. (2019). In vivo–mimicking microfluidic perfusion culture of pancreatic islet spheroids. *Science Advances*, *5*(11), 1–13. https://doi.org/10.1126/sciadv.aax4520

Juturu, V., & Wu, J. C. (2014). Microbial cellulases: Engineering, production and applications. *Renewable and Sustainable Energy Reviews*, *33*, 188–203. https://doi.org/10.1016/j.rser.2014.01.077

Ka-ming Chan, F., Moriwaki, K., & De Rosa, M. J. (2013). Detection of Necrosis by Release of Lactate Dehydrogenase (LDH) Activity. *Methods in Molecular Biology*, *979*, 65–70. https://doi.org/10.1007/978-1-62703-290-2_7

Kailemia, M. J., Ruhaak, L. R., Lebrilla, C. B., & Amster, I. J. (2014). Oligosaccharide Analysis By Mass Spectrometry: A Review Of Recent Developments. *Anal Chem*, *86*(1), 196–212. https://doi.org/10.1021/ac403969n

Kaja, S., Payne, A. J., Naumchuk, Y., & Koulen, P. (2017). Quantification of lactate dehydrogenase for cell viability testing using cell lines and primary cultured astrocytes. *Current Protocols in Toxicology*, *72*(1), 2.26.1–2.26.10. https://doi.org/10.1002/cptx.21

Kaneto, H., Kajimoto, Y., Miyagawa, J. ichiro, Matsuoka, T. aki, Fujitani, Y., Umayahara, Y., Hanafusa, T., Matsuzawa, Y., Yamasaki, Y., & Hori, M. (1999). Beneficial effects of antioxidants in diabetes: Possible protection of pancreatic β-cells against glucose toxicity. *Diabetes*, *48*(12), 2398–2406. https://doi.org/10.2337/diabetes.48.12.2398

Karaoz, E., Genç, Z. S., Demircan, P. Ç., Aksoy, A., & Duruksu, G. (2010). Protection of rat pancreatic islet function and viability by coculture with rat bone marrow-derived mesenchymal stem cells. *Cell Death and Disease*, *1*(4), 1–9. https://doi.org/10.1038/cddis.2010.14

Kelly, C., McClenaghan, N. H., & Flatt, P. R. (2011). Role of islet structure and cellular interactions in the control of insulin secretion. *Islets*, *3*(2), 41–47. https://doi.org/10.4161/isl.3.2.14805

Kim, A., Miller, K., Jo, J., Kilimnik, G., Wojcik, P., & Hara, M. (2009). Islet architecture: A comparative study. *Islets*, *1*(2), 129–136. https://doi.org/10.4161/isl.1.2.9480

Kim, J., Shim, I. K., Hwang, D. G., Lee, Y. N., Kim, M., Kim, H., Kim, S. W., Lee, S., Kim, S. C., Cho, D. W., & Jang, J. (2019). 3D cell printing of islet-laden pancreatic tissue-derived extracellular matrix bioink constructs for enhancing pancreatic functions. *Journal of Materials Chemistry B*, *7*(10), 1773–1781. https://doi.org/10.1039/c8tb02787k

Kin, T., & Korbutt, G. S. (2007). Delayed functional maturation of neonatal porcine islets in recipients under strict glycemic control. *Xenotransplantation*, *14*(4), 333–338. https://doi.org/10.1111/j.1399-3089.2007.00414.x

Kin, T., Senior, P., O'Gorman, D., Richer, B., Salam, A., & Shapiro, A. M. J. (2008). Risk factors for islet loss during culture prior to transplantation. *Transplant International*, *21*(11), 1029–1035. https://doi.org/10.1111/j.1432-2277.2008.00719.x

Kitzmann, J. P., Law, L., Shome, A., Muzina, M., Elliott, R. B., Mueller, K. R., Schuurman, H. J., & Papas, K. K. (2012). Real-time assessment of encapsulated neonatal porcine islets prior to clinical xenotransplantation. *Xenotransplantation*, *19*(6), 333–336. https://doi.org/10.1111/xen.12005

Klein, J., Stock, J., & Vorlop, K. D. (1983). Pore Size and Properties of Spherical Ca-Alginate Biocatalysts. *European Journal of Applied Microbiology and Biotechnology*, *18*(2), 86–91. https://doi.org/10.1007/BF00500829

Klöck, G., Frank, H., Houben, R., Zekorn, T., Horcher, A., Siebers, U., Wöhrle, M., Federlin, K., & Zimmermann, U. (1994). Production of purified alginates suitable for use in immunoisolated transplantation. *Applied Microbiology and Biotechnology*, *40*(5), 638–643. https://doi.org/10.1007/BF00173321

Knarr, M. (2003). *Rheologische Untersuchung und Modellierung der Sol-Gel-Charakteristika von Methylcellulose und κ-Carrageenan* [book]. Universität Hamburg.

Koch, H. H., & Pimsler, M. (1987). Evaluation of Uvitex 2B: A Nonspecific Fluorescent Stain for Detecting and Identifying Fungi and Algae in Tissue. *Laboratory Medicine*, *18*(9), 603–606. https://doi.org/10.1093/labmed/18.9.603

Köllmer, M., Appel, A. A., Somo, S. I., & Brey, E. M. (2016). Long-Term Function of Alginate-Encapsulated Islets. *Tissue Engineering Part B: Reviews*, *22*(1), 34–46. https://doi.org/10.1089/ten.teb.2015.0140

Komatsu, H., Cook, C., Wang, C. H., Medrano, L., Lin, H., Kandeel, F., Tai, Y. C., & Mullen, Y. (2017). Oxygen environment and islet size are the primary limiting factors of isolated pancreatic islet survival. *PLoS ONE*, *12*(8), 1–17. https://doi.org/10.1371/journal.pone.0183780

Korbutt, G. S., Elliott, J. F., Ao, Z., Smith, D. K., Warnock, G. L., & Rajotte, R. V. (1996). Large scale isolation, growth, and function of porcine neonatal islet cells. *Journal of Clinical Investigation*, *97*(9), 2119–2129. https://doi.org/10.1172/JCI118649

Korsgren, O. (2017). Islet encapsulation: Physiological possibilities and limitations. *Diabetes*, *66*(7), 1748–1754. https://doi.org/10.2337/db17-0065

Kumagai-Braesch, M., Jacobson, S., Mori, H., Jia, X., Takahashi, T., Wernerson, A., Flodström-Tullberg, M., & Tibell, A. (2013). The theracyte™ device protects against islet allograft rejection in immunized hosts. *Cell Transplantation*, *22*(7), 1137–1146. https://doi.org/10.3727/096368912X657486

Kundu, J., Shim, J.-H., Jang, J., Kim, S.-W., & Cho, D.-W. (2015). An additive manufacturing-based PCL-alginate-chondrocyte bioprinted scaffold for cartilage tissue engineering. *Journal of Tissue Engineering and Regenerative Medicine*, *9*(11), 1286–1297. https://doi.org/10.1002/term.1682

Kuo, C. K., & Ma, P. X. (2008). Maintaining dimensions and mechanical properties of ionically crosslinked alginate hydrogel scaffolds in vitro. *Journal of Biomedical Materials Research - Part A*, *84*(4), 899–907. https://doi.org/10.1002/jbm.a.31375

Lacy, P. E., Hegre, O. D., Gerasimidi-Vazeou, A., Gentile, F. T., & Dionne, K. E. (1991). Maintenance of Normoglycemia in Diabetic Mice by Subcutaneous Xenografts of Encapsulated Islets. *Technology*, *254*, 2–4. https://doi.org/10.1126/science.1763328

Lamb, M., Storrs, R., Li, S., Liang, O., Laugenour, K., Dorian, R., Chapman, D., Ichii, H., Imagawa, D., Foster, C., King, S., & Lakey, J. R. T. (2011). Function and viability of human islets encapsulated in alginate sheets: In vitro and in vivo culture. *Transplantation Proceedings*, *43*(9), 3265–3266. https://doi.org/10.1016/j.transproceed.2011.10.028

Lang, F., & Lang, P. (2007). *Basiswissen Physiologie* (2nd ed.). Springer Medizin Verlag.

Langlois, G., Dusseault, J., Bilodeau, S., Tam, S. K., Magassouba, D., & Hallé, J. P. (2009).

Direct effect of alginate purification on the survival of islets immobilized in alginate-based microcapsules. *Acta Biomaterialia, 5*(9), 3433–3440. https://doi.org/10.1016/j.actbio.2009.05.029

Lanza, R. P., Kühtreiber, W. M., Ecker, D., Staruk, J. E., & Chick, W. L. (1995). Xenotransplantation of Porcine and Bovine Islets Without Immunosuppression Using Uncoated Alginate Microspheres. *Transplantation, 59*(10), 1377–1384. https://doi.org/10.1097/00007890-199505270-00003

Lee, E.-M., Lee, Y.-E., Lee, E., Ryu, G. R., Ko, S.-H., Moon, S.-D., Song, K.-H., & Ahn, Y.-B. (2011). Protective Effect of Heme Oxygenase-1 on High Glucose-Induced Pancreatic β-Cell Injury. *Diabetes & Metabolism Journal, 35*(5), 469. https://doi.org/10.4093/dmj.2011.35.5.469

Lee, K. Y., & Mooney, D. J. (2012). Alginate: Properties and biomedical applications. *Progress in Polymer Science (Oxford), 37*(1), 106–126. https://doi.org/10.1016/j.progpolymsci.2011.06.003

Lehmann, R., Zuellig, R. A., Kugelmeier, P., Baenninger, P. B., Moritz, W., Perren, A., Clavien, P. A., Weber, M., & Spinas, G. A. (2007). Superiority of small islets in human islet transplantation. *Diabetes, 56*(3), 594–603. https://doi.org/10.2337/db06-0779

Li, H., Tan, Y. J., Leong, K. F., & Li, L. (2017). 3D Bioprinting of Highly Thixotropic Alginate/Methylcellulose Hydrogel with Strong Interface Bonding. *ACS Applied Materials & Interfaces, 9*(23), 20086–20097. https://doi.org/10.1021/acsami.7b04216

Li, X., Meng, Q., & Zhang, L. (2019). Overcoming Immunobiological Barriers Against Porcine Islet Xenografts: What Should Be Done? *Pancreas 48*(3), 299–308. https://doi.org/10.1097/MPA.0000000000001259

Liang, H. F., Hong, M. H., Ho, R. M., Chung, C. K., Lin, Y. H., Chen, C. H., & Sung, H. W. (2004). Novel method using a temperature-sensitive polymer (methylcellulose) to thermally gel aqueous alginate as a pH-sensitive hydrogel. *Biomacromolecules, 5*(5), 1917–1925. https://doi.org/10.1021/bm049813w

Lin, Y. F., Jan, Y. N., & Jan, L. Y. (2000). Regulation of ATP-sensitive potassium channel function by protein kinase A-mediated phosphorylation in transfected HEK293 cells. *EMBO Journal, 19*(5), 942–955. https://doi.org/10.1093/emboj/19.5.942

Liu, J., Zheng, H., Poh, P. S. P., Machens, H. G., & Schilling, A. F. (2015). Hydrogels for engineering of perfusable vascular networks. *International Journal of Molecular Sciences, 16*(7), 15997–16016. https://doi.org/10.3390/ijms160715997

Liu, X., Carter, S. S. D., Renes, M. J., Kim, J., Rojas-Canales, D. M., Penko, D., Angus, C., Beirne, S., Drogemuller, C. J., Yue, Z., Coates, P. T., & Wallace, G. G. (2019). Development of a Coaxial 3D Printing Platform for Biofabrication of Implantable Islet-Containing Constructs. *Advanced Healthcare Materials, 8*(7), 1–12.

https://doi.org/10.1002/adhm.201801181

Livingstone, S. J., Levin, D., Looker, H. C., Lindsay, R. S., Wild, S. H., Joss, N., Leese, G., Leslie, P., McCrimmon, R. J., Metcalfe, W., McKnight, J. A., Morris, A. D., Pearson, D. W. M., Petrie, J. R., Philip, S., Sattar, N. A., Traynor, J. P., & Colhoun, H. M. (2015). Estimated life expectancy in a scottish cohort with type 1 diabetes, 2008-2010. *JAMA - Journal of the American Medical Association*, *313*(1), 37–44. https://doi.org/10.1001/jama.2014.16425

Llacua, L. A., Hoek, A., de Haan, B. J., & de Vos, P. (2018). Collagen type VI interaction improves human islet survival in immunoisolating microcapsules for treatment of diabetes. *Islets*, *10*(2), 60–68. https://doi.org/10.1080/19382014.2017.1420449

Lode, A., Krujatz, F., Brüggemeier, S., Quade, M., Schütz, K., Knaack, S., Weber, J., Bley, T., & Gelinsky, M. (2015). Green bioprinting: Fabrication of photosynthetic algae-laden hydrogel scaffolds for biotechnological and medical applications. *Engineering in Life Sciences*, *15*(2), 177–183. https://doi.org/10.1002/elsc.201400205

Luca, G., Nastruzzi, C., Calvitti, M., Becchetti, E., Baroni, T., Neri, L. M., Capitani, S., Basta, G., Brunetti, P., & Calafiore, R. (2005). Accelerated functional maturation of isolated neonatal porcine cell clusters: In vitro and in vivo results in NOD mice. *Cell Transplantation*, *14*(5), 249–261. https://doi.org/10.3727/000000005783983034

Ludwig, B., Ludwig, S., Steffen, A., Knauf, Y., Zimerman, B., Heinke, S., Lehmann, S., Schubert, U., Schmid, J., Bleyer, M., Schönmann, U., Colton, C. K., Bonifacio, E., Solimena, M., Reichel, A., Schally, A. V., Rotem, A., Barkai, U., Grinberg-Rashi, H., … Bornstein, S. R. (2017). Favorable outcome of experimental islet xenotransplantation without immunosuppression in a nonhuman primate model of diabetes. *Proceedings of the National Academy of Sciences of the USA*, *114*(44), 11745–11750. https://doi.org/10.1073/pnas.1708420114

Ludwig, B., Ludwig, S., Steffen, A., Saeger, H. D., & Bornstein, S. R. (2010). Islet versus pancreas transplantation in type 1 diabetes: Competitive or complementary? *Current Diabetes Reports*, *10*(6), 506–511. https://doi.org/10.1007/s11892-010-0146-y

Ludwig, B., Reichel, A., Steffen, A., Zimerman, B., Schally, A. V., Block, N. L., Colton, C. K., Ludwig, S., Kersting, S., Bonifacio, E., Solimena, M., Gendler, Z., Rotem, A., Barkai, U., & Bornstein, S. R. (2013). Transplantation of human islets without immunosuppression. *Proceedings of the National Academy of Sciences of the USA*, *110*(47), 19054–19058. https://doi.org/10.1073/pnas.1317561110

Ludwig, B., Rotem, A., Schmid, J., Weir, G. C., Colton, C. K., Brendel, M. D., Neufeld, T., Block, N. L., Yavriyants, K., Steffen, A., Ludwig, S., Chavakis, T., Reichel, A., Azarov, D., Zimermann, B., Maimon, S., Balyura, M., Rozenshtein, T., Shabtay, N., … Barkai, U. (2012). Improvement of islet function in a bioartificial pancreas by enhanced oxygen supply and growth hormone releasing hormone agonist. *Proceedings of the National Academy of Sciences of the USA*, *109*(13), 5022–5027. https://doi.org/10.1073/pnas.1201868109

MacGregor, R. R., Williams, S. J., Tong, P. Y., Kover, K., Moore, W. V., & Stehno-Bittel, L. (2006). Small rat islets are superior to large islets in in vitro function and in transplantation outcomes. *American Journal of Physiology - Endocrinology and Metabolism*, *290*(5), 771–779. https://doi.org/10.1152/ajpendo.00097.2005

MacKenzie, D. A., Hullett, D. A., & Sollinger, H. W. (2003). Xenogeneic transplantation of porcine islets: An overview. *Transplantation 76*(6), 887–891. https://doi.org/10.1097/01.TP.0000087114.18315.17

Malda, J., Visser, J., Melchels, F. P., Jüngst, T., Hennink, W. E., Dhert, W. J. A., Groll, J., & Hutmacher, D. W. (2013). 25th anniversary article: Engineering hydrogels for biofabrication. *Advanced Materials*, *25*(36), 5011–5028. https://doi.org/10.1002/adma.201302042

Mallett, A. G., & Korbutt, G. S. (2009). Alginate modification improves long-term survival and function of transplanted encapsulated islets. *Tissue Engineering - Part A*, *15*(6), 1301–1309. https://doi.org/10.1089/ten.tea.2008.0118

Malusis, M. A., Shackelford, C. D., & Olsen, H. W. (2001). A Laboratory Apparatus to Measure Chemico-Osmotic Efficiency Coefficients for Clay Soils. *Geotechnical Testing Journal*, *24*(3), 229–242. https://doi.org/10.1520/gtj11343j

Manell, E., Hedenqvist, P., Svensson, A., & Jensen-Waern, M. (2016). Establishment of a refined oral glucose tolerance test in pigs, and assessment of insulin, glucagon and glucagon-like peptide-1 responses. *PLoS ONE*, *11*(2), 1–14. https://doi.org/10.1371/journal.pone.0148896

Mansur, H. S., Lobato, Z. P., Oréfice, R. L., Vasconcelos, W. L., Oliveira, C., & Machado, L. J. (2000). Surface functionalization of porous glass networks: Effects on bovine serum albumin and porcine insulin immobilization. *Biomacromolecules*, *1*(4), 789–797. https://doi.org/10.1021/bm0056198

Marchioli, G., Van Gurp, L., Van Krieken, P. P., Stamatialis, D., Engelse, M., Van Blitterswijk, C. A., Karperien, M. B. J., De Koning, E., Alblas, J., Moroni, L., & Van Apeldoorn, A. A. (2015). Fabrication of three-dimensional bioplotted hydrogel scaffolds for islets of Langerhans transplantation. *Biofabrication*, *7*(2), 025009. https://doi.org/10.1088/1758-5090/7/2/025009

Marshall, W., Lapsley, M., Day, A., & Ayling, R. (2014). *Clinical Biochemistry: Metabolic and Clinical Aspects* (3rd ed.). Churchill Livingstone Elsevier. https://doi.org/10.1016/B978-0-7020-5140-1.00015-8

Martinsen, A., Skjåk-Braek, G., & Smidsrød, O. (1989). Alginate as immobilization material: I.

Correlation between chemical and physical properties of alginate gel beads. *Biotechnology and Bioengineering*, *33*(1), 79–89. https://doi.org/10.1002/bit.260330111

Matai, I., Kaur, G., Seyedsalehi, A., McClinton, A., & Laurencin, C. T. (2020). Progress in 3D bioprinting technology for tissue/organ regenerative engineering. *Biomaterials*, *226*(September 2019), 119536. https://doi.org/10.1016/j.biomaterials.2019.119536

Matsumoto, S., Tan, P., Baker, J., Durbin, K., Tomiya, M., Azuma, K., Doi, M., & Elliott, R. B. (2014). Clinical porcine islet xenotransplantation under comprehensive regulation. *Transplantation Proceedings*, *46*(6), 1992–1995. https://doi.org/10.1016/j.transproceed.2014.06.008

Matsumoto, S., Abalovich, A., Wechsler, C., Wynyard, S., & Elliott, R. B. (2016). Clinical Benefit of Islet Xenotransplantation for the Treatment of Type 1 Diabetes. *EBioMedicine*, *12*, 255–262. https://doi.org/10.1016/j.ebiom.2016.08.034

Mazzini, V., & Craig, V. S. J. (2017). What is the fundamental ion-specific series for anions and cations? Ion specificity in standard partial molar volumes of electrolytes and electrostriction in water and non-aqueous solvents. *Chemical Science*, *8*(10), 7052–7065. https://doi.org/10.1039/c7sc02691a

McCall, M., & Shapiro, A. M. J. (2012). Update on islet transplantation. *Cold Spring Harbor Perspectives in Medicine*, *2*(7). https://doi.org/10.1101/cshperspect.a007823

Melander, C., Adden, R., Brinkmalm, G., Gorton, L., & Mischnick, P. (2006). New approaches to the analysis of enzymatically hydrolyzed methyl cellulose. Part 2. Comparison of various enzyme preparations. *Biomacromolecules*, *7*(5), 1410–1421. https://doi.org/10.1021/bm0509422

Miller, K. M., Foster, N. C., Beck, R. W., Bergensta, R. M., DuBose, S. N., DiMeglio, L. A., Maahs, D. M., & Tamborlane, W. V. (2015). Current State of Type 1 Diabetes Treatment in the U.S.: Updated Data From the T1D Exchange Clinic Registry. *Diabetes Care*, *38*(6), 971–978. https://doi.org/10.2337/dc15-0078

Montanucci, P., Terenzi, S., Santi, C., Pennoni, I., Bini, V., Pescara, T., Basta, G., & Calafiore, R. (2015). Insights in behavior of variably formulated alginate-based microcapsules for cell transplantation. *BioMed Research International*, *2015*. https://doi.org/10.1155/2015/965804

Mørch, Ý. A., Donati, I., Strand, B. L., & Skjåk-Bræk, G. (2006). Effect of Ca2+, Ba2+, and Sr2+ on alginate microbeads. *Biomacromolecules*, *7*(5), 1471–1480. https://doi.org/10.1021/bm060010d

Morini, S., Braun, M., Onori, P., Cicalese, L., Elias, G., Gaudio, E., & Rastellini, C. (2006). Morphological changes of isolated rat pancreatic islets: A structural, ultrastructural and morphometric study. *Journal of Anatomy*, *209*(3), 381–392. https://doi.org/10.1111/j.1469-7580.2006.00620.x

Mourad, N. I., & Gianello, P. (2019). Long-term culture and in vitro maturation of macroencapsulated adult and neonatal porcine islets. *Xenotransplantation, 26*(2), 22–26. https://doi.org/10.1111/xen.12461

Mourad, N. I., Perota, A., Xhema, D., Galli, C., & Gianello, P. (2017). Transgenic Expression of Glucagon-Like Peptide-1 (GLP-1) and Activated Muscarinic Receptor (M3R) Significantly Improves Pig Islet Secretory Function Nizar. *Cell Transplantation, 26*(5), 901–911. https://doi.org/10.3727/096368916X693798

Musuc, A. M., Dumitru, R., Stan, A., Munteanu, C., Birjega, R., & Carp, O. (2015). Synthesis, characterization and thermoreactivity of some methylcellulose-zinc composites. *Journal of Thermal Analysis and Calorimetry, 120*(1), 85–94. https://doi.org/10.1007/s10973-015-4415-5

Nafea, E. H., Poole-Warren, A. M. L. A., & Martens, P. J. (2011). Immunoisolating semi-permeable membranes for cell encapsulation: Focus on hydrogels. *Journal of Controlled Release, 154*(2), 110–122. https://doi.org/10.1016/j.jconrel.2011.04.022

Najdahmadi, A., Lakey, J. R. T., & Botvinick, E. (2018). Diffusion coefficient of alginate microcapsules used in pancreatic islet transplantation, a method to cure type 1 diabetes. *Proc. SPIE, 10506*. https://doi.org/10.1117/12.2318565

Narang, A. S., & Mahato, R. I. (2006). Biological and Biomaterial Approaches for Improved Islet Transplantation. *Pharmacological Reviews, 58*(2), 194–243. https://doi.org/10.1124/pr.58.2.6.194

Nasatto, P. L., Pignon, F., Silveira, J. L. M., Duarte, M. E. R., Noseda, M. D., & Rinaudo, M. (2015). Methylcellulose, a cellulose derivative with original physical properties and extended applications. *Polymers, 7*(5), 777-803. DOI: 10.3390/polym7050777

Nesher, R., & Cerasi, E. (2002). Modeling phasic insulin release: Immediate and time-dependent effects of glucose. *Diabetes, 51*(SUPPL.), 53–59. https://doi.org/10.2337/diabetes.51.2007.s53

Nielsen, S. P. (2004). The biological role of strontium. *Bone, 35*(3), 583–588. https://doi.org/10.1016/j.bone.2004.04.026

Nielsen, T. B., Yderstraede, K. B., Schrøder, H. D., Holst, J. J., Brusgaard, K., & Beck-Nielsen, H. (2003). Functional and immunohistochemical evaluation of porcine neonatal islet-like cell clusters. *Cell Transplantation, 12*(1), 13–25. https://doi.org/10.3727/000000003783985142

Noguchi, H., Miyagi-shiohira, C., Kurima, K., Kobayashi, N., Saitoh, I., Watanabe, M., Noguchi, Y., & Matsushita, M. (2015). Islet Culture/Preservation Before Islet Transplantation. *Cell Medicine, 8*, 25–29. https://doi.org/http://dx.doi.org/10.3727/215517915X689047

Olack, B. J., Jaramillo, A., Benshoff, N. D., Kaleem, Z., Swanson, C. J., Lowell, J. A., & Mohanakumar, T. (2002). Rejection of porcine islet xenografts mediated by CD4+ T cells activated through the indirect antigen recognition pathway. *Xenotransplantation*, *9*(6), 393–401. https://doi.org/10.1034/j.1399-3089.2002.01070.x

Omer, A., Duvivier-Kali, V. F., Trivedi, N., Wilmot, K., Bonner-Weir, S., & Weir, G. C. (2003). Survival and maturation of microencapsulated porcine neonatal pancreatic cell clusters transplanted into immunocompetent diabetic mice. *Diabetes*, *52*(1), 69–75. https://doi.org/10.2337/diabetes.52.1.69

Omer, A., Duvivier-Kali, V., Fernandes, J., Tchipashvili, V., Colton, C. K., & Weir, G. C. (2005). Long-term normoglycemia in rats receiving transplants with encapsulated islets. *Transplantation*, *79*(1), 52–58. https://doi.org/10.1097/01.TP.0000149340.37865.46

Opara, E. C., & Kendall, W. F. (2002). Immunoisolation techniques for islet cell transplantation. *Expert Opinion on Biological Therapy*, *2*(5), 503–511. https://doi.org/10.1517/14712598.2.5.503

Orive, G., Ponce, S., Hernández, R. M., Gascón, A. R., Igartua, M., & Pedraz, J. L. (2002). Biocompatibility of microcapsules for cell immobilization elaborated with different type of alginates. *Biomaterials*, *23*(18), 3825–3831. https://doi.org/10.1016/S0142-9612(02)00118-7

Otonkoski, T., Ustinov, J., Rasilainen, S., Kallio, E., Korsgren, O., & Häyry, P. (1999). Differentiation and maturation of porcine fetal islet cells in vitro and after transplantation. *Transplantation*, *68*(11), 1674–1683. https://doi.org/10.1097/00007890-199912150-00010

Pape, H.-C., Kurtz, A., & Silbernagl, S. (Eds.). (2018). *Physiologie* (8th ed.). Thieme.

Paredes Juárez, G. A., Spasojevic, M., Faas, M. M., & de Vos, P. (2014). Immunological and Technical Considerations in Application of Alginate-Based Microencapsulation Systems. *Frontiers in Bioengineering and Biotechnology*, *2*(AUG). https://doi.org/10.3389/fbioe.2014.00026

Park, J. Y., Choi, Y. J., Shim, J. H., Park, J. H., & Cho, D. W. (2017). Development of a 3D cell printed structure as an alternative to autologs cartilage for auricular reconstruction. *Journal of Biomedical Materials Research - Part B Applied Biomaterials*, *105*(5), 1016–1028. https://doi.org/10.1002/jbm.b.33639

Park, S. J., Shin, S., Koo, O. J., Moon, J. H., Jang, G., Ahn, C., Lee, B. C., & Yoo, Y. J. (2012). Functional improvement of porcine neonatal pancreatic cell clusters via conformal encapsulation using an air-driven encapsulator. *Experimental and Molecular Medicine*, *44*(1), 20–25. https://doi.org/10.3858/emm.2012.44.1.001

Pellegrini, S., Cantarelli, E., Sordi, V., Nano, R., & Piemonti, L. (2016). The state of the art of islet transplantation and cell therapy in type 1 diabetes. *Acta Diabetologica*, *53*(5), 683–691. https://doi.org/10.1007/s00592-016-0847-z

Pepper, A. R., Bruni, A., & Shapiro, A. M. J. (2018). Clinical islet transplantation: Is the future finally now? *Current Opinion in Organ Transplantation*, 23(4), 428–439. https://doi.org/10.1097/MOT.0000000000000546

Pepper, A. R., Pawlick, R., Gala-Lopez, B., MacGillivary, A., Mazzuca, D. M., White, D. J. G., Toleikis, P. M., & James Shapiro, A. M. (2015). Diabetes is reversed in a murine model by marginal mass syngeneic islet transplantation using a subcutaneous cell pouch device. *Transplantation*, 99(11), 2294–2300. https://doi.org/10.1097/TP.0000000000000864

Petersen, M. C., & Shulman, G. I. (2018). Mechanisms of insulin action and insulin resistance. *Physiological Reviews*, 98(4), 2133–2223. https://doi.org/10.1152/physrev.00063.2017

Pileggi, A., Molano, R. D., Ricordi, C., Zahr, E., Collins, J., Valdes, R., & Inverardi, L. (2006). Reversal of diabetes by pancreatic islet transplantation into a subcutaneous, neovascularized device. *Transplantation*, 81(9), 1318–1324. https://doi.org/10.1097/01.tp.0000203858.41105.88

Polonsky, K. S., Licinio-Paixao, J., Given, B. D., Pugh, W., Rue, P., Galloway, J., Karrison, T., & Frank, B. (1986). Use of biosynthetic human C-peptide in the measurement of insulin secretion rates in normal volunteers and type I diabetic patients. *Journal of Clinical Investigation*, 77(1), 98–105. https://doi.org/10.1172/JCI112308

Portha, B., Giroix, M. H., Serradas, P., Welsh, N., Hellerstrom, C., Sener, A., & Malaisse, W. J. (1988). Insulin production and glucose metabolism in isolated pancreatic islets of rats with NIDDM. *Diabetes*, 37(9), 1226–1233. https://doi.org/10.2337/diab.37.9.1226

Qi, M., Mørch, Y., Lacík, I., Formo, K., Marchese, E., Wang, Y., Danielson, K. K., Kinzer, K., Wang, S., Barbaro, B., Kolláriková, G., Chorvát, D., Hunkeler, D., Skjåk-Braek, G., Oberholzer, J., & Strand, B. L. (2012). Survival of human islets in microbeads containing high guluronic acid alginate crosslinked with Ca2+ and Ba2+. *Xenotransplantation*, 19(6), 355–364. https://doi.org/10.1111/xen.12009

Rackham, C. L., Dhadda, P. K., Le Lay, A. M., King, A. J. F., & Jones, P. M. (2014). Preculturing Islets with Adipose-Derived Mesenchymal Stromal Cells is an Effective Strategy for Improving Transplantation Efficiency at the Clinically Preferred Intraportal Site. *Cell Medicine*, 7(1), 37–47. https://doi.org/10.3727/215517914x680047

Rackham, C. L., Jones, P. M., & King, A. J. F. (2013). Maintenance of Islet Morphology Is Beneficial for Transplantation Outcome in Diabetic Mice. *PLoS ONE*, 8(2). https://doi.org/10.1371/journal.pone.0057844

Rasconi, S., Jobard, M., Jouve, L., & Sime-Ngando, T. (2009). Use of calcofluor white for detection, identification, and quantification of phytoplanktonic fungal parasites. *Applied and Environmental Microbiology*, 75(8), 2545–2553. https://doi.org/10.1128/AEM.02211-08

Rayat, G. R., Rajotte, R. V., Hering, B. J., Binette, T. M., & Korbutt, G. S. (2003). In vitro and in vivo expression of Galα-(1,3)Gal on porcine islet cells is age dependent. *Journal of*

Endocrinology, 177(1), 127–135. https://doi.org/10.1677/joe.0.1770127

Rayat, G. R., Rajotte, R. V., Ao, Z., & Korbutt, G. S. (2000). Microencapsulation of neonatal porcine islets: Protection from human antibody/complement-mediated cytolysis in vitro and long-term reversal of diabetes in nude mice. *Transplantation, 69*(6), 1084–1090. https://doi.org/10.1097/00007890-200003270-00011

Remuñán-López, C., & Bodmeier, R. (1997). Mechanical, water uptake and permeability properties of crosslinked chitosan glutamate and alginate films. *Journal of Controlled Release, 44*(2–3), 215–225. https://doi.org/10.1016/S0168-3659(96)01525-8

Rezania, A., Bruin, J. E., Arora, P., Rubin, A., Batushansky, I., Asadi, A., O'Dwyer, S., Quiskamp, N., Mojibian, M., Albrecht, T., Yang, Y. H. C., Johnson, J. D., & Kieffer, T. J. (2014). Reversal of diabetes with insulin-producing cells derived in vitro from human pluripotent stem cells. *Nature Biotechnology, 32*(11), 1121–1133. https://doi.org/10.1038/nbt.3033

Ribalet, B., & Beigelman, P. M. (1981). Effects of divalent cations on beta-cell electrical activity. *The American Journal of Physiology, 241*(1). https://doi.org/10.1152/ajpcell.1981.241.1.c59

Richards, N. J., & Williams, D. G. (1970). Complex formation between aqueous zinc chloride and cellulose-related D-glucopyranosides. *Carbohydrate Research, 12*(3), 409–420. https://doi.org/10.1016/S0008-6215(00)80621-7

Richter, B., Neises, G., & Bergerhoff, K. (2002). Human versus animal insulin in people with diabetes mellitus: A systematic review. *Endocrinology and Metabolism Clinics of North America, 31*(3), 723–749. https://doi.org/10.1016/S0889-8529(02)00020-8

Rickels, M. R., & Robertson, R. P. (2019). Pancreatic Islet Transplantation in Humans: Recent Progress and Future Directions. *Endocrine Reviews, 40*(2), 631–668. https://doi.org/10.1210/er.2018-00154

Riddl, M. C., Bakris, G., Blonde, L., Boulton, A. J. M., D'Alessio, D., Groot, M. de, Greene, E. L., Hu, F. B., Kahn, S. E., Kaul, S., LeRoith, D., Moses, R. G., Rich, S., Rosenstock, J., Tamborlane, W. V., & Wylie-Rosett, J. (Eds.). (2018). Microvascular Complications and Foot Care. In *Standards of Medical Care in Diabetes - 2018* (Vol. 41, Issue Supplement 1, pp. 105–118). American Diabetes Association. https://doi.org/doi.org/10.2337/dc18-S010

Robitaille, R., Leblond, F. A., Bourgeois, Y., Henley, N., Loignon, M., & Hallé, J.-P. (2000). Studies on small (<350 µm) alginate-poly-L-lysine microcapsules. V. Determination of carbohydrate and protein permeation through microcapsules by reverse-size exclusion chromatography. *Journal of Biomedical Materials Research, 50*(3), 420–427. https://doi.org/10.1002/(SICI)1097-4636(20000605)50:3<420::AID-JBM17>3.0.CO;2-S

Rock, K. L., & Kono, H. (2011). The inflammatory response to cell death Kenneth. *Annu Rev*

Pathol, 3, 99–126. https://doi.org/10.1146/annurev.pathmechdis.3.121806.151456.The

Rokstad, A. M. A., Lacík, I., de Vos, P., & Strand, B. L. (2014). Advances in biocompatibility and physico-chemical characterization of microspheres for cell encapsulation. *Advanced Drug Delivery Reviews, 67–68*, 111–130. https://doi.org/10.1016/j.addr.2013.07.010

Rokstad, A. M., Brekke, O. L., Steinkjer, B., Ryan, L., Kolláriková, G., Strand, B. L., Skjåk-Bræk, G., Lacík, I., Espevik, T., & Mollnes, T. E. (2011). Alginate microbeads are complement compatible, in contrast to polycation containing microcapsules, as revealed in a human whole blood model. *Acta Biomaterialia, 7*(6), 2566–2578. https://doi.org/10.1016/j.actbio.2011.03.011

Rorsman, P., & Braun, M. (2013). Regulation of Insulin Secretion in Human Pancreatic Islets. *Annual Review of Physiology, 75*(1), 155–179. https://doi.org/10.1146/annurev-physiol-030212-183754

Rosales, I. A., & Colvin, R. B. (2019). The pathology of solid organ xenotransplantation. *Current Opinion in Organ Transplantation, 24*(5), 535–542. https://doi.org/10.1097/MOT.0000000000000681

Rush, B. T., Fraga, D. W., Kotb, M. Y., Sabek, O. M., Lo, A., Gaber, L. W., Halim, A. B., & Gaber, A. O. (2004). Preservation of human pancreatic islet in vivo function after 6-month culture in serum-free media. *Transplantation, 77*(8), 1147–1154. https://doi.org/10.1097/01.TP.0000116769.94299.F4

Ryan, A. J., O'Neill, H. S., Duffy, G. P., & O'Brien, F. J. (2017). Advances in polymeric islet cell encapsulation technologies to limit the foreign body response and provide immunoisolation. *Current Opinion in Pharmacology, 36*, 66–71. https://doi.org/10.1016/j.coph.2017.07.013

Saake, B., Lebioda, S., & Puls, J. (2004). Analysis of the substituent distribution along the chain of water-soluble methyl cellulose by combination of enzymatic and chemical methods. *Holzforschung, 58*(1), 97–104. https://doi.org/10.1515/HF.2004.013

Sagvolden, G., Giaever, I., & Feder, J. (1998). Characteristic protein adhesion forces on glass and polystyrene substrates by atomic force microscopy. *Langmuir, 14*(21), 5984–5987. https://doi.org/10.1021/la980271b

Salg, G. A., Giese, N. A., Schenk, M., Hüttner, F. J., Felix, K., Probst, P., Diener, M. K., Hackert, T., & Kenngott, H. G. (2019). The emerging field of pancreatic tissue engineering: A systematic review and evidence map of scaffold materials and scaffolding techniques for insulin-secreting cells. *Journal of Tissue Engineering, 10*, 1–25. https://doi.org/10.1177/2041731419884708

Sannino, A., Demitri, C., & Madaghiele, M. (2009). Biodegradable cellulose-based hydrogels: Design and applications. *Materials, 2*(2), 353–373. https://doi.org/10.3390/ma2020353

Santos, E., Zarate, J., Orive, G., Hernández, R. M., & Pedraz, J. L. (2010). Biomaterials in Cell

Microencapsulation. In J. L. Pedraz & G. Orive (Eds.), *Therapeutic Applications of Cell Microencapsulation* (Vol. 640, pp. 5–21). Springer Science+Business Media, LLC Landes Bioscience.

Saqib, A. A. N., & Whitney, P. J. (2011). Differential behaviour of the dinitrosalicylic acid (DNS) reagent towards mono- and di-saccharide sugars. *Biomass and Bioenergy, 35*(11), 4748–4750. https://doi.org/10.1016/j.biombioe.2011.09.013

Sarkar, N. (1979). Thermal gelation properties of methyl and hydroxypropyl methylcellulose. *Journal of Applied Polymer Science, 24*(4), 1073–1087. https://doi.org/10.1002/app.1979.070240420

Schagerlöf, U., Schagerlöf, H., Momcilovic, D., Brinkmalm, G., & Tjerneld, F. (2007). Endoglucanase Sensitivity for Substituents in Methyl Cellulose Hydrolysis Studied Using MALDI-TOFMS for Oligosaccharide Analysis and Structural Analysis of Enzyme Active Sites. *Biomacromolecules, 8*(8), 2358–2365. https://doi.org/10.1021/bm0701200

Scharp, D. W., & Marchetti, P. (2014). Encapsulated islets for diabetes therapy: History, current progress, and critical issues requiring solution. *Advanced Drug Delivery Reviews, 67–68*, 35–73. https://doi.org/10.1016/j.addr.2013.07.018

Scheen, A. J. (2004). Pathophysiology of insulin secretion. *Annales d'Endocrinologie, 65*(1), 29–36. https://doi.org/10.1016/S0003-4266(04)95627-2

Schmied, B. M., Ulrich, A., Matsuzaki, H., Ding, X., Ricordi, C., Moyer, M. P., Batra, S. K., Adrian, T. E., & Pour, P. M. (2000). Maintenance of human islets in long term culture. *Differentiation, 66*, 173–180. https://doi.org/10.1046/j.1432-0436.2000.660403.x

Schneider, S., Feilen, P. J., Brunnenmeier, F., Minnemann, T., Zimmermann, H., Zimmermann, U., & Weber, M. M. (2005). Long-term graft function of adult rat and human islets encapsulated in novel alginate-based microcapsules after transplantation in immunocompetent diabetic mice. *Diabetes, 54*(3), 687–693. https://doi.org/10.2337/diabetes.54.3.687

Schumacher, M. (2014). *Entwicklung und Charakterisierung Strontium-modifizierter CaP-Knochenzemente zur Behandlung osteoporotischer Knochendefekte* [book]. Technische Universität Dresden.

Schütz, K., Placht, A. M., Paul, B., Brüggemeier, S., Gelinsky, M., & Lode, A. (2017). Three-dimensional plotting of a cell-laden alginate/methylcellulose blend: towards biofabrication of tissue engineering constructs with clinically relevant dimensions. *Journal of Tissue Engineering and Regenerative Medicine, 11*(5), 1574–1587. https://doi.org/10.1002/term.2058

Schweiger, R. G. (1962). Acetylation of Alginic Acid. II. Reaction of Algin Acetates with Calcium and Other Divalent Ions. *Journal of Organic Chemistry, 27*(5), 1789–1791. https://doi.org/10.1021/jo01052a073

Sefton, M. V., & Antonacci, G. M. (1984). Adsorption isotherms of insulin onto various materials. *Diabetes, 33*(7), 674–680. https://doi.org/10.2337/diab.33.7.674

Shapiro, A. M. J., Lakey, J. R. T., Ryan, E. A., Korbutt, G. S., Toth, E., Warnock, G. L., Kneteman, N. M., & Rajotte, R. V. (2000). Islet transplantation in seven patients with type 1 diabetes mellitus using a glucocorticoid-free immunosuppressive regimen. *New England Journal of Medicine, 343*(4), 230–238. https://doi.org/10.1056/NEJM200007273430401

Shapiro, A. M. J., Pokrywczynska, M., & Ricordi, C. (2017). Clinical pancreatic islet transplantation. *Nature Reviews Endocrinology, 13*(5), 268–277. https://doi.org/10.1038/nrendo.2016.178

Shin, J. S., Kim, J. M., Kim, J. S., Min, B. H., Kim, Y. H., Kim, H. J., Jang, J. Y., Yoon, I. H., Kang, H. J., Kim, J., Hwang, E. S., Lim, D. G., Lee, W. W., Ha, J., Jung, K. C., Park, S. H., Kim, S. J., & Park, C. G. (2015). Long-term control of diabetes in immunosuppressed nonhuman primates (NHP) by the transplantation of adult porcine islets. *American Journal of Transplantation, 15*(11), 2837–2850. https://doi.org/10.1111/ajt.13345

Shintaku, H., Okitsu, T., Kawano, S., Matsumoto, S., Suzuki, T., Kanno, I., & Kotera, H. (2008). Effects of fluid dynamic stress on fracturing of cell-aggregated tissue during purification for islets of Langerhans transplantation. *Journal of Physics D: Applied Physics, 41*(11). https://doi.org/10.1088/0022-3727/41/11/115507

Shoichet, M. S., Li, R. H., White, M. L., & Winn, S. R. (1996). Stability of hydrogels used in cell encapsulation: An in vitro comparison of alginate and agarose. *Biotechnology and Bioengineering, 50*(4), 374–381. https://doi.org/10.1002/(SICI)1097-0290(19960520)50:4<374::AID-BIT4>3.0.CO;2-I

Silva, P. N., Green, B. J., Altamentova, S. M., & Rocheleau, J. V. (2013). A microfluidic device designed to induce media flow throughout pancreatic islets while limiting shear-induced damage. *Lab on a Chip, 13*(22), 4374–4384. https://doi.org/10.1039/c3lc50680k

Skelin, M., Rupnik, M., & Cencic, A. (2010). Pancreatic beta cell lines and their applications in diabetes mellitus research. *Altex, 27*(2), 105–113. https://doi.org/10.14573/altex.2010.2.105

Smidsrød, O., & Skjåk-Braek, G. (1990). Alginate as immobilization matrix for cells. *Trends in Biotechnology, 8*(4), 71–78. https://doi.org/10.1016/0167-7799(90)90139-O

Smidsrød, O. (1974). Molecular basis for some physical properties of alginates in the gel state. *Faraday Discuss. Chem. Soc., 57*, 263–274. https://doi.org/10.1039/DC9745700263

Smith, L. F. (1966). Species variation in the amino acid sequence of insulin. *The American Journal of Medicine, 40*(5), 662–666. https://doi.org/10.1016/0002-9343(66)90145-8

Soltanian, A., Ghezelayagh, Z., Mazidi, Z., Halvaei, M., Mardpour, S., Ashtiani, M. K.,

Hajizadeh-Saffar, E., Tahamtani, Y., & Baharvand, H. (2019). Generation of functional human pancreatic organoids by transplants of embryonic stem cell derivatives in a 3D-printed tissue trapper. *Journal of Cellular Physiology*, *234*(6), 9564–9576. https://doi.org/10.1002/jcp.27644

Song, J., & Millman, J. R. (2017). Economic 3D-printing approach for transplantation of human stem cell-derived β-like cells. *Biofabrication*, *9*(1). https://doi.org/10.1088/1758-5090/9/1/015002

Soria, B., Tudurí, E., González, A., Hmadcha, A., Martin, F., Nadal, A., & Quesada, I. (2010). Pancreatic islet cells: A model for calcium-dependent peptide release. *HFSP Journal*, *4*(2), 52–60. https://doi.org/10.2976/1.3364560

Squires, P. E., Harris, T. E., Persaud, S. J., Curtis, S. B., Buchan, A. M. J., & Jones, P. M. (2000). The extracellular calcium-sensing receptor on human β-cells negatively modulates insulin secretion. *Diabetes*, *49*(3), 409–417. https://doi.org/10.2337/diabetes.49.3.409

Stabenfeldt, S. E., García, A. J., & LaPlaca, M. C. (2006). Thermoreversible laminin-functionalized hydrogel for neural tissue engineering. *Journal of Biomedical Materials Research Part A*, *79*(4), 963–973. https://doi.org/10.1002/jbm.a

Steffens, A. B. (1970). Plasma insulin content in relation to blood glucose level and meal pattern in the normal and hypothalamic hyperphagic rat. *Physiology and Behavior*, *5*(2), 147–151. https://doi.org/10.1016/0031-9384(70)90058-2

Stokke, B. T., Smidsrød, O., Bruheim, P., & Skjåk-Bræk, G. (1991). Distribution of Uronate Residues in Alginate Chains in Relation to Alginate Gelling Properties. *Macromolecules*, *24*(16), 4637–4645. https://doi.org/10.1021/ma00016a026

Strand, B. L., Coron, A. E., & Skjåk-Bræk, G. (2017). Current and future perspectives on alginate encapsulated pancreatic islet. *Stem Cells Translational Medicine*, *6*(4), 1053–1058. https://doi.org/10.1002/sctm.16-0116

Sun, Y., Ma, X., Zhou, D., Vacek, I., & Sun, A. M. (1996). Normalization of diabetes in spontaneously diabetic cynomologus monkeys by xenografts of microencapsulated porcine islets without immunosuppression. *Journal of Clinical Investigation*, *98*(6), 1417–1422. https://doi.org/10.1172/JCI118929

Tack, P., Victor, J., Gemmel, P., & Annemans, L. (2016). 3D-printing techniques in a medical setting: A systematic literature review. *BioMedical Engineering Online*, *15*(1), 1–21. https://doi.org/10.1186/s12938-016-0236-4

Tal, M., Liang, Y., Najafi, H., Lodish, H. F., & Matschinsky, F. M. (1992). Expression and function of GLUT-1 and GLUT-2 glucose transporter isoforms in cells of cultured rat pancreatic islets. *The Journal of Biological Chemistry*, *267*(24), 17241–17247. https://www.jbc.org/content/267/24/17241.short?related-urls=yes&legid=jbc;267/24/17241

Tam, S. K., Dusseault, J., Polizu, S., Ménard, M., Hallé, J. P., & Yahia, L. (2006). Impact of residual contamination on the biofunctional properties of purified alginates used for cell encapsulation. *Biomaterials, 27*(8), 1296–1305. https://doi.org/10.1016/j.biomaterials.2005.08.027

Tan, Y. H., Liu, M., Nolting, B., Go, J. G., Gervay-Hague, J., & Liu, G. (2008). A Nanoengineering Approach for Investigation and Regulation of Protein Immobilization. *ACS Nano, 2*(11), 2374–2384. https://doi.org/10.1021/nn800508f

Tatarkiewicz, K., Garcia, M., Lopez-Avalos, M., Bonner-Weir, S., & Weir, G. C. (2001). Porcine neonatal pancreatic cell clusters in tissue culture: Benefits of serum and immobilization in alginate hydrogel. *Transplantation, 71*(11), 1518–1526. https://doi.org/10.1097/00007890-200106150-00007

Teixeira, R. S. S., Da Silva, A. S. A., Ferreira-Leitão, V. S., & Da Silva Bon, E. P. (2012). Amino acids interference on the quantification of reducing sugars by the 3,5-dinitrosalicylic acid assay mislead carbohydrase activity measurements. *Carbohydrate Research, 363*, 33–37. https://doi.org/10.1016/j.carres.2012.09.024

Tengholm, A., & Gylfe, E. (2017). cAMP signalling in insulin and glucagon secretion. *Diabetes, Obesity and Metabolism, 19*(April), 42–53. https://doi.org/10.1111/dom.12993

Thirumala, S., Gimble, J., & Devireddy, R. (2013). Methylcellulose Based Thermally Reversible Hydrogel System for Tissue Engineering Applications. *Cells, 2*(3), 460–475. https://doi.org/10.3390/cells2030460

Thompson, P., Cardona, K., Russell, M., Badell, I. R., Shaffer, V., Korbutt, G., Rayat, G. R., Cano, J., Song, M., Jiang, W., Strobert, E., Rajotte, R., Pearson, T., Kirk, A. D., & Larsen, C. P. (2011). CD40-specific costimulation blockade enhances neonatal porcine islet survival in nonhuman primates. *American Journal of Transplantation, 11*(5), 947–957. https://doi.org/10.1111/j.1600-6143.2011.03509.x

Trivedi, N., Keegan, M., Steil, G. M., Hollister-Lock, J., Hasenkamp, W. M., Colton, C. K., Bonner-Weir, S., & Weir, G. C. (2001). Islets in alginate macrobeads reverse diabetes despite minimal acute insulin secretory responses. *Transplantation, 71*(2), 203–211. https://doi.org/10.1097/00007890-200101270-00006

Tuch, B. E., Keogh, G. W., Williams, L. J., Wu, W., Foster, J., Vaithilingam, V., & Phlips, R. (2009). Safety and Viability of Microencapsulated Human Islets Transplanted Into Diabetic Humans. *Diabetes Care, 32*(10), 1887–1889. https://doi.org/10.2337/dc09-0744.Clinical

Twardowski, Z. J., Nolph, K. D., McGary, T. J., & Moore, H. L. (1983). Nature of insulin binding to plastic bags. *American Journal of Hospital Pharmacy, 40*(4), 579–582. https://doi.org/10.1093/ajhp/40.4.579

Uludag, H., De Vos, P., & Tresco, P. A. (2000). Technology of mammalian cell encapsulation. *Advanced Drug Delivery Reviews, 42*(1–2), 29–64. https://doi.org/10.1016/S0169-409X(00)00053-3

Urban, P. L. (2016). Quantitative mass spectrometry: An overview. *Philosophical Transactions of the Royal Society A: Mathematical, Physical and Engineering Sciences, 374*(2079). https://doi.org/10.1098/rsta.2015.0382

U.S. Food and Drug Administration. (2020). *Inactive Ingredient Search for Approved Drug Products.* Website. https://www.accessdata.fda.gov/scripts/cder/iig/index.cfm

Van Der Windt, D. J., Bottino, R., Casu, A., Campanile, N., & Cooper, D. K. C. (2007). Rapid loss of intraportally transplanted islets: An overview of pathophysiology and preventive strategies. *Xenotransplantation, 14*(4), 288–297. https://doi.org/10.1111/j.1399-3089.2007.00419.x

Van Der Windt, D. J., Marigliano, M., He, J., Votyakova, T. V., Echeverri, G. J., Ekser, B., Ayares, D., Lakkis, F. G., Cooper, D. K. C., Trucco, M., & Bottino, R. (2012). Early islet damage after direct exposure of pig islets to blood: Has humoral immunity been underestimated? *Cell Transplantation, 21*(8), 1791–1802. https://doi.org/10.3727/096368912X653011

Van Schilfgaarde, R., & De Vos, P. (1999). Factors influencing the properties and performance of microcapsules for immunoprotection of pancreatic islets. *Journal of Molecular Medicine, 77*(1), 199–205. https://doi.org/10.1007/s001090050336

Veiseh, O., Doloff, J. C., Ma, M., Vegas, A. J., Tam, H. H., Bader, A. R., Li, J., Langan, E., Wyckoff, J., Loo, W. S., Jhunjhunwala, S., Chiu, A., Siebert, S., Tang, K., Hollister-Lock, J., Aresta-Dasilva, S., Bochenek, M., Mendoza-Elias, J., Wang, Y., … Anderson, D. G. (2015). Size- and shape-dependent foreign body immune response to materials implanted in rodents and non-human primates. *Nature Materials, 14*(6), 643–651. https://doi.org/10.1038/nmat4290

Vériter, S., Gianello, P., Igarashi, Y., Beaurin, G., Ghyselinck, A., Aouassar, N., Jordan, B., Gallez, B., & Dufrane, D. (2014). Improvement of subcutaneous bioartificial pancreas vascularization and function by coencapsulation of pig islets and mesenchymal stem cells in primates. *Cell Transplantation, 23*(11), 1349–1364. https://doi.org/10.3727/096368913X663550

Wang, Y., Qi, M., McGarrigle, J. J., Rady, B., Davis, M., Vaca, P., & Oberholzer, J. (2013). Use of Glucagon-Like Peptide-1 Agonists to Improve Islet Graft Performance. *Curr Diab Rep, 13*(5), 723–732. https://doi.org/10.1007/s11892-013-0402-z

Warshauer, J. T., Bluestone, J. A., & Anderson, M. S. (2020). New Frontiers in the Treatment of Type 1 Diabetes. *Cell Metabolism, 31*(1), 46–61. https://doi.org/10.1016/j.cmet.2019.11.017

Wei, L., Jiang, Y., Zhou, W., Liu, S., Liu, Y., Rausch-Fan, X., & Liu, Z. (2018). Strontium ion attenuates lipopolysaccharide-stimulated proinflammatory cytokine expression and lipopolysaccharide-inhibited early osteogenic differentiation of human periodontal ligament cells. *Journal of Periodontal Research*, *53*(6), 999–1008. https://doi.org/10.1111/jre.12599

Weiss, M., Steiner, D. F., & Philipson, L. H. (2014). Insulin Biosynthesis, Secretion, Structure, and Structure-Activity Relationships. In K. R. Feingold, B. Anawalt, A. Boyce, G. Chrousos, K. Dungan, A. Grossman, J. M. Hershman, G. Kaltsas, C. Koch, P. Kopp, M. Korbonits, R. McLachlan, J. E. Morley, M. New, L. Perreault, J. Purnell, R. Rebar, F. Singer, D. L. Trence, … D. P. Wilson (Eds.), *Endotext [Internet]*. MDText.com, Inc.

Welsch, C. A., Rust, W. L., & Csete, M. (2019). Concise Review: Lessons Learned from Islet Transplant Clinical Trials in Developing Stem Cell Therapies for Type 1 Diabetes. *Stem Cells Translational Medicine*, *8*(3), 209–214. https://doi.org/10.1002/sctm.18-0156

Wikipedia. (2007). *Human insulin hexamer*. Website. https://de.wikipedia.org/wiki/Datei:Human-insulin-hexamer-3D-ribbons.png%0A

Wikipedia. (2020a). *Carboxymethylcellulosen*. Website. https://de.wikipedia.org/wiki/Carboxymethylcellulosen

Wikipedia. (2020b). *Cellulose*. Website. https://de.wikipedia.org/wiki/Cellulose

Wikipedia. (2020c). *Methylcellulose*. Website. https://de.wikipedia.org/wiki/Methylcellulose

Wollheim, C. B., & Sharp, G. W. (1981). Regulation of insulin release by calcium. *Physiological Reviews*, *61*(4), 914–973. https://doi.org/10.1152/physrev.1981.61.4.914

Wüstenberg, T. (2015). Fundamentals of Water-Soluble Cellulose Ethers and Methylcellulose. In T. Wüstenberg (Ed.), *Cellulose and Cellulose Derivatives in the Food Industry* (pp. 185–274). Wiley-VCH Verlag GmbH & Co. KGaA. https://doi.org/10.1002/9783527682935

Xu, Q., & Chen, L.-F. (1994). Characterization of cellulose film prepared from zinc-cellulose complexes. *Biomass and Bioenergy*, *6*(5), 415–417. https://doi.org/10.1016/0961-9534(94)E0023-L

Xu, Y., Wang, C., Tam, K. C., & Li, L. (2004). Salt-assisted and salt-suppressed sol-gel transitions of methylcellulose in water. *Langmuir*, *20*(3), 646–652. https://doi.org/10.1021/la0356295

Yan, Q., Dong, H., Su, J., Han, J., Song, B., Wei, Q., & Shi, Y. (2018). A Review of 3D Printing Technology for Medical Applications. *Engineering*, *4*(5), 729–742. https://doi.org/10.1016/j.eng.2018.07.021

Yoon, K. H., Quickel, R. R., Tatarkiewicz, K., Ulrich, T. R., Hollister-Lock, J., Trivedi, N., Bonner-Weir, S., & Weir, G. C. (1999). Differentiation and expansion of beta cell mass in porcine neonatal pancreatic cell clusters transplanted into nude mice. *Cell*

Transplantation, *8*(6), 673–689. https://doi.org/10.1177/096368979900800613

You, J. O., Park, S. B., Park, H. Y., Haam, S., Chung, C. H., & Kim, W. S. (2001). Preparation of regular sized Ca-alginate microspheres using membrane emulsification method. *Journal of Microencapsulation*, *18*(4), 521–532. https://doi.org/10.1080/02652040010018128

Yousefi, R., Taheri, B., Alavi, P., Shahsavani, M. B., Asadi, Z., Ghahramani, M., Niazi, A., Alavianmehr, M. M., & Moosavi-Movahedi, A. A. (2016). Aspirin-mediated acetylation induces structural alteration and aggregation of bovine pancreatic insulin. *Journal of Biomolecular Structure and Dynamics*, *34*(2), 362–375. https://doi.org/10.1080/07391102.2015.1039584

Yue, Z., Liu, X., Coates, P. T., & Wallace, G. G. (2016). Advances in printing biomaterials and living cells: Implications for islet cell transplantation. *Current Opinion in Organ Transplantation*, *21*(5), 467–475. https://doi.org/10.1097/MOT.0000000000000346

Zekorn, T., Siebers, U., Horcher, A., Schnettler, R., Zimmermann, U., Bretzel, R. G., & Federlin, K. (1992). Alginate coating of islets of Langerhans: in vitro studies on a new method for microencapsulation for immuno-isolated transplantation. *Acta Diabetologica*, *29*(1), 41–45. https://doi.org/10.1007/BF00572829

Zhao, F., Lei, B., Li, X., Mo, Y., Wang, R., Chen, D., & Chen, X. (2018). Promoting in vivo early angiogenesis with sub-micrometer strontium-contained bioactive microspheres through modulating macrophage phenotypes. *Biomaterials*, *178*, 36–47. https://doi.org/10.1016/j.biomaterials.2018.06.004

Zhu, H., Li, W., Liu, Z., Li, W., Chen, N., Lu, L., Zhang, W., Wang, Z., Wang, B., Pan, K., Zhang, X., & Chen, G. (2018). Selection of Implantation Sites for Transplantation of Encapsulated Pancreatic Islets. *Tissue Engineering - Part B: Reviews*, *24*(3), 191–214. https://doi.org/10.1089/ten.teb.2017.0311

Zimmermann, H., Hillgärtner, M., Manz, B., Feilen, P., Brunnenmeier, F., Leinfelder, U., Weber, M., Cramer, H., Schneider, S., Hendrich, C., Volke, F., & Zimmermann, U. (2003). Fabrication of homogeneously cross-linked, functional alginate microcapsules validated by NMR-, CLSM- and AFM-imaging. *Biomaterials*, *24*(12), 2083–2096. https://doi.org/10.1016/S0142-9612(02)00639-7

Addendum

A.1 Supplementary data for the results

Supplementary data for "4.1.1. Paste viscosity and scaffold stability"

Ion release

Figure 61 depicts the third repetition of the release of Sr^{2+} ions from plotted Alg/MC scaffolds, which had been crosslinked in 70 mM $SrCl_2$ for 10 min, into RPMI+.

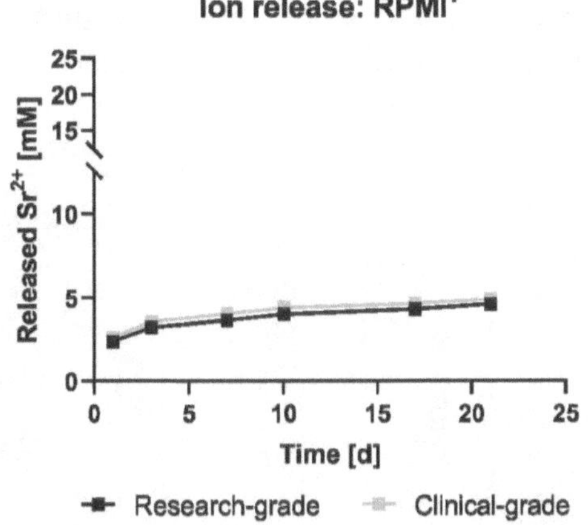

Figure 61: Release of crosslinking ions in different cell culture media. Cumulative release of Sr^{2+} ions from plotted Alg/MC scaffolds prepared with research-grade and clinical-grade alginate into RPMI+ over 21 d. Mean ± SD, n = 6.

Supplementary data for "4.1.2 Scaffold composition during incubation under cell culture conditions"

Precipitation of crosslinking ions in cell culture media

As mentioned in the results, the overall release of Sr^{2+} ions measured was lower in RPMI+ than in DMEM+ despite stability data predicting the opposite. To investigate the possibility of released crosslinking ions precipitating from the supernatant, 100 mM $CaCl_2$ or 70 mM $SrCl_2$ were added to DMEM+ and RPMI+ in a ratio of 1:1. In all variants tested, the formation of a white precipitate was observed (Figure 12, page 39, results). Visual estimation of the quantity of precipitate revealed a decreasing order of Ca^{2+}-RPMI+ > Sr^{2+}-RPMI+ > Ca^{2+}-DMEM+ > Sr^{2+}-DMEM+. The most likely cause of this is the formation of calcium or strontium phosphate depending on the ion used for crosslinking.

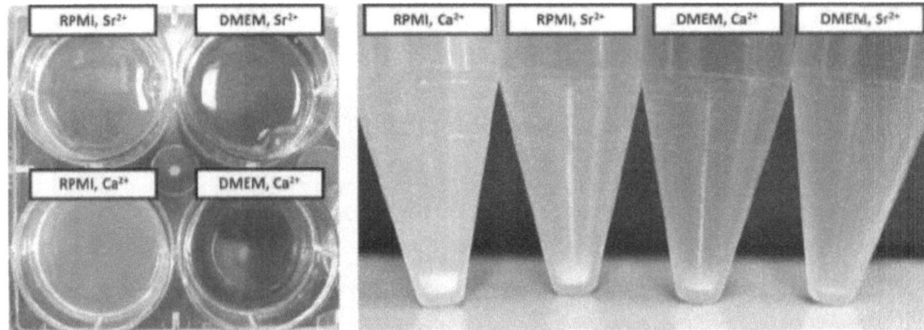

Figure 62: Formation of a white precipitate after addition of crosslinking ions into the cell culture media. 100 mM $CaCl_2$ or 70 mM $SrCl_2$ were added to DMEM+ and RPMI+ in a ratio of 1:1.

Quantitative MC release

Figure 63 depicts the release of MC also depicted in Figure 13 (page 41, results), but without error bars for better visibility.

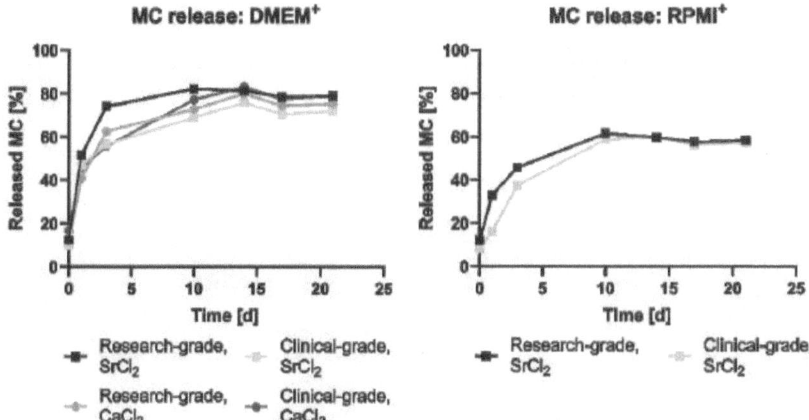

Figure 63: Release of MC in different media. Cumulative release of MC from plotted Alg/MC scaffolds prepared with research-grade or clinical-grade alginate over 21 days of culture. Release of MC from scaffolds crosslinked with 70 mM SrCl$_2$ or 100 mM CaCl$_2$ and incubated in DMEM$^+$ (left), and release from scaffolds crosslinked with 70 mM SrCl$_2$ and incubated in RPMI$^+$ (right). Mean ± SD, n = 6 for each.

Supplementary data for "4.1.3 Permeability for glucose & insulin"

Prior versions of the diffusion chamber

Within the scope of this book, different versions of a diffusion chamber system were developed and analysed. The versions analysed prior to the chosen osmosis chamber were 3D
prin-ted in-house (Figure 64 A) or based on commercially available syringes (Figure 64 B).
The 3D printed version was tight initially but tightness could not be guaranteed for more than
6 h run-time, and despite a moulded lid some evaporation and a large amount of condensation
could not be avoided.

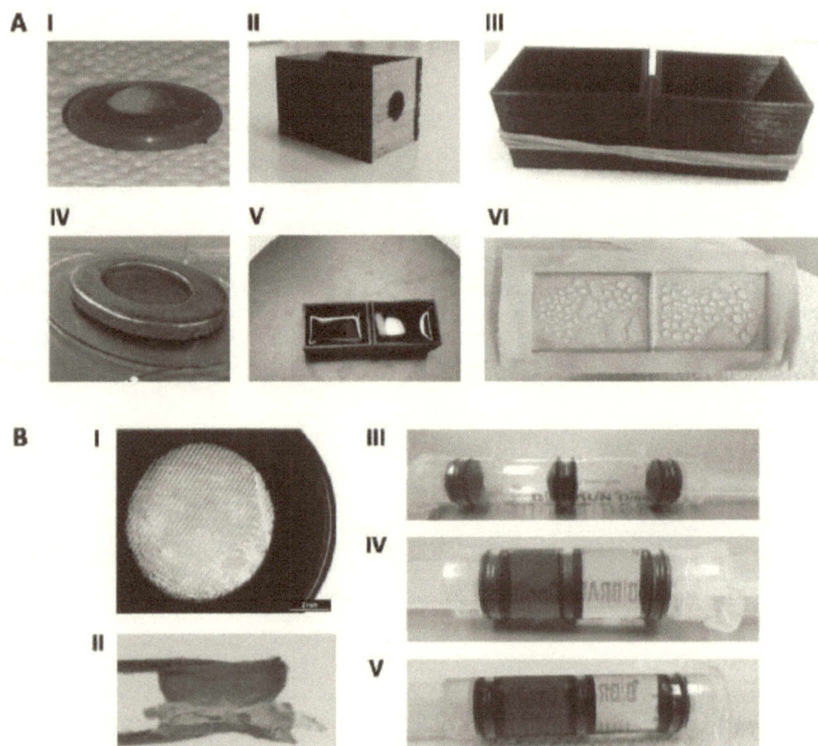

Figure 64: Prior versions of the diffusion chamber. A) A 3D printed chamber system. I&IV: Different
methods for gel reparation, retrospectively wedged into a rubber seal ring or prepared within a metal
washer. II&III: one chamber half and the empty assembled chamber. V: the filled assembled chamber
showing tightness with phenol red. VI: A moulded lid to reduce evaporation. B) A syringe-based chamber
system whereby the gels were directly prepared within the rubber seal ring of such syringes. I: Light
microscopic image of a plain alginate gel within the rubber seal ring, pattern caused by the mesh used
during preparation to enable crosslinking from the underside. Prior to preparation the mesh had been
wetted with 70 mM $SrCl_2$. II: A plain alginate gel removed from the seal ring depicting diffusion through
the gel as a proof of tightness. III-V: The assembled chamber system empty, freshly filled with HBSS
containing phenol red on the left and plain HBSS on the right, and beginning diffusion of phenol red from
left to right.

The syringe-based system required gel preparation directly within the seal rings which was challenging to realise with plain alginate and could only be achieved with roughening the inner surface of the seal ring. Tightness of research-grade plain alginate gels could only be achieved with a specific batch, while tightness of clinical-grade alginate gels was not batch-dependent. Improvements over the prior chamber system were tightness, and that evaporation could be avoided completely. The main disadvantage which resulted in the choice of the osmosis chamber (Figure 17, page 46, results) was that gels for the syringe-based system had a very small surface-to-volume ratio, which interfered strongly with the diffusion through Alg/MC gels.

Permeability for glucose

Figure 65 depicts the diffusion of glucose through research-grade and clinical-grade alginate and Alg/MC gels, in a comparison by incubation time for each gel type. The data shown here corresponds to Figure 23 & Figure 24 (page 53 & 54, results).

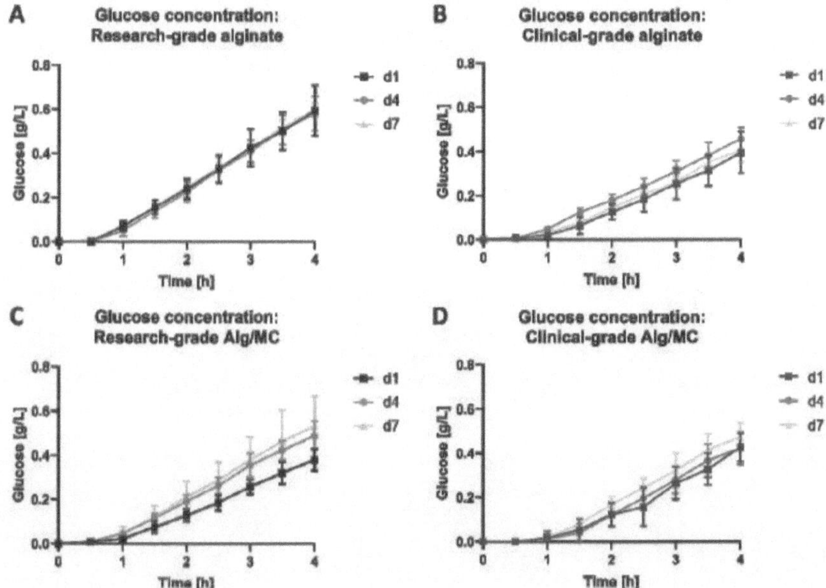

Figure 65 Glucose concentration compared by incubation time. Glucose concentration is depicted for the acceptor compartment. Alginate (top) and Alg/MC (bottom) gel discs were prepared with research-grade (left) or clinical-grade (right) alginate and crosslinked with 70 mM SrCl$_2$. Incubation of discs in 10 mM SrCl$_2$ under cell culture conditions for 1, 4, or 7 days before mounting in the chamber filled with 10 mM SrCl$_2$. Samples of 200 µl were taken from both compartments every 30 min during a period of 4 h. Mean ± SD, n = 3, data were adjusted for gel height.

Figure 66 depicts the diffusion of glucose through research-grade Alg/MC gels incubated in either 10 mM $SrCl_2$ or Krebs-Ringer buffer solution for up to 7 days, in a comparison by incubation time for each gel type. The data depicted here corresponds to Figure 25 (page 55, results).

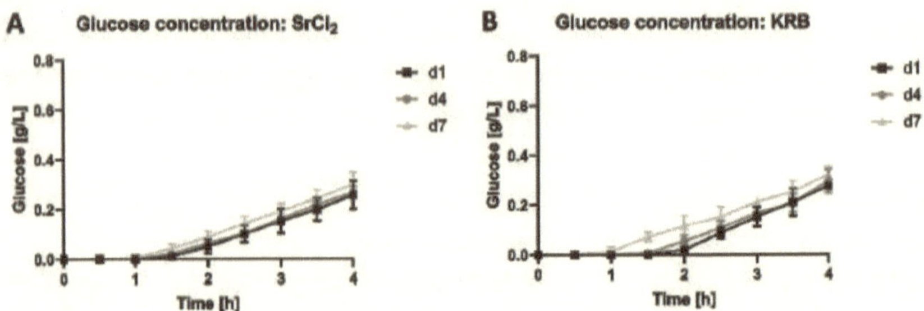

Figure 66: Glucose concentration in different diffusion media compared by incubation time. Glucose concentration is depicted for the acceptor compartment. Alg/MC gel discs were prepared with research-grade alginate and crosslinked with 70 mM $SrCl_2$. Incubation of discs in 10 mM $SrCl_2$ (left) or Krebs-Ringer buffer (right) for 1, 4, or 7 days before mounting in the chamber filled with 10 mM $SrCl_2$ or Krebs-Ringer buffer. Samples of 200 µl were taken from both compartments every 30 min during a period of 4 h. Mean ± SD, n = 3, data were adjusted for gel height.

Supplementary data for "4.2.1 Sterilisation of MC: influence on β-cell survival and behaviour"

Determination of cell number from 3D plotted Alg/MC scaffolds

During development of this blend, cell survival was measured by the enzyme activity of the lactate dehydrogenase (LDH) content after mechanical disruption of scaffolds, i.e. the lysis protocol was optimised for gentle lysis so as not to destroy the LDH (Schütz et al., 2017). The LDH content of cells is a relatively variable parameter though (Ka-ming Chan et al., 2013; Kaja et al., 2017), whereas readout from DNA measurements is more consistent. The precise determination of cell count, especially from plotted islets, therefore required a complete dissolution of scaffolds, complete lysis of cells and measurement of DNA content.

Dissolution of alginate-based scaffolds can be achieved with the chelating agent sodium citrate by binding the divalent crosslinking ions, the presence of sodium citrate needed to be cross-checked for interference with the quantitative DNA-measurement though. The standard lysis buffer with a high content of Triton-X 100, which interferes with the assay according to the manufacturer, was used as a control for interference. De-ionised water was used as a control for non-interference. In combination with different protocols for cell lysis, these three solutions were compared according to their effectiveness of cell lysis (Figure 67 A). Following this, lysis in sodium citrate vs standard lysis buffer were compared as to the DNA-content measured from 2D hTERT-MSC samples (Figure 67 B). Analysis of single cells grown on tissue culture plastic (TCP) revealed a strong difference in the ratio of lysed cells when lysis protocols were performed in either sodium citrate, lysis buffer or de-ionised water, with by far the most remaining cells in lysis buffer and the highest lysis after the use of sodium citrate (Figure 67 A). With sodium citrate as solvent, lysis efficiency improved with the use of three freeze-thaw cycles or incubation at 60°C over night instead, and was absolute with a combination of those as analysed qualitatively. Quantitatively, DNA-content of cells grown on TCP was compared between the use of sodium citrate and lysis buffer (Figure 67 B) which confirmed that lysis in lysis buffer is less efficient, but also displayed stronger differences between the lysis methods than could be detected in the qualitative analysis. Measured DNA-content was higher after overnight incubation at 60°C than after the application of three freeze-thaw cycles. In contrast to the microscopic analysis, the quantitative measurements did not reveal an additional benefit of the combination of overnight incubation and freeze-thaw cycles. All three methods led to a higher measured DNA-content than an incubation of 30 min at 37°C.

For an analysis of DNA-content of plotted scaffolds (Figure 67 C), only sodium citrate was used and gentle lysis at 37°C was excluded. Plotted scaffolds containing 5×10^6 hTERT-MSC or 3×10^7 INS-1 per gram material were dissolved in sodium citrate and cells were lysed with three freeze-thaw cycles, at 60°C over night, or with a combination of both. Results from plotted scaffolds corroborate results from cells cultured on TCP and measured DNA-content is proportional to the ratio of cells incorporated.

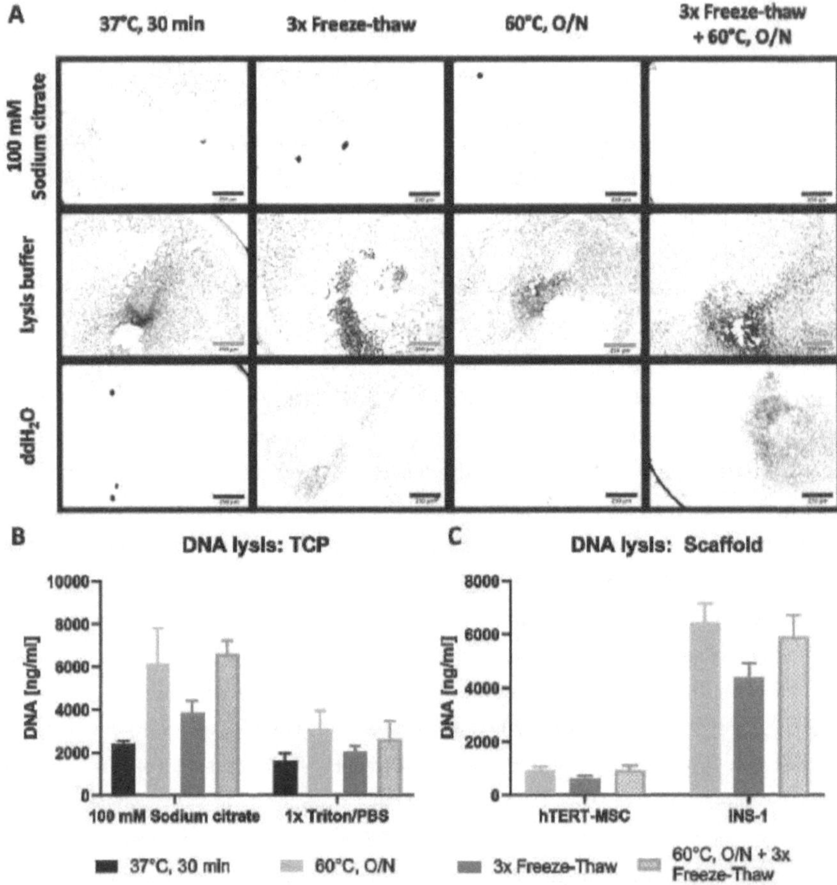

Figure 67: Optimisation of the cell lysis for quantitative DNA measurements. A) Representative images of remaining nuclei after lysis stained with Hoechst, scale bars = 250 µm. B) Quantitative analysis of DNA after lysis of hTERT-MSC grown on tissue culture plastic (TCP) of 6-well plates. Mean ± SD, n = 6. C) Quantitative analysis of DNA from 5×10^6 hTERT-MSC or 3×10^7 INS-1 per gram material incorporated into plotted Alg/MC scaffolds. Scaffolds had been dissolved in sodium citrate prior to cell lysis. Mean ± SD, n = 5.

Live/dead staining of INS-1

Figure 68-Figure 70 depict INS-1 stained for live and dead cells, in plotted in Alg/MC scaffolds, whereby the pastes were prepared with MC which had been exposed to autoclaving, scCO$_2$ treatment or UV irradiation,. Live cells depicted in green, and dead cells depicted in red, are represented in the middle and lower row respectively. The top row depicts an overlay of both channels. The data depicted here corresponds to Figure 28 (page 59, results) where only the overlay is shown.

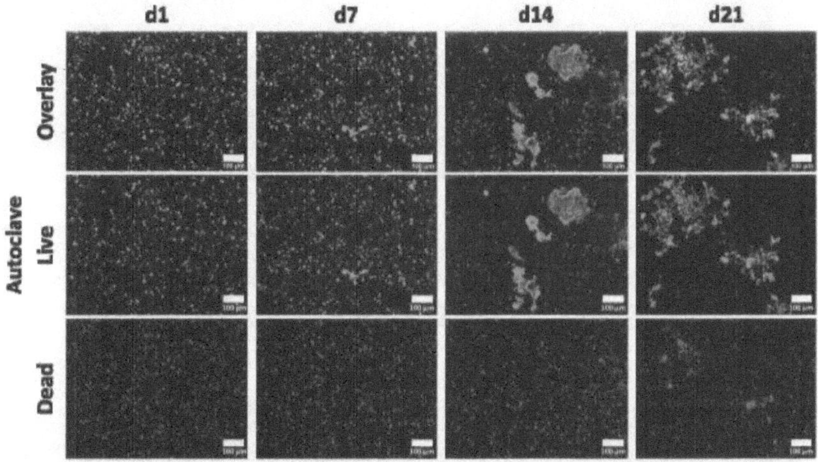

Figure 68: Qualitative depiction of the influence of different sterilisation methods applied to MC on the viability of INS-1 cells: Autoclave. Plotted INS-1 in research-grade Alg/MC scaffolds cross-linked with 70 mM SrCl$_2$ and incubated in RPMI$^+$ under cell culture conditions for up to 21 days. Representative images of INS-1 stained for live (green) and dead (red) cells in the middle and lower row respectively. An overlay of both channels is depicted in the top row. Scale bars = 100 µm.

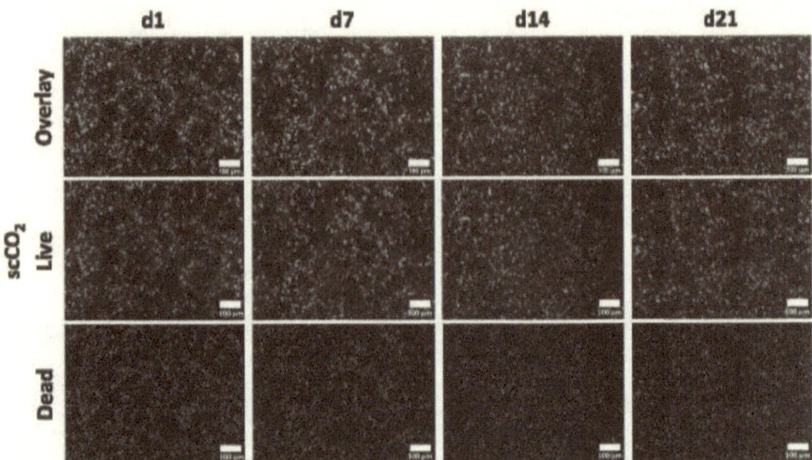

Figure 69: Qualitative depiction of the influence of different sterilisation methods applied to MC on the viability of INS-1 cells: scCO₂. Plotted INS-1 in research-grade Alg/MC scaffolds crosslinked with 70 mM SrCl$_2$ and incubated in RPMI$^+$ under cell culture conditions for up to 21 days. Representative images of INS-1 stained for live (green) and dead (red) cells in the middle and lower row respectively. An overlay of both channels is depicted in the top row. Scale bars = 100 µm.

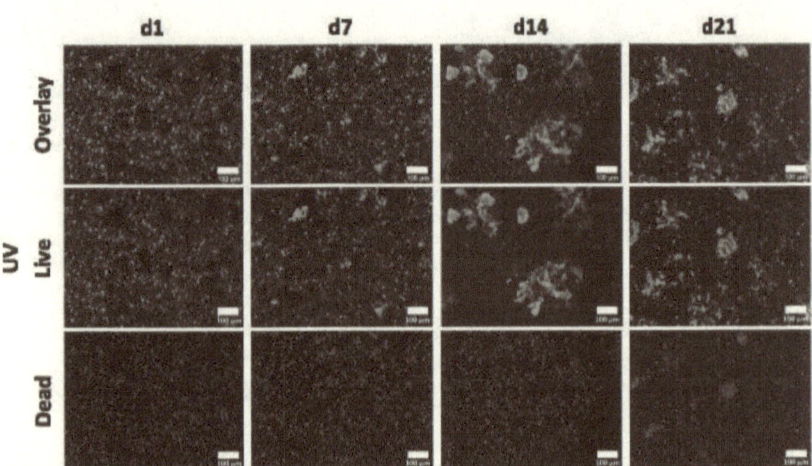

Figure 70: Qualitative depiction of the influence of different sterilisation methods applied to MC on the viability of INS-1 cells: UV. Plotted INS-1 in research-grade Alg/MC scaffolds crosslinked with 70 mM SrCl$_2$ and incubated in RPMI$^+$ under cell culture conditions for up to 21 days. Representative images of INS-1 stained for live (green) and dead (red) cells in the middle and lower row respectively. An overlay of both channels is depicted in the top row. Scale bars = 100 µm.

Supplementary data for "4.3.2 Functionality of bioplotted murine islets"

Glucose-stimulated insulin release of adult murine islets

For scaffolds prepared with clinical-grade alginate, the functional response of murine islets is depicted for all 7 isolations plotted with these parameters. The data is divided into two figures for better visibility (Figure 71 & Figure 72), whereby Figure 71 corresponds to Figure 43 (page 77, results) and Figure 72 depicts the remaining four isolations.

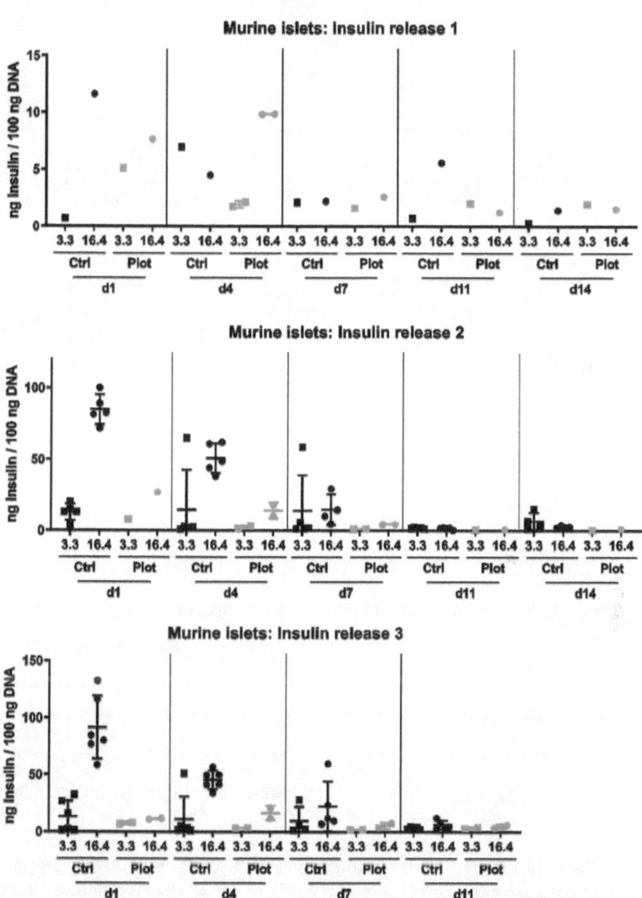

Figure 71: Insulin release of murine islets in clinical-grade Alg/MC. Plotted islets in clinical-grade Alg/MC scaffolds crosslinked with 70 mM SrCl2 and control islets in suspension culture incubated in RPMI+ under cell culture conditions for up to 7 days. Single values of ng insulin released in response to either low (3.3 mM) or high (16.4 mM) glucose stimulation normalised to 100 ng DNA. Stimulation over a cultivation time of 14 days depicted for isolations 1-3. Data points for each isolation depict replicate samples. For an overview over the calculated values refer to Table 3-Table 5.

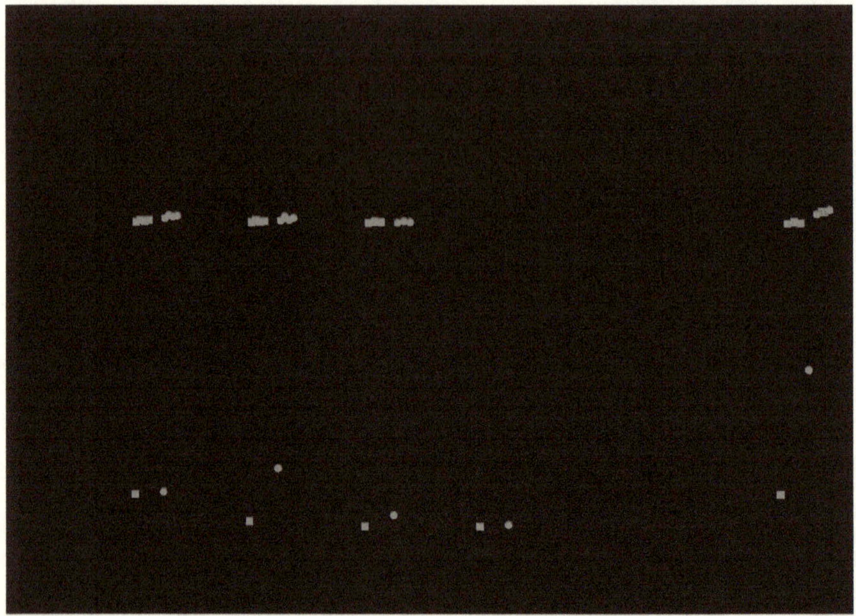

Figure 72: Insulin release of murine islets in clinical-grade Alg/MC. Plotted islets in clinical-grade Alg/MC scaffolds crosslinked with 70 mM SrCl$_2$ and control islets in suspension culture incubated in RPMI$^+$ under cell culture conditions for up to 7 days. Single values of ng insulin released in response to either low (3.3 mM) or high (16.4 mM) glucose stimulation normalised to 100 ng DNA. Stimulation over a cultivation time of 14 days depicted for isolations 4-7. Data points for each isolation depict replicate samples. For an overview over the calculated values refer to Table 6-Table 9.

The following tables show the calculated values for ng insulin per 100 ng DNA which are graphically depicted in Figure 71 & Figure 72. All values in Table 3-Table 10 are from plotted islets in clinical-grade Alg/MC scaffolds crosslinked with 70 mM SrCl$_2$ and from control islets in suspension culture incubated in RPMI$^+$ under cell culture conditions for up to 14 days. Samples in isolation 1-7 were exposed to either low or high glucose stimulation, samples in isolation 8 (Figure 45, page 79, results) were exposed to successive low-high-low glucose stimulation.

Table 3: Insulin release of murine islets in clinical-grade Alg/MC, isolation 1. Single values of ng insulin released in response to either low (3.3 mM) or high (16.4 mM) glucose stimulation normalised to 100 ng DNA.

	d1	d4	d7	d11	d14
Ctrl, 3.3 mM	0.71	6.99	2.14	0.74	0.28
Ctrl, 16.4 mM	11.63	4.53	2.25	5.62	1.46
Plot, 3.3 mM	5.14	1.78 2.20	1.67	2.06	2.02
Plot, 16.4 mM	7.68	9.86 9.90	2.64	1.27	1.56

Table 4: Insulin release of murine islets in clinical-grade Alg/MC, isolation 2. Single values of ng insulin released in response to either low (3.3 mM) or high (16.4 mM) glucose stimulation normalised to 100 ng DNA.

	d1	d4	d7	d11	d14
Ctrl, 3.3 mM	20.00	0.81	58.81	2.03	15.16
	3.92	2.71	1.37	1.63	6.75
	12.90	2.24	1.55	2.25	3.82
	12.91	65.10	1.73	1.41	1.47
	14.50	1.62	5.73	1.39	
Ctrl, 16.4 mM	71.91	48.73	29.59	1.88	2.16
	81.52	38.26	14.45	0.47	2.72
	82.52	62.04	4.77	1.65	2.38
	89.01	44.22		1.77	3.87
	100.17	61.10	10.18	2.19	
Plot, 3.3 mM	7.86	3.03	1.37	0.73	0.49
		1.48	1.06		
Plot, 16.4 mM	27.06	18.09	4.28	0.78	1.22
		10.21	4.59		

Table 5: Insulin release of murine islets in clinical-grade Alg/MC, isolation 3. Single values of ng insulin released in response to either low (3.3 mM) or high (16.4 mM) glucose stimulation normalised to 100 ng DNA.

	d1	d4	d7	d11
Ctrl, 3.3 mM	1.37	51.44	28.01	2.22
	32.44	1.95	1.53	4.06
	26.75	4.75	2.62	4.53
	16.04	1.33	6.00	2.54
	2.28	3.68		3.28
	1.35	2.86		
Ctrl, 16.4 mM	58.83	41.51	9.82	3.03
	132.73	49.75	60.09	7.98
	76.98	49.54	12.06	3.68
	116.40	41.42	6.91	4.37
	84.77	57.06	23.52	11.90
	80.39	34.13		
Plot, 3.3 mM	8.23	3.66	2.12	3.03
	6.85	3.34	2.02	3.94
Plot, 16.4 mM	11.76	21.09	7.61	3.29
	11.03	12.32	3.63	5.98

Table 6: Insulin release of murine islets in clinical-grade Alg/MC, isolation 4. Single values of ng insulin released in response to either low (3.3 mM) or high (16.4 mM) glucose stimulation normalised to 100 ng DNA.

	d1	d4	d7
Ctrl, 3.3 mM	2.38	1.95	59.76
	0.11	1.32	7.93
	2.94		2.08
	1.04	30.38	2.87
	1.51	8.49	5.10
	0.71	6.22	1.53
Ctrl, 16.4 mM	231.81	3.74	4.02
	3.38	3.66	5.04
	12.74		1.83
	59.96	4.49	3.40
	13.02	40.79	2.77
	269.72	9.40	1.33
Plot, 3.3 mM	6.23	4.59	4.40
	6.35	4.39	5.02
	5.25	6.05	3.50
	4.64	5.21	
Plot, 16.4 mM	10.09	5.70	5.25
	10.77	6.35	4.57
	9.37	9.52	3.83
	7.72	8.07	

Table 7: Insulin release of murine islets in clinical-grade Alg/MC, isolation 5. Single values of ng insulin released in response to either low (3.3 mM) or high (16.4 mM) glucose stimulation normalised to 100 ng DNA.

	d1	d4
Ctrl, 3.3 mM		12.68
		4.00
		2.91
		1.92
		2.85
		11.83
Ctrl, 16.4 mM		48.85
		55.61
		186.85
		122.60
		48.78
		57.69
Plot, 3.3 mM		6.48
		4.66
		4.08
Plot, 16.4 mM		20.44
		15.45

Table 8: Insulin release of murine islets in clinical-grade Alg/MC, isolation 6. Single values of ng insulin released in response to either low (3.3 mM) or high (16.4 mM) glucose stimulation normalised to 100 ng DNA.

	d1	d4	d7	d11
Ctrl, 3.3 mM	47.44			
Ctrl, 16.4 mM	30.69	32.32	8.99	1.90
Plot, 3.3 mM	10.91	2.94	1.56	1.57
Plot, 16.4 mM	11.57	18.30	4.71	1.97

Table 9: Insulin release of murine islets in clinical-grade Alg/MC, isolation 7. Single values of ng insulin released in response to either low (3.3 mM) or high (16.4 mM) glucose stimulation normalised to 100 ng DNA.

	d1	d4
Ctrl, 3.3 mM		
Ctrl, 16.4 mM		
Plot, 3.3 mM		5.4
Plot, 16.4 mM		23.55

Table 10: Insulin release of murine islets in clinical-grade Alg/MC, isolation 8. Single values of ng insulin released in response to successive low (3.3 mM), high (16.4 mM), and low (3.3 mM) glucose stimulation normalised to 100 ng DNA.

	Ctrl, 3.3 mM I	Ctrl, 16.4 mM	Ctrl, 3.3 mM II	Plot, 3.3 mM I	Plot, 16.4 mM	Plot, 3.3 mM II
d1	0.48	3.38	2.38	6.62	10.09	6.23
	32.55	12.74	0.11	6.73	10.77	6.35
	3.18	59.96	2.94	8.23	9.37	5.25
	1.66	13.02	1.04	6.85	7.72	4.64
	1.45		1.51		11.76	6.41
	1.61		0.71		11.03	6.73
	1.37	58.83	3.51			
	32.44	132.73	7.89			
	26.75	76.98	5.81			
	16.04	116.40	11.04			
	2.28	84.77	13.54			
	1.35	80.39	8.21			
d4		3.74	1.95	3.10	5.70	4.59
	40.21	3.66	1.32	3.60	6.35	4.39
		4.49	30.38	6.07	9.52	6.05
	2.09	40.79	8.49	3.58	8.07	5.21
	51.44	9.40	6.22	3.66	21.09	6.68
	1.95	41.51	10.76	3.34	12.32	4.66
	4.75	49.75	13.58			
	1.33	49.54	6.90			
	3.68	41.42	17.04			
	2.86	57.06	5.45			
		34.13				
	0.48	3.38	2.38			

Supplementary data for "4.4.2 Functionality of bioplotted NICC"

The following tables show the calculated values for ng insulin per 100 ng DNA, released from NICC, which are graphically depicted in Figure 54 (page 90, results). All values in Table 11 & Table 12 are from plotted islets in clinical-grade Alg/MC scaffolds crosslinked with 70 mM $SrCl_2$ and from control islets in suspension culture incubated in $RPMI^+$ under cell culture conditions for up to 21 days. Samples were exposed to successive low and high glucose stimulation, whereby samples listed in Table 12 were additionally exposed to 100 nM liraglutide per ml medium during high-glucose stimulation.

Table 11: Insulin release of NICC in clinical-grade Alg/MC. Single values of ng insulin released in response to successive low (3.3 mM) and high (16.4 mM) glucose stimulation normalised to 100 ng DNA. Plot 1-3 denote different isolations.

	d1, Plot 1	d4, Plot 1	d4, Plot 2	d4, Plot 3	d7, Plot 1
Ctrl, 3.3 mM	0.05	0.02	0.05	0.04	0.03
	0.02	0.10	0.05	0.07	0.08
	0.01	0.03	0.03	0.08	0.04
	0.06	0.05	0.03	0.10	0.04
	0.02	0.02	0.02	0.05	
	0.04		0.02		
			0.03		
			0.03		
Ctrl, 16.4 mM	0.04	0.03	0.03	0.06	0.06
	0.03	0.02	0.05	0.09	
	0.10	0.03	0.04	0.08	0.05
	0.03	0.04	0.03	0.08	0.07
	0.04	0.04	0.03	0.08	
	0.03		0.04		
			0.02		
			0.03		
Plot, 3.3 mM	0.02	0.02	0.01	0.02	0.04
	0.01	0.02	0.00	0.02	0.03
			0.01	0.02	
				0.02	
Plot, 16.4 mM	0.01	0.01	0.00	0.04	0.03
	0.01	0.02	0.01	0.03	0.02
			0.01	0.03	
				0.03	

Table 12: Insulin release of NICC in clinical-grade Alg/MC, with liraglutide. Single values of ng insulin released in response to successive low (3.3 mM) and high (16.4 mM) glucose stimulation normalised to 100 ng DNA. Plot 1 & 2 denote different isolations.

	d1, Plot 2	d4, Plot 1	d7, Plot 1	d7, Plot 2	d10, Plot 1	d14, Plot 1	d21, Plot 1
Ctrl, 3.3 mM	0.01	0.10	0.21	0.03	3.61	3.88	0.29
	0.02	0.26	0.23	0.03	1.80	3.24	0.26
	0.02	0.20	0.42	0.04	2.15	1.33	0.24
	0.04						
	0.03						
	0.03						
Ctrl, 16.4 mM	0.13	1.19	2.23	0.22	21.87	11.49	1.21
	0.21	0.84	1.37	0.20	6.52	6.62	0.79
	0.16	1.12	1.92	0.25	5.82	3.64	1.37
	0.33						
	0.29						
	0.26						
Plot, 3.3 mM	0.03	0.03	0.03	0.03	0.05	0.06	0.62
	0.03	0.03	0.03	0.05	0.03	0.22	0.61
	0.03	0.02	0.06	0.04	0.03	0.05	0.45
	0.03	0.03	0.02		0.02	0.06	0.13
	0.03						
	0.03						
Plot, 16.4 mM	0.32	0.20	0.16	0.20	0.18	0.18	1.11
	0.36	0.23	0.22	0.31	0.19	0.16	0.98
	0.28	0.17	0.22	0.24	0.21	0.18	0.87
	0.26	0.21	0.22		0.21	0.18	0.59
	0.22						
	0.29						

A.2 Supplementary data for the discussion

Supplementary data for "5.1.1. Gel viscosity and crosslinking of alginate"

Swelling of hydrogel strands

Addition of MC to alginate hydrogels results in stable constructs with minimal swelling over time. Figure 73 depicts the strand width of Alg/MC scaffolds in DMEM$^+$ over an incubation time of 21 days. Strand width was analysed from images taken on a stereo light microscope and measured with ImageJ.

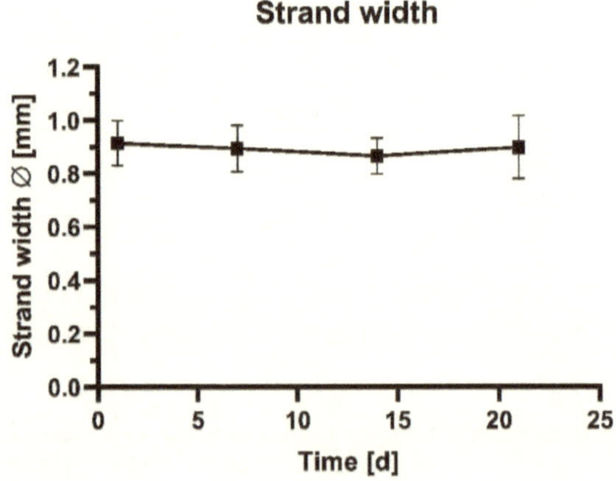

Figure 73: Strand width of plotted Alg/MC scaffolds. Scaffolds prepared with research-grade alginate, crosslinked with 100 mM CaCl$_2$ and incubated in DMEM$^+$ over 21 days under cell culture conditions. Mean ± SD, n = 3.

Viability of murine islets after repeated crosslinking

Figure 74 depicts the viability of adult murine islets in plotted research-grade Alg/MC scaffolds crosslinked with 70 mM $SrCl_2$ and incubated in $RPMI^+$ for up to 14 days under cell culture conditions. Viability of islets in scaffolds re-crosslinked with 70 mM $SrCl_2$ every other day was compared to viability of control islets in suspension culture. Repeated exposure to $SrCl_2$ slightly reduced viability compared to the control islets over 14 days of incubation.

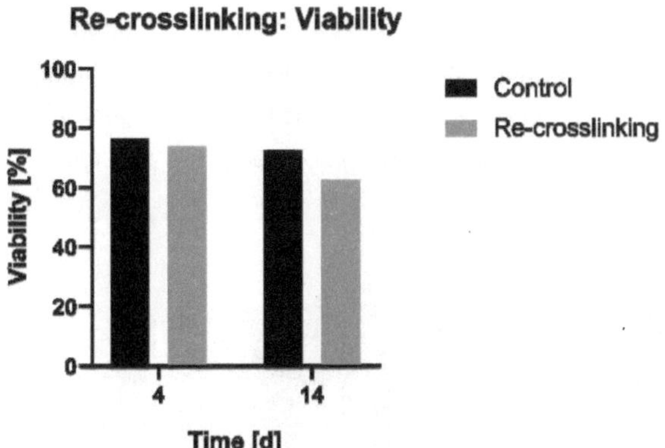

Figure 74: Quantitative viability of murine islets after repeated crosslinking. Plotted islets in clinical-grade Alg/MC scaffolds crosslinked with 70 mM $SrCl_2$ and control islets in suspension culture incubated in $RPMI^+$ under cell culture conditions for up to 14 days. Scaffolds were re-crosslinked every other day. Semi-quantitative assessment of islet viability on the basis of live/dead stainings. Mean ± SD, n = 1 isolation, 24-62 islets.

Supplementary data for "5.1.2. MC release"

Probable deposition of MC fibres

Figure 75 depicts the probable deposition of MC fibres within scaffold strands. Sr^{2+}-crosslinked research-grade Alg/MC scaffolds were incubated in $RPMI^+$ for 14 days. Scaffolds were either stored at 4°C or 37°C for the entire duration. In light-microscopic images (Figure 75), fibre-like structures became visible after 7 days of incubation at 37°C and decreased again until 14 days of incubation. No structures could be observed in scaffolds incubated at 4°C. The same structures had previously been observed for scaffolds incubated in $DMEM^+$, except for MC with a strongly reduced Mw after sterilisation with γ-irradiation (data not shown). Hypothetically the observed structures could be gelled MC fibres, as the range of geometries observed largely correlates with the different stages of MC swelling proposed by Grosse & Klaus (Grosse & Klaus, 1972).

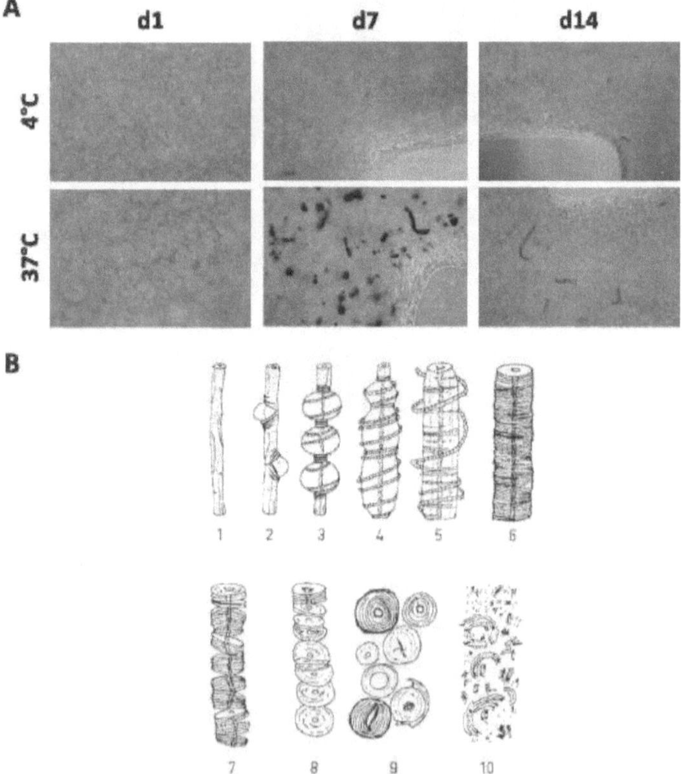

Figure 75: MC fibre deposition. A) Scaffolds prepared with research-grade alginate, crosslinked with 70 mM $SrCl_2$ and incubated in $RPMI^+$ over 14 days at 4°C or 37°C. Representative images of scaffolds incubated for 1, 4, or 7 days after plotting. Probable MC fibre deposition distinctly visible after 7 days of incubation at 37°C. B) Schematic depiction of the different stages of the swelling of MC fibres as proposed by Grosse & Klaus (Grosse & Klaus, 1972).

Temperature-dependent release of MC

To analyse temperature dependent release of MC, scaffolds were prepared with research-grade alginate, crosslinked with 70 mM $SrCl_2$ and incubated in $RPMI^+$ over 14 days at 4°C or 37°C (Figure 76).

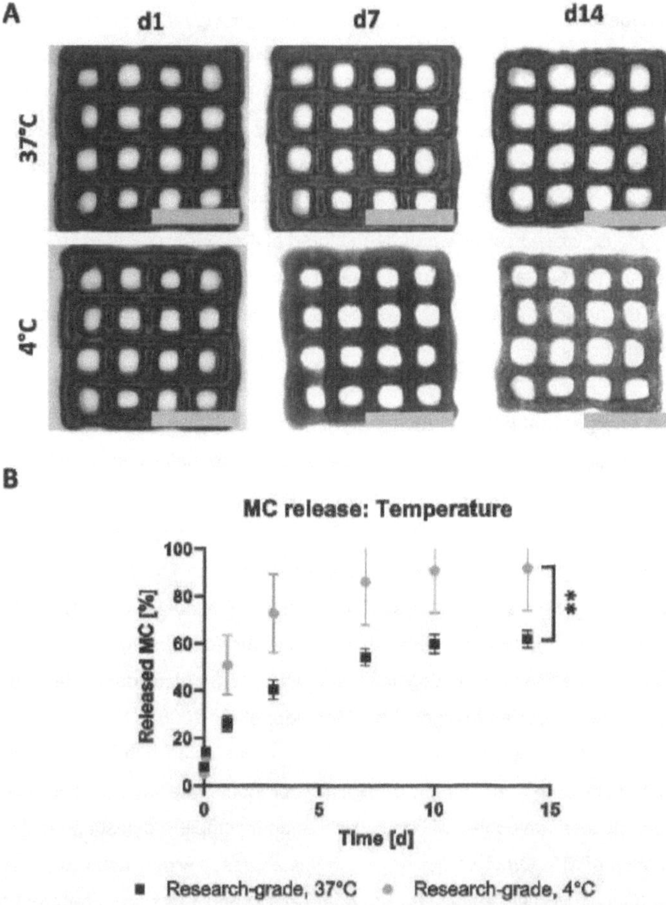

Figure 76: Temperature-dependent release of MC. Scaffolds prepared with research-grade alginate, crosslinked with 70 mM $SrCl_2$ and incubated in $RPMI^+$ over 14 days at 4°C or 37°C. A) Representative images of scaffolds incubated for 1, 4, or 7 days after plotting stained with for the presence of MC with chlorine-zinc-iodine solution. Scale bars = 5 mm. B) Cumulative release of MC into the supernatant over 14 days. Mean ± SD, n = 6 for each, significances indicate **$p<0.01$.

MC remaining within the scaffolds was visualised qualitatively via staining with a CZI solution (Roth). Prior to staining, the CZI was diluted 1:10 in distilled water and scaffolds were incubated in the staining solution for exactly 1 min at constant rotation. Images were taken using a stereo light microscope. The presence of a high amount of MC was observed as black staining over the entire time of observation when scaffolds were incubated under cell culture conditions, whereas incubation at 4°C led to a lighter brown staining after 7-14 days of incubation (Figure 76 A). Quantitative release of MC was measured from the supernatant with Mykoval™ (Figure 76 B). As had been the case for all analyses performed with Mykoval™ (Figure 13, page 41, results), a burst release of MC was observed within the first day (specifically during crosslinking, washing and the first 24 h of incubation). Independent of the incubation temperature, release of MC entered a plateau around day 10 of incubation, but overall release was significantly higher when scaffolds had been stored at 4°C.

Taken together, the CZI and Mykoval™ measurements give a strong indication that the MC used for the present book does indeed partly gelate at 37°C which decreases its release from plotted scaffolds.

Mechanism of digestion with cellulase

Figure 77 schematically depicts the different cleaving sites for cellulases in cellulose molecules with the β-1,4-glycosidic linkage also depicted in carboxy-methylcellulose and methylcellulose. The cellulases tested within the scope of this book were isolated from three different sources, *Aspergillus niger*, *Trichoderma species*, and *Trichoderma reesei*. Of those *Aspergillus niger* is described to catalyse the hydrolysis of endo-1,4-β-D-glycosidic linkages by the manufacturer. *Trichoderma reesei* has been reported as being comprised of two exoglucanases, more than four endoglucanases, and one β-glucosidase (Henriksson et al., 1996) and has been reported to digest MC (Melander et al., 2006).

For the detection of digestion products, the DNS-assay which detects reducing ends was chosen. With increasing chain length of digestion products, the ratio of reducing ends to de facto present glucose molecules will be lower, i.e. an incomplete digestion would result in an underestimation of MC. On the other hand, DNS is an assay widely used to assess digestion of cellulose (Gusakov et al., 2011; Teixeira et al., 2012) and it has been reported that at least cellobiose and cellotriose (short chains of two and three glucose molecules respectively) are hydrolysed partially during the DNS assay (Saqib & Whitney, 2011). The presence of amino acids in the medium could interfere with this assay (Teixeira et al., 2012) but since glucose measurements in medium were established for permeability measurements and no over-estimation was detected, this factor was considered negligible.

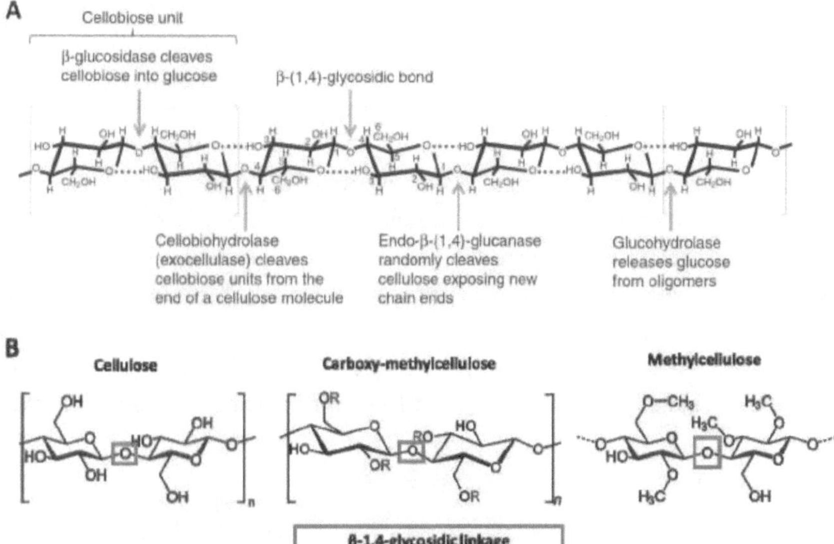

Figure 77: Mechanism of cellulase digestion. A) Schematic depiction of the cleaving sites in cellulose molecules for different cellulases (Byrt et al., 2013). B) Schematic depiction of the β-1,4-glycosidic linkage cellulases recognise present in cellulose (Wikipedia, 2020b), carboxy-methylcellulose (Wikipedia, 2020a) and methylcellulose (Wikipedia, 2020c).

Concentration-dependent digestion of MC with cellulases

Figure 78 exemplarily depicts a standard curve for the amount of reducing sugars measured after digestion of MC with *Trichoderma reesei*. While the measured emission was dependent on the concentration of MC originally present in the sample, the digestion efficacy was very low and the vast majority of samples were below the detection limit of the glucose assays used.

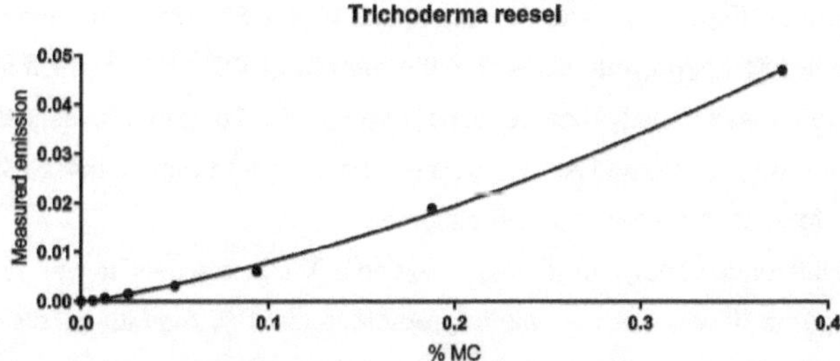

Figure 78: Exemplary standard curve for the concentration-dependent digestion of MC with cellulases. Digestion was performed with MC dissolve in RPMI⁺ and measured via DNS-assay for reducing sugars. The values were fitted with 2ⁿᵈ order polynomial equations in GraphPad Prism.

Supplementary data for "5.1.3 Permeability for glucose & insulin"

Gel curvature during chamber assembly

As a result of the pressure applied to the gel discs during chamber assembly, the thin planar discs distorted irregularly. This did not impact the tightness of the chamber, but it prevents the accurate measurement of area for the diffusion. Attempts to prevent the distortion were a change in crosslinking ions, storage conditions and the addition of meshes to add mechanical stability, neither of which could completely prevent curving of the gels during chamber assembly. The addition of two stiff meshes on either side of the disc before assembly and the incorporation of melt-electro-written polycaprolactone meshes during disc preparation are exemplarily depicted in Figure 79 A&B respectively.

Since curving was of irregular geometry, thereby not affecting filling level and present in all gels to some degree, this factor was neglected for the comparison of average concentrations.

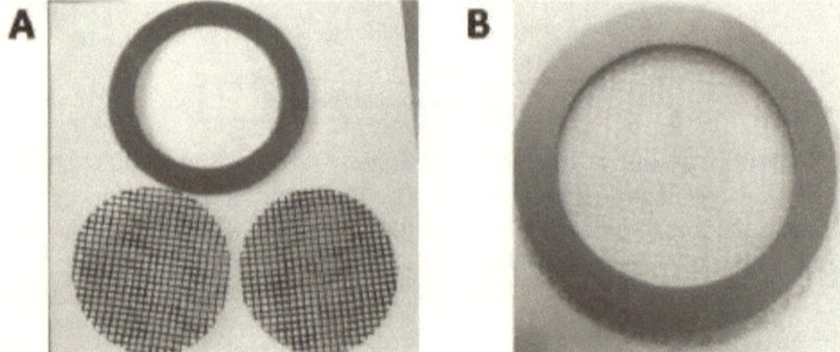

Figure 79: Addition of meshes to the discs before assembly of the diffusion chamber. A) Stiff meshes on either side of the disc before assembly. B) Incorporation of a melt-electro-written polycaprolactone mesh during disc preparation.

Influence of mesh density

The trend towards quicker diffusion visible between research-grade Alg/MC gels that had been incubated for longer (Figure 23, page 53, results and Figure 65, page 176, addendum) might be attributed to a different polymer content or the release of MC, both of which hypothetically result in a different mesh density (chapter 5.1.1, page 93 ff.). To further investigate this possibility, research-grade alginate and Alg/MC gels were crosslinked with 70 mM $SrCl_2$ and stored in 10 mM $SrCl_2$ for 4 days before chamber assembly.

To analyse the influence of polymer density, 1 % and 2 % alginate gels as well as 2 % Alg/MC gels were compared. It was not possible to prepare stable 1 % Alg/MC gel discs. For these lower alginate percentages, a trend towards quicker diffusion and a difference between plain alginate and Alg/MC was visible. It is of further note that the lag-phase of plain alginate gels lasted for 30 min, but that of the 2 % Alg/MC gels for 1 h (Figure 80 A).

To further analyse the influence of presence of MC, 3 % Alg/MC gels were stored at 37°C to mimic cell culture conditions, and at 4°C, a temperature at which the solubility of MC is increased (see also Figure 76, page 192). For permeability for glucose, no difference between the gels stored at different temperatures could be observed (Figure 80 B).

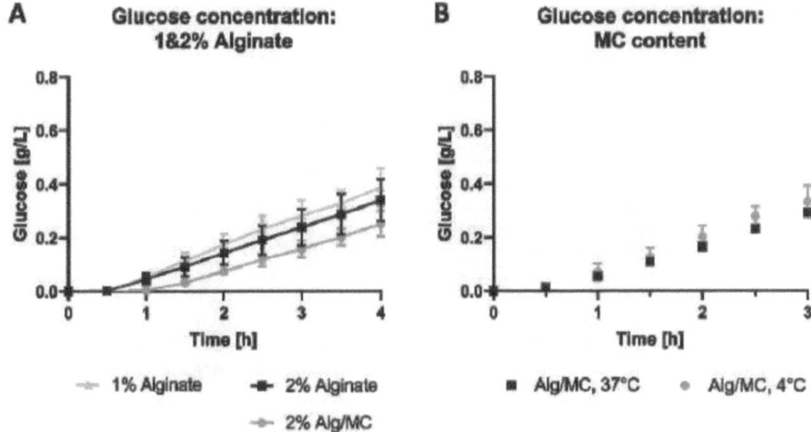

Figure 80: Dependence of glucose diffusion on mesh density. Glucose concentration is depicted for the acceptor compartment. Alginate and Alg/MC gel discs were prepared with research-grade alginate and crosslinked with 70 mM $SrCl_2$. Incubation of discs in 10 mM $SrCl_2$ under cell culture conditions for 1 day before mounting in the chamber filled with 10 mM $SrCl_2$. Samples of 200 µl were taken from both compartments every 30 min during a period of 4 h. Mean ± SD, n = 3, data were adjusted for gel height. A) Glucose diffusion through research-grade plain alginate gels prepared with 1 % & 2 % alginate, and research-grade Alg/MC gels prepared with 2 % alginate. B) Glucose diffusion through research-grade Alg/MC gels stored at 37°C and 4°C for 4 days.

Supplementary data for "5.2.1 Incorporation of β-cells"

Metabolic activity of hTERT-MSC and INS-1

Compared to other cell types such as hTERT-MSC, which tolerate the embedding and plotting in Alg/MC very well, INS-1 seem to be more sensitive to this process. Figure 81 depicts a comparison between hTERT-MSC and INS-1 in plotted research-grade Alg/MC scaffolds after 1 day of incubation under cell culture conditions.

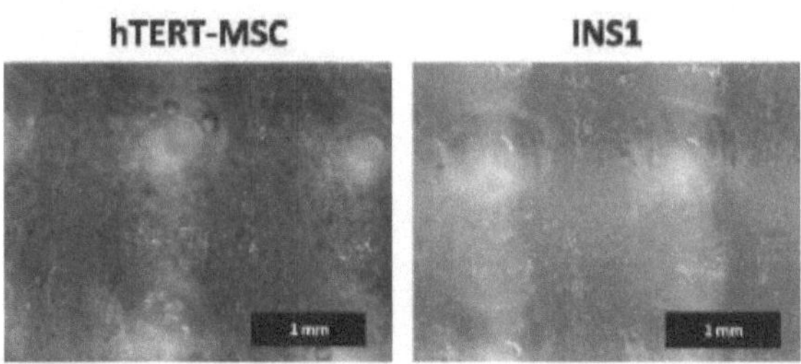

Figure 81: Exemplary depiction of metabolic activity of plotted hTERT-MSC and INS-1. 5×10^6 hTERT or 1×10^7 INS-1 cells in plotted research-grade Alg/MC scaffolds crosslinked with 70 mM $SrCl_2$ and incubated in RPMI+ under cell culture conditions. Exemplary depiction of scaffolds stained with MTT on day 1 after plotting. Scale bars = 1 mm.

Supplementary data for "5.4.1 Plotting of neonatal porcine islet-like cell clusters (NICC)"

DNA content of NICC over time

Table 13 depicts the decrease of DNA content in the suspension culture used as control, and in plotted clinical-grade Alg/MC scaffolds with NICC observed over of 7 days.

Table 13: DNA content of control and plotted Alg/MC scaffolds containing NICC. DNA content over time was normalised to the DNA content measured on day 1 after plotting. Clinical-grade Alg/MC scaffolds were crosslinked with 70 mM $SrCl_2$ and incubated under cell culture conditions for up to 7 days. n = 1 isolation, 6 samples for control, 4 samples for plotted NICC.

	d1	d4	d7
Control	100	90.7	29.8
Plotted	100	98.1	74.1

List of tables

List of publications

(* resulting from this book)

* **Duin, S.**, Schütz, K., Ahlfeld, T., Lehmann, S., Lode, A., Ludwig, B., & Gelinsky, M. (2019). 3D Bioprinting of Functional Islets of Langerhans in an Alginate/Methylcellulose Hydrogel Blend. *Advanced Healthcare Materials*, *8*(7), 1801631. https://doi.org/10.1002/adhm.201801631

* Hodder, E.[#], **Duin, S.**[#], Kilian, D., Ahlfeld, T., Seidel, J., Nachtigall, C., Bush, P., Covill, D., Gelinsky, M., & Lode, A. (2019). Investigating the effect of sterilisation methods on the physical properties and cytocompatibility of methyl cellulose used in combination with alginate for 3D-bioplotting of chondrocytes. *Journal of Materials Science: Materials in Medicine*, *30*(1). https://doi.org/10.1007/s10856-018-6211-9
[#] Shared first co-authorship

* Ahlfeld, T., Guduric, V., **Duin, S.**, Akkineni, A. R., Schütz, K., Kilian, D., Emmermacher, J., Cubo-Mateo, N., Dani, S., von Witzleben, M., Spangenberg, J., Abdelgaber, R., Richter, R. F., Lode, A., & Gelinsky, M. (2020). Methylcellulose – a versatile printing material that enables biofabrication of tissue equivalents with high shape fidelity. *Biomaterials Science*, *8*(8), 2102–2110. https://doi.org/10.1039/D0BM00027B

Quade, M., Münch, P., Lode, A., **Duin, S.**, Vater, C., Gabrielyan, A., Rösen-Wolff, A., & Gelinsky, M. (2020). The Secretome of Hypoxia Conditioned hMSC Loaded in a Central Depot Induces Chemotaxis and Angiogenesis in a Biomimetic Mineralized Collagen Bone Replacement Material. *Advanced Healthcare Materials*, *9*(2). https://doi.org/10.1002/adhm.201901426

Wieduwild, R., Wetzel, R., Husman, D., Bauer, S., El-Sayed, I., **Duin, S.**, Murawala, P., Thomas, A. K., Wobus, M., Bornhäuser, M., & Zhang, Y. (2018). Coacervation-Mediated Combinatorial Synthesis of Biomatrices for Stem Cell Culture and Directed Differentiation. *Advanced Materials*, *30*(22), 1–9. https://doi.org/10.1002/adma.201706100

Ahlfeld, T., Cidonio, G., Kilian, D., **Duin, S.**, Akkineni, A. R., Dawson, J. I., Yang, S., Lode, A., Oreffo, R. O. C., & Gelinsky, M. (2017). Development of a clay based bioink for 3D cell printing for skeletal application. *Biofabrication*, *9*(3), 34103. https://doi.org/10.1088/1758-5090/aa7e96

Sadovskaya, I., Souissi, A., Souissi, S., Grard, T., Lencel, P., Greene, C. M., **Duin, S.**, Dmitrenok, P. S., Chizhov, A. O., Shashkov, A. S., & Usov, A. I. (2014). Chemical structure and biological activity of a highly branched $(1 \rightarrow 3, 1 \rightarrow 6)$-β-D-glucan from Isochrysis galbana. *Carbohydrate Polymers*, *111*, 139–148. https://doi.org/10.1016/j.carbpol.2014.04.077

Conference contributions resulting from this book

S. Duin, S. Lehmann, C. Paßkönig, E. Kemter, E. Wolf, A. Lode, M. Gelinsky, B. Ludwig. *3D Bioprinting of neonatal porcine islet cluster (NICC) in an alginate/ methylcellulose (Alg/MC) hydrogel-blend.* 30th Annual Conference of the European Society for Biomaterials ESB, Dresden, Germany (09.09.2019-13.09.2019).

S. Duin, K. Schütz, A. Lode, B. Ludwig, M. Gelinsky. *3D Bioprinting of functional islets of Langerhans in an alginate/methylcellulose hydrogel-blend.* International Conference on Biofabrication, Würzburg, Germany (28-10.2018-31.10.2018).

S. Duin, K. Schütz, A. Lode, B. Ludwig, M. Gelinsky. *3D Bioprinting of functional islets of Langerhans in an alginate/methylcellulose (Alg/MC) hydrogel-blend.* 29th Annual Conference of the European Society for Biomaterials ESB, Maastricht, Netherlands (09.09.2018-13.09.2018).

S. Duin, K. Schütz, A. Steffen, A. Lode, B. Ludwig, M. Gelinsky. *Embedding of pancreatic islets in structured alginate-based hydrogels by 3D bioprinting.* 11th CRTD Summer Conference, Dresden, Germany (02.06.2017).

S. Duin, K. Schütz, A. Steffen, A. Lode, B. Ludwig, M. Gelinsky. *Embedding of pancreatic islets in structured alginate-based hydrogels by 3D bioprinting.* International Conference on Biofabrication, Winston-Salem, North Carolina, USA (29-10.2016-31.10.2016).

S. Duin, K. Schütz, A. Steffen, A. Lode, B. Ludwig, M. Gelinsky. *Embedding of pancreatic islets in structured alginate-based hydrogels by 3D bioprinting.* 10th CRTD Summer Conference, Dresden, Germany, Germany (04.06.2016).

www.ingramcontent.com/pod-product-compliance
Lightning Source LLC
LaVergne TN
LVHW040016200726

843493LV00005B/1277